JOURNEY

Robert and Suzanne Massie

LONDON
VICTOR GOLLANCZ LTD
1975

ISBN 0 575 02055 5

Portions of the book were first published in *Family Health*
and *Ladies' Home Journal*

Grateful acknowledgment is made to Warner Bros. Music for
permission to reprint eight lines of lyrics from "Weave
Me the Sunshine" by Peter Yarrow. Copyright © 1972 by Mary
Beth Music. All Rights Reserved. Also, the authors wish to
thank Mr. Hy Zaret and Argosy Music Corporation for permission
to reprint lyrics from records in their "Ballads For the Age
of Science" Collection: Lyrics from "Vibrations" from the record
"Experiment Songs" Copyright © 1961, lyrics from "Metamorphosis"
from the record "More Nature Songs" Copyright © 1961, and lyrics
from "Jets (Action and Reaction)" from the record "Energy and
Motion Songs" Copyright © 1961. All lyrics by Hy Zaret, music
by Lou Singer.

Printed in Great Britain by
Lowe & Brydone (Printers) Ltd, Thetford, Norfolk

JOURNEY

For our children

Illustrations follow page 178

Acknowledgments

Many people who touched our lives importantly over the past eighteen years are not mentioned in this book. Some are doctors, nurses, and people who work in hospitals. Others are teachers, neighbors, colleagues, and friends. We want them to know that we have not forgotten any of them and we shall never forget what they have done.

Also, there are the blood donors, many of whom we shall never know. But they have given us what is most precious. Bobby could not be alive today without the web of human compassion and generosity created by thousands of human beings. Beyond any capacity to express our feeling in words, we are grateful to them.

Finally there are six people whose devoted support helped us during the writing of this book: Robert Gottlieb, Janet and Richard Dowling, Leslie Kitchell Bullock, Thérèse Doll, and Louis Mild.

Preface

Every 73 seconds a child who is not quite perfect—who is chronically ill or mentally or physically handicapped—is born in America. There are 1,177 more of these children every day, 8,241 every week, 428,571 every year. In all, more than 9 million youthful Americans under twenty-one are sufficiently impaired to need serious help.

Some of these children get the help they need; others don't. Most of them live outside the mainstream of our health-worshipping society. Within the family when they are very young the tenderness of their parents protects them. But when they begin to grow up and have to face the world, the battle begins.

This book is the story of one of these battles. The disease we have fought is hemophilia. The details of this struggle are personal, but the story itself is not unique. Every family with a handicapped or chronically ill child shares the same problems: lack of money, isolation from the community of the healthy, prejudice, misunderstanding in the schools, loneliness, boredom, depression.

For many years, we did not feel that we could write about such intense and intimate personal experience. We worried too, about the effect a book like this might have on our son while he was growing up. But now Bobby is eighteen. His adjustments to the world and to his disease are made. He hopes, as we do, that telling this story may give some measure of new strength to those who are fighting similar battles every day, and also perhaps provide some new element of understanding for those watching from outside.

Having decided to write this book together, we faced the practical editorial problem of "How?" We did not want to merge ourselves into an artificial "We." "We" are a woman and a man, a mother and a father; our emotions and reactions have sometimes been very different. And so we decided that each of us should write his or her part of the story in his or her own way. The authorship of each chapter or sub-chapter is indicated by the initials *R M* or *S M* on the right-hand pages.

For eighteen years, hemophilia has dominated our lives. It has molded our relationships with people and our attitude toward the world. It has determined our work, affected our philosophy, and deepened our faith. Above all, it has widened our perspective. During these years, we have learned to look differently at illness and to ask ourselves, Who is the more seriously handicapped—the child trying to lead a normal life despite his defects or the physically healthy person who is unable to accept him? In a world whose moral disabilities are far greater than its physical imperfections, the question deserves thought.

Robert Massie
Suzanne Massie

JOURNEY

Chapter 1

There was no sign that we were to be singled out for any particularly dramatic experience in life. When I think back to those faraway days, I can recall only with difficulty that youthful stranger who looked so eagerly toward the future. Then life seemed to spread before me like a flower-filled garden in which I had only to choose the most beautiful flowers. Had I not done well in my studies and won scholarships? Now, armed with shiny new knowledge and the unshakable conviction that hard work and honesty would inevitably be crowned with success, I bubbled with optimism.

Even in childhood, I had always yearned for a dramatic life. Sometimes at night, lying awake and staring at the ceiling dappled with the shadows of the street light, I felt certain that something extraordinary was going to happen to me. It seemed unlikely, but I was sure . . . and I nestled the knowledge close to my heart like a wonderful secret. I remember in college thinking how sad it would be to have an ordinary, humdrum existence where nothing unexpected ever happened. When I looked at the adult world, I grieved to see faces snuffed out like candles by the pressure of responsibility. I vowed that this would never happen to me. Always, I seem to have craved strong emotions and experiences. But nothing prepared me for the way they were to come.

Bob and I met in Paris. He was a bright, fiery boy from an old Southern family; I was the eldest of three daughters of the Swiss consul posted in Philadelphia. Bob was at Oxford on a Rhodes scholarship; I was spending my junior year at the Sorbonne. We met when an English team, including Bob, came for a whimsical debate with a French team on which was more important: Good

Cooking or Good Table Manners. I was in the audience, and was impressed with his wit and the cool way he handled words. I arranged to meet him. He had wonderful blue eyes. His letters were marvelous.

We had an up-and-down courtship which lasted four years. During this time I was graduated from Vassar and went to work as an editorial trainee at Time Inc., and he went into the navy. Just when it appeared that our story was over, Bob decided it was just beginning. He had arranged to be assigned to the naval legal school in Newport, Rhode Island, for six weeks. With a decisive spurt of energy, he smothered me in roses, and we decided to get married immediately.

I worked at *Life* magazine until the day before the wedding. I posed for my wedding picture against a huge piece of white paper tacked on the back of the rickety set for a superefficient kitchen that had been temporarily created in the *Life* studio (we were doing an elaborate picture story called "The Perfect Kitchen"). With my still unfinished wedding gown pinned behind me, Martha Holmes took my picture. There I am, clutching a slightly wilted gardenia that we had managed to extract from the corner florist, trying to look like the serene society brides I had admired in the newspapers.

We were married a week before Christmas, in the obligatory style of those conservative days of the mid-1950's, with the correct number of bridesmaids and flowers, and as many monogrammed towels and pieces of silver as our family and friends could provide. There was no time for a proper honeymoon. Bob had to report back to the Jacksonville Naval Air Station immediately. He was an air intelligence officer for a squadron assigned to the aircraft carrier *Coral Sea*, which was leaving for the Mediterranean. In those days, the "Med" cruise was considered pleasant and easy duty for the pilots and other officers. A number of wives went along to be with husbands when the ship came into port. As a navy lieutenant j.g.'s pay did not cover the cost of a traveling wife, Bob's brother Kim offered to lend us $500 to make the trip. Deciding to live now and pay later, we accepted. So I spent the first six months of our marriage following the fleet, or, more precisely, trying to find and extract Bob from the fleet in ten Mediterranean ports. The reality of the Med cruise was somewhat less glamorous than the promise; I crisscrossed Italy thirteen times in third-class coaches, stayed in flea-bag hotels brewing Nescafé from rusty tap water, and scanned the horizon for the silhouette of the huge carrier. By the time we returned, we had spent every penny we had. We owned a few silver platters, assorted cookbooks, and little else. But what did it matter? We knew the future was bright.

After that rollicking and exhausting beginning to our married life, we settled down for the last two months of Bob's service in Jacksonville. The night air was like velvet, the flowers perfumed, and the beaches deliciously smooth.

We had not planned to have a baby. But one sunny day, like all the other sunny days in Florida, I went to the dentist. The dentist took one look at my teeth and asked, "Don't you think you might be pregnant?" It turned out he was right. We were overwhelmed. This did not figure in our plans at all. I was planning to go back to work at *Life*, and although Bob did not know exactly what he wanted to do, we had always assumed that a man of his abilities would be needed somewhere; it was only a matter of presenting himself with his résumé. Then we would make some money, pay back Kim, and buy some furniture and a nice little house, the way all our friends were doing. And soon after that, we would fulfill my deepest wish by going back to live a pleasant life in Paris for a while.

Still . . . a baby. It was a wonderful idea. I thought it must be a little like getting a puppy. I mean, it changed your life, but not that much. In Jacksonville, in those remaining days before Bob got out of the navy, I pampered myself.

We came back north. Bob began to look for a job. It turned out to be a lot harder than we had anticipated. When I called *Life* about returning to my old job, I got cheery words of congratulations, but personnel was hardly anxious to take me back in my interesting condition. We had nowhere to live. We went to stay a while with my family in Philadelphia, and then Bob's aunt put us up in her small apartment in Summit, New Jersey. Bob was gone all day looking for work. I grew lonely and depressed. I felt awful.

I longed to have a place of our own, a nest. Where was my little house with its shiny towel racks on which to hang the mono-grammed towels?

Bob kept commuting back and forth to New York or Phila-delphia looking for jobs. He was turned down in many places, despite the fact that he had graduated with honors from Yale, won a Rhodes scholarship, and spent three and a half years as an officer in the navy. When he went to *The New York Times* he was turned away by a personnel woman who stared at him coldly and said, "Frankly, Mr. Massie, we are suspicious of people like you, who have reached the age of twenty-seven and never done anything."

We began to understand how difficult our financial situation really was. Our parents weren't in a position to help us. There was no more pay coming in, and the time before the baby's arrival was growing short. In desperation, Bob decided to accept the only solid offer he had: as a trainee in a bank in Philadelphia. This was far from the sort of job he had in mind (the salary was even less than his navy pay), but we were not in a position to be proud.

Then at the last minute, as it has so many times in our life, the unexpected intervened. The night before Bob was to start working at the bank, a Yale friend called from New York to ask if Bob would be interested in taking over his job as administrative assistant to a quixotic and colorful character named Paul C. Smith, who was then trying to resuscitate the *Collier's* magazine empire. Bob ac-cepted on the phone and the next day went to work, not at the bank but as private secretary to this very dramatic man. It was an oblique approach to a journalistic career, but at least it was closer than a bank in Philadelphia.

We had no money, so we lived in a furnished room on a run-down street on the Lower West Side. Our room had paper curtains and a moldy-looking shower curtain which covered an even more uncertain-looking shower stall regularly overrun with cockroaches. I cooked on a hot plate. There was a communal pay phone out on the hall landing and a double lock on our door. Fierce-looking people came in and out, the smell of garbage hung in the air, and an occasional wino huddled morosely on the doorstep.

Paul Smith was given to sudden changes of plans. He would pick up and leave New York without giving any warning and take

Bob with him. Often I would say good-bye to Bob in the morning, and then around dinnertime get a call from him from Minneapolis or somewhere, telling me he wouldn't be home that night. I would sit alone and melancholy behind the double-locked door looking at the one tree that grew in the courtyard and trying not to be afraid when at night I heard crying and fighting in the rooms downstairs.

We never could find any apartment in New York City that we could afford. Eventually my father was able to help us find a very inexpensive two-and-a-half-room apartment in a development in the town of Eastchester, in Westchester County. It was tiny, but it was a home. We settled in. A bed was our only piece of furniture. We used a packing crate as a table. We unpacked the silver platters and piled them on the floor of the hall closet. I was growing bigger. We had found a nest just in time.

Because of our wanderings, I had not had an obstetrician. I had stopped in a doctor's office once in Jacksonville and once in Philadelphia, but no one had really followed my case. In New York, on the advice of a college friend, I happened to find a fashionable doctor who showed very little interest in me. During my regular visits he scarcely emitted more than a few gruff sounds. I was afraid of him, but was too unsure to know what to do about it. And, as bad luck would have it, my baby was due to arrive on the day he was to begin his summer vacation.

Bobby was born on August 17, 1956. It was an unusually hot summer. One sweltering morning I felt a great urge to clean up the house and bake a peach cobbler. I didn't know it then, but it was what the doctors refer to as the prebirth spurt of activity. The contractions became frequent. We left for the hospital, taking the peach cobbler with us. To my extreme disappointment, I stayed there for eight hours, having contractions every five minutes and was released—false labor. I was advised to stay close to the hospital, so Bob and I went to the apartment of our best man, Jack May, and ate the peach cobbler and watched the Democratic Convention, which was nominating Adlai Stevenson. Late that evening the contractions began again. We went back to the hospital.

It was a long, difficult birth. I was already tired from the hours of false labor. During the last twelve long hours of labor I was very conscious of the increasing impatience of the doctor: the time for his vacation departure was approaching. I remember that I kept apologizing to him. I had wanted very much to have a natural childbirth; Bob and I had proudly completed the required course. But as the doctor was in a hurry and I was having such a difficult time, he finally had me knocked out with drugs from which I did not recover easily. I think he delivered the baby. I don't know because I never saw him again.

The baby had finally arrived precisely at twelve noon. Astrologically, it was a most propitious time. When I woke up, through the haze of gas, I saw a tiny blond creature with the bright eyes of a bird. He was nestled in the arms of a dark, pretty nurse whose name I could make out by concentrating hard on her lapel pin: Miss Spain. Standing next to her was a very proud and awed Bob. We had never planned to name Bobby after his father. Bob and I had always thought it a little old-fashioned and vain to name a son after the father. We had toyed with the idea of Nathaniel, but at that moment I heard him ask rather hesitantly, "You don't mind if maybe we call him Robert, do you?" I remember answering groggily, "Oh, no. No." Which is how he was named Bobby.

Bobby was really very nice looking, except that he had such a lot of bruises, including a very big swollen one behind the back of his skull which they called a hematoma. But as I had had a difficult birth and forceps had been necessary, no one paid much attention to these marks of a bumpy road into life. Nurses would comment, "Well, you had a hard time, didn't you?" and pass on. We called the pediatrician in Eastchester to announce the birth and arrange for a future visit. He thought our description of these bruises strange, and commented, "That's a funny place to have a hematoma," but left it at that.

It took me a long time to recover from the birth. My stitches became infected, causing me much pain, so I had to stay in the hospital ten days. It was terribly hot. But it was a wonderful room. As it turned out, I have rested from the birth of all three of my babies in that same room in the same bed. It is a sunshine-filled rotunda of New York Hospital, looking out over the East River. At night, as I lay sweltering on my rubber sheets hardly able to move from pain, it was pleasant and soothing to hear the boats throbbing busily on the East River.

Two days after birth, Bobby was routinely taken away to be circumcised. In the distance I heard him cry and scream. These screams wrenched my heart. He was returned to me, but later he was still bleeding from his wound. I pointed this out to the nurse. Neither resident nor nurses took it as anything unusual. They simply said, "We must have forgotten to tie off a little vein." They took him away again, and when he came back this time, everything was fine. And when we took him home, the pediatrician examined him and looked carefully at the hematoma. In ten days it had diminished considerably, and the doctor did nothing more than note it on his records.

From the beginning Bobby was a wonderful, happy baby who loved everybody. I thought him very handsome with his fuzz of blond hair, his round rosy cheeks, and his bright-eyed, curious look. He was extremely active very early. He wanted to go everywhere, explore everything. He managed to roll off the bed long before Dr. Spock predicts such a possibility. I was so proud! He was strong. How was I to know that these were the last carefree months I was to enjoy; that the sun was soon to go behind a cloud, never to shine with full brightness again.

I did not appreciate these months enough, because shortly after Bobby's birth we began to have very severe professional problems. Bob had managed to extricate himself from his wild and difficult life with Paul Smith and to have himself assigned to the editorial staff of *Collier's* magazine, which was where he had wanted to be from the beginning. He was working for Theodore H. White as a research assistant, making story suggestions and beginning to write. Although he wasn't making much money, he was happy. But the future at *Collier's* grew blacker and blacker. As the autumn wore on, one convulsion followed another. Finally, in mid-December the magazine went down for good. One Sunday, the employees received telegrams telling them that since the previous Friday they had been out of work. There was no severance pay. It was ruthless and heartbreaking.

We were left without any money at all. We had to go on welfare, which was then $36 a week. It was the week before Christmas; it was our wedding anniversary. We took refuge with my family in Philadelphia over the holidays while Bob went out to look for another job. It wasn't easy; there were dozens of trained writers, reporters, and researchers all out looking at the same time. Luckily, a few weeks before, in the fall, an editor at *Newsweek* had asked Bob if he might be interested in coming there. Now he immediately went over to talk to them. Of course, nobody was thinking of hiring anybody during the holidays. Discouraged, we thought that life had reached its lowest ebb.

Sometime during those weeks, two strange things happened. I went into a vegetable store. On the counter, near the cash register, there was a small can. I had seen cans like this everywhere, collecting coins for one disease or another. This one was for hemophilia. I exclaimed something then that has remained to haunt me to this day. "Oh, my goodness," I said, "what will they be collecting for next?" The other thing was a terrible nightmare, from which I woke up trembling. In my dream I had seen Bobby wasting away.

Bob went back to *Newsweek* in January and, to our immense relief, was offered a job writing book reviews. He was to start work the following week. One day when Bobby was five months old, Bob's brother Kim came out to see us and was playing joyfully with Bobby—throwing him up in the air and rolling him around in his play pen. Bobby chuckled and gurgled happily. But afterward, I noticed a small bruise, about the size of a marble, under his left upper forearm. I was taking Bobby to the doctor for his usual monthly checkup, and I pointed it out to him. The doctor studied the bruise and said, "Hmm, that's kind of strange. He may have a vitamin deficiency or something. Maybe we'd better have a blood count."

On an icy winter day I went to a laboratory in White Plains. Bobby was wrapped up in his little blue snowsuit with red and white stripes. His face and cheeks were all rosy from the cold. It was very late in the afternoon and the technician was in a hurry to go home. She stuck Bobby, taking blood from his toe.

When I got home, I found that something strange had happened. His tiny sock was soaked with blood. I took it off and put him back in the little wicker bed. He lay there, dandling his toes and cooing. The blood was oozing slowly but regularly from his toe. I took out my hair dryer and tried to dry the wound. But it went right on bleeding. In the depth of my soul I felt a terrible premonition. The only thing that sprang to my mind was that strange bleeding disease that kings had. That can—in the vegetable store—what did it say? I rushed to the dictionary. There it was written:

> he·mo·phil·i·a: from the Greek *hemo-* blood + *philia* a fondness for or an affection for. *Medical:* a tendency, usually hereditary, to profuse bleeding from slight wounds.

With growing alarm, I rushed to the telephone to call the doctor. He paused, but then said reassuringly, "Well, it is strange, but it's probably some sort of vitamin deficiency. I think you had better take him to the hospital for tests." Time has mercifully erased some of the painful details of these hours. Bob was already on his way home from New York. I called my mother in Philadelphia. She said she would come in a day or two.

The next morning, we found ourselves once again in New York Hospital, only this time it was a very different part of the hospital. The hospital personnel treated us with that blend of condescension and coldness that I have now learned to know well, and to hate. They took Bobby away. No one would explain what was happening or what was going to be done to him. Mysteriously, they said only, "We are going to take some blood." He was taken from my arms, my roly-poly jolly baby, and rolled away down the hall. Then, chillingly, I heard from far down that hall some terrible screams. I was filled with panic. The screaming went on and on. We asked what was happening. "They must not be finished yet," was the curt answer. After nearly an hour I was so agitated that Bob said, "I'm taking you downstairs so you don't have to hear it anymore." We went to the cafeteria. When I came up I could still hear his screams; by now they were hoarse. Beside myself, ignoring the nurses who called after me, "You can't go down there," I ran down the hall in the direction of the noise and into a room filled with other babies in cribs. I found Bobby, still screaming, exhausted from crying so long. He was all alone. I snatched him up, rocked him, and kissed him. In a few moments his crying stopped. I found out later that the procedure itself had taken only ten minutes. They had taken blood from the jugular vein and then dumped him back in his crib, leaving him to cry, although we had been only a few yards away down the hall and could have calmed him quickly. It was the first of many such experiences. In the years ahead I was seared by the lack of understanding, the lack of compassion—yes, the cruelty—that comes from the rigid and arbitrary rules practiced in some of the best hospitals we have. Even now, when I think of this moment, I am filled with a terrible rage.

A day had gone by. We still knew nothing. Increasingly alarmed, we hovered over the head nurse's desk, asking anxiously, "But can't you tell us anything? What is the matter with him?" The head nurse would put on what I call now the head-nurse smirk and say, "Oh, no, there is nothing I can tell you. I think you will want to wait to hear what Doctor has to say." I particularly loathe nurses who use that expression, Doctor, without a name.

So we went on waiting. Doctor did not come. In this case, Doctor was one of the most renowned hematologists of New York Hospital. Neither he nor any one of his assistants ever took a moment to call the head nurse's desk to give us a word of advice or hope. The agony of waiting by terrified parents was simply not considered. We tried to get in touch with Doctor himself; we were put off by secretaries. Over and over again the same cold phrase was repeated. "Wait." My mother arrived and kept vigil with us.

On the evening of the second day we were still waiting in a stifling, overheated waiting room with hospital-green walls and antiseptic furniture of cheap chrome and plastic. I smoked cigarette after cigarette. Bob was exhausted. It had been his first day on the new job. He had just joined us again. Suddenly a man entered. It was at last the long-awaited Eminence, "Doctor" himself. He was wearing a gray suit, and his eyes looked down at the floor as he hurriedly came in. There were no preliminaries. He announced, coldly and matter-of-factly, "The child has classical hemophilia. There will be compensations, you may be sure." And with these enigmatic words, he turned on his heel and walked out.

I don't know what we did then. My baby was returned to me. I cannot remember leaving the hospital or finding the car in the parking lot. Somehow, we reached the safe haven of the tiny apartment with its packing crate and kitchen chair. In one cataclysmic moment, our world had been shattered; we only numbly recognized our familiar surroundings. We wept there, the three of us—Bob, my mother, and I—clinging to each other, helpless and alone. Without warning, as surely as if we had been abandoned on the bleak surface of the moon, our lives had changed. We had no idea what lay ahead.

The creation of a child is a miracle. I remember once hearing a doctor say that he never lost his sense of wonder at what happens in the delivery room. "There are four people in the room and then, suddenly, there is a fifth person, a brand-new, freshly minted human being."

New, pure, perfect, filled with infinite potential, a newborn child is a miracle of God. I believe this. Who created it, if not God? Where did it come from, if not from God?

A few months before, two of us had gone to the hospital and three of us had come home. We had with us our perfect child. Now we had gone back to the same hospital and come home again with the same child. But this time was different. This time our child was no longer perfect.

If a healthy child is a perfect miracle of God, who created the imperfect child? Why would God create imperfection? Especially in a child? Especially in our child?

The doctor had said, "The child has classical hemophilia." And yet, there in his crib next to our bed, cooing happily, lay this beautiful little boy. A classical hemophiliac. My son. Bobby. Two thoughts raced in circles through my brain. It can't be true. It is. It can't be. It is.

I wasn't ready. We weren't ready. But everything important in life happens before you are ready.

I would have given everything I had to make him well. I still would. But I had nothing, and still have nothing to give.

Hemophilia. It was a frightening word, but so far it was still only a word. So far, Bobby was still a blond, happy baby. Except for the blood oozing from his toe and the bruise under his arm, nothing had happened to him. I vowed that nothing would. I would shield him and ward off danger. If anything came near to threaten him, I would attack it ferociously. Whatever was necessary to defeat this disease and protect this child, I would do.

I vowed to fight. But how? What weapons did I have? I was a young man, bookish, romantic, wary of the real world and unsure of my place in it, accustomed for most of my life to thinking mainly of self. Already, I was changing; in a dizzyingly rapid sequence, I had become a husband and a father. I was just discovering the felicity of these two new roles. There was a new weight on my shoulders, but it was not entirely the oppressive burden I had thought it would be. Instead, it was pleasant to be doing something for people I loved, people who made my life happier and more interesting than it had been before.

For Bobby had been a joy. Those early months in New York were difficult, but he made everything worthwhile. In the evenings when I came home tired from New York, Sue would have Bobby bathed and smelling of baby powder and she would be wearing something fresh and together we would play with him, roll him over, tickle him and make him laugh, and laugh ourselves. It washed away all the stains on my spirit. The world was in that tiny apartment. Here, no matter how disappointing the day had been or how foolish or mediocre what I seemed to be doing with my life, here was a unique, radiant little human being whose every gurgle and every gesture seemed significant. Here, in this sunny child, all blond and pink, was reason enough for life. And here, beyond life, was our immortality.

Help us! Help us! But who could help us? My mother and stepfather in Tennessee were far away; and besides, psychologically they were not equipped to provide the kind of enfolding warmth that was all, really, that anyone could give us then. Sue's parents were closer, both in distance and in spirit, but now they were as fearful as we were. Sue's father, a good man who has done his best all his life to cope with every family problem, tried to comfort us. But his face was gray with worry. Who was there to comfort him?

The news spread rapidly among our family and friends. Some were too busy or too shocked to do anything except gasp, telepathically. But many sent love and hope ("In these days of medical miracles, surely something will be discovered soon . . ."). A generous older man, a friend of Sue's father, understood that a chronic disease was likely to be expensive. "When my own son died," he wrote, "he left some money which I intend to use in a manner that I feel sure would have pleased him. I am sure he would heartily approve of my sending the enclosed check. He was particularly fond of small children."

Our own friends, most of them still single or recently married, organized to give what they knew we would need most: blood. Valerie Vondermuhll, who was Bobby's godmother and a *Life* editor, sat down with another *Life* reporter, Susan Neuberger, and wrote a memo to the entire staff:

> We at the magazine who know Sue and are extremely fond of her, her husband and little boy, decided to see if we could do something to help. Sue and Bob have been very brave and have been carrying on almost as though nothing had happened to their child. . . . If you would like to help young Bob Massie and his parents, would you give a pint of blood?

Barbara Rowe, one of Sue's classmates at Vassar, wrote a similar appeal to everyone in the class. Jack May, our best man and Bobby's godfather, dragooned everyone he knew: "Dear Chum: Robert Kinloch Massie IV has hemophilia. . . ." Jack asked them to donate blood, adding, "Do not go if you are under eighteen or over sixty, if you have had jaundice, if you have a cold, weigh under 107 pounds, or have had a Salk shot within two weeks. Or given blood within eight weeks. Or are just rotten to the core."

Of all the letters, there were two whose authors had looked into our future and tried to confront the essential question: Philosophically or psychologically, how are Sue and Bob going to be able to cope with this catastrophe?

One of these letters came from one of Sue's aunts in Switzerland. She was a woman who had seen—and was still to see—great sadness in her life. For her, doctors were only part of the answer:

> Nature sometimes does much better than medicine and as you will be a very vigilant young mother, this little baby will be well cared for. The influence of the mother on the infant is of such power that perhaps you will be able to create a miracle. The greatest doctors can be wrong. It is necessary to believe in something higher than doctors, not in fanatical mysticism, but to keep a hope so grand that it leaves no place for doubt. I have seen a photograph of your son and this little baby has such a ravishing air and appears so well! Concentrate on the little jewel, give him your love, you have so much character and power of persuasion.
>
> You will think I am perhaps talking nonsense, but believe me, Sue, we often see extraordinary things. Who knows? Life has extraordinary surprises in reserve for us all.

And then came another letter which touched us deeply but which at the time we simply did not understand. It came from Arnold Lewis, an old friend and a bishop of the Episcopal Church.

Other people had advised us to pray and we had prayed. Not for strength to accept and wisdom to understand, but for Bobby to be well. We had been told that through suffering comes character, but we were not interested in that. We did not want Bobby to suffer and grow in character; we wanted him to be well. We did not want to suffer ourselves and grow in character; we wanted him to be well. We wanted desperately for this affliction to be taken away. By medicine; by prayer; by a miracle; we didn't care how. What we really wanted, and dreamed of, and prayed for, was

that one morning we would wake up and look in Bobby's crib and
see that it had happened, a re-creation of the original miracle: a
perfect child.

We had known Arnold Lewis in Jacksonville where he was
dean of St. John's Cathedral. He was a husky, gray-haired man
whose great appeal for me lay in the admirable balance of faith,
reason, and experience on which he based his belief. His view of
God and man had been tempered, literally by fire, during his years
as a front-line military chaplain in the Second World War. In
Jacksonville, for the first time I went to church eagerly; Arnold's
sermons, crunchy with intellectual argument, crystalline with insight, were the best I had ever heard. In early January 1957, during
a visit to New York, Arnold had come to Eastchester to baptize
Bobby. This had been scarcely a month before, in that now un-
imaginable prehistory of our lives before we had known about
Bobby's hemophilia. Before I could write to thank him, the blow
had fallen. My subsequent letter must have told him and mirrored
our confusion and desperation. In any case, as soon as he received
my letter, Arnold Lewis wrote to us:

> I can well imagine the mental turmoil you are both going through.
> It's one thing for me to stand on the sidelines and tell you to have
> faith. It's quite another thing to have it strike home with you and
> have to face it. I know one thing, though. God doesn't do these
> things to punish us. I believe that He set in motion certain laws of
> nature. It is perfectly possible for these laws to be upset. Disease
> interferes with the normal health of a person. Sometimes disease
> can be cured, sometimes not. All medicine can do is to assist.
> Beyond that, it is up to nature. Yet, nature recognizes growth and
> change, life and death. The trouble is that we set up in our minds
> a picture of perfection, as far as nature is concerned: so many
> years of life; such and such a standard of health; etc. Then, when
> something happens, we ask "why?"
>
> No one has ever given an answer to that question that is
> satisfactory. The problem is not why these things happen; rather
> it is what are we going to do about it when they do happen, how
> are we going to take it. That is where faith comes in. Bobby's
> difficulty is no one's fault. You can't go around looking for some-
> one to blame. Your task now is to accept it, adjust to it, and try to

make something out of it. People are doing that every day and rising to heights that they never thought possible.

What I have said may not make sense at this point. But I know that both of you are strong enough to accept it. In your love for him and for each other, in whatever sacrifice will be called for, you will find a new faith, a stronger faith, knowing that God is good. I like that phrase in the Prayer Book that says He "does not willingly afflict or grieve the children of men."

Days passed. Perhaps they were weeks. And then, gradually, we began to face the facts. What were they?

New York Hospital had sent us the medical report of Bobby's diagnosis:

Hemoglobin—11.4 gm. per cent
RBC—4.6 million
Platelets—500,000
WBC—12,850
Polys:
    Seg.—36
Lymphocytes—59
Monocytes—4
Eosinophiles—1

COAGULATION STUDIES:

Clotting time—40 minutes (normal 5 to 10 minutes)
Clotting retraction—good
Prothrombin consumption—15.5 seconds (normal over 20 seconds)
Prothrombin time—17.5 seconds (control 14.5 seconds)
Recalcification time—8 minutes (normal less than 180 seconds)
Thromboplastin generation tests with the patient's plasma and serum and alternately substituting normal plasma and serum confirmed the diagnosis of classical hemophilia.

We read most of these words and numbers uncomprehendingly, as if they were hieroglyphics. The only part that made sense was that normal clotting time was five to ten minutes and Bobby's was forty minutes. But at the bottom of the page, standing out as if the words

were written in crimson, was the statement "confirmed the diagnosis of classical hemophilia."

How could this be true? Leaving aside all philosophical and
religious issues, how medically could this have happened? We had
only the vaguest knowledge about hemophilia. We knew, dimly,
that it was hereditary. We had heard, somewhere, that it was very
rare, a disease of kings, "the curse of the Hapsburgs." How could
it happen that Sue Rohrbach, whose forebears were sturdy Swiss,
and Bob Massie, whose clan came from the Highlands to farm in
Virginia, had produced a child with a hereditary "royal" disease?

We tried a second diagnosis. This time the tests were performed by Dr. Leandro Tocantins, a famous hematologist at Jeffer-
son Hospital in Philadelphia. Dr. Tocantins, a friend of Sue's parents since her childhood, had written to her: "Dear Suzy . . . I am
sorry that our paths have to cross again under such unfortunate
circumstances. I hope, however, that we may be able to reassure
you that things are not as dark as they seem."

Again, when the tests were completed, we did not understand
the results, but the comparisons were ominous. In one test, Bobby
was only 35 per cent normal; in another, he was 60 per cent normal;
in a third, he was 75 per cent normal. There was "no clotting in 24
hours." "One part of the patient's plasma significantly delays clotting time of two parts normal plasma" . . . and so forth. Dr.
Tocantins' conclusions: "The child has Hemophilia A (Classical
Hemophilia), Grade II, Moderate." The word "moderate" was a
single ray of hope.

But still, why us? We began to read, to ask questions, to learn.
We learned that hemophilia preceded the Hapsburgs, preceded
even kings. As I have already written elsewhere, it is as old as man.
In ancient Egypt, a woman whose first-born son bled to death from
a minor wound was forbidden to bear further children. The Tal-
mud barred circumcision in a family if two successive male children
had suffered fatal hemorrhages.

The genetic pattern by which hemophilia is transmitted was
discovered in 1803 by Dr. John Conrad Otto of Philadelphia. But
even seventy years after that, no one knew what caused the disease.
Some believed it was caused by too much blood, others thought it

was a nervous disease, still others thought it was infectious. The only treatment known was to elevate the afflicted limb, put it in a splint or cast, and put ice on it. "These children should not be punished," advised one doctor in 1905, "and their play with other children should be supervised. If possible, they should have the advantages of a warm, dry climate, country life, and sea bathing. Bleeders with means should take up some learned profession and, if they are students, dueling should be forbidden."

This was putting much too rosy a face on it. In fact, the prognosis was grim. Fifty-four per cent died before the age of five, and only 11 per cent lived to twenty-one. For these boys and young men who survived, it was an appalling existence: bedridden or in wheelchairs, their limbs twisted and locked by bleeding, most of them were hopelessly addicted to the drugs they took to dull their pain.

Today, despite the rapid advance of medical science in other fields, hemophilia remains one of the most mysterious and malicious of the genetic chronic diseases. The cause and the cure are still unknown.

We began to grapple with dozens of new medical terms. Hemophilia, we read, is an inherited coagulation deficiency, transmitted according to the sex-linked recessive Mendelian pattern. Thus, while women carry the defective gene, they almost never suffer from the disease. With rare exceptions, it strikes only males. Yet it does not necessarily strike all the males in a family. Genetically as well as clinically, hemophilia is capricious. Members of a family in which hemophilia has appeared never know, on the birth of a new son, whether or not the child will have hemophilia. If a woman who carries the hemophilia gene has a daughter, the family cannot know with certainty whether the daughter is a hemophilia carrier until she grows and has children of her own. The secret is locked inside the structure of the chromosomes.

For at the heart of the problem of hemophilia are the genes that issue the biochemical instructions that tell the body how to grow and nourish itself. Gathered in curiously shaped agglomerations of matter called chromosomes, they are probably the most intricate bundles of information known. They determine the nature of every one of the trillions of highly specialized cells that make up a human being. Scientists know that the defective gene that causes hemophilia appears on one of the female sex chromosomes, known as X chromosomes, but they have never precisely pinpointed the location of the faulty gene or determined the nature of the flaw. All they know is that once the hemophilic gene is present, it is passed, like some primeval curse, from a mother to her child.*

Still, this did not answer our question, Why us? There was no hemophilia in Sue's family history. Switzerland is a medical researcher's paradise because careful records, kept in town and village churches, usually list the cause of death. By chance, a distant cousin still lived in the small town of Sue's family origin. His job was Keeper of the Records. Faithfully, he set to work, going through the archives, looking not only for descriptions of illness but for any sudden, unexplained infant deaths. In time, he traced the line back through nine generations and forty-two male antecedents. He found no record of anything suggesting hemophilia.

By then, in any case, we had learned that there was no need to search the past for an answer. What had happened to us was not so unusual. In 40 per cent of the cases of hemophilia—two hemophiliacs out of five—there has been no previous hemophiliac in the family. The small victim and his parents are struck as if by a bolt of lightning from a cloudless sky. Something new has happened; a gene has just been changed; no one knows how or why. Doctors speak of this phenomenon as "spontaneous mutation."

This is what happened to us.

Nor, we learned, was the disease exclusively royal or even so terribly rare. It certainly was not the "disease of the Hapsburgs," for no prince of the Austrian house ever suffered from hemophilia. Rather, it was the lethal gift of Queen Victoria to a dozen royal princes scattered through the ruling dynasties of Russia, Spain, Germany, and England. The Queen herself was the most famous case of spontaneous mutation. One of her sons, Prince Leopold, had hemophilia, and two of her daughters, Princess Alice and Princess Beatrice, were hemophilia carriers. When the daughters of Alice

* For an explanation of the genetic transmission of hemophilia, see Appendix, page 415.

and Beatrice—Queen Victoria's granddaughters—married into the royal houses of Russia and Spain, their sons, the heirs to those two thrones, were born with hemophilia.

But the disease is broadly democratic. It appears on every continent, following no geographical or racial pattern, turning up at a more or less constant statistical rate of one hemophiliac in twenty thousand males. (In 1972, the first carefully conducted census of severely afflicted American hemophiliacs—those who, like Bobby, require constant transfusions—produced a figure of 25,500.) In time, I discovered a Michigan congressman who had three sons with hemophilia and a Bronx fireman with hemophiliac triplets. The disease has appeared in the family of A. P. Giannini, founder of the world's largest bank, the Bank of America, the family of a New York fashion designer, a family of Chinese immigrants newly arrived from Hong Kong, and the family of a black Salvation Army worker in Miami.

Just as most of what we had vaguely known about the genetic nature of hemophilia was wrong, so most of our smattering of knowledge about the clinical side of the disease was wrong, too. Bobby had hemophilia. Therefore, according to the nightmarish folklore that has come down through the centuries, he should bleed to death from the slightest scratch. If he cut himself or tore a hole anywhere in the intricate, elaborate human tubing system of arteries, veins, or even infinitesimal capillaries, then his blood, the marvelous, crimson, life-carrying fluid, should flow out unchecked.

But this was not true. Bobby had not bled to death from the pinprick on his toe, even though, because a vein had been torn, the wound had oozed for almost twelve hours. We learned quickly that the correct procedure for dealing with small cuts and scratches was simply to bind the wound tightly with a bandage or even a Band-Aid. Pressure alone would pinch off the blood; the healing process, as distinct from the clotting process, would take over and, within a day or so, a glaze of new tissue would form over the wound.

Understanding this, we breathed a cautious sigh of relief. But we did so too quickly. Suppose Bobby suffered something worse than a tiny cut on his finger or his toe? What about those areas of the body where pressure would be difficult to apply: the face? the throat? inside the nose? inside the mouth? Worse, what if the bleeding was not external at all, but entirely internal? What happened when internal bleeding started in the confined space of a knee, or ankle, or elbow joint? Suppose, after a kick from a playmate, bleeding began in a kidney? Suppose, as a toddler, he fell and hit his head and bleeding began in the brain?

Sue and I did not learn everything at once. Instead, we had to grope from fact to fact, learning what questions to ask and whom to ask, sometimes anxious to hear more, sometimes fearful to pile up too many anticipated horrors. At one point in those early weeks, we sat down together and made a list of specific questions. I still have it, eighteen years later, written in her hand in pencil on a yellowing piece of notebook paper. The questions come in no particular order; we were simply trying to peer ahead into this vast and forbidding unknown territory:

> Who is greatest specialist?
> Where is best research being done?
> Where can we get books?
> What about bruises? Are they dangerous?
> Why transfusions? Are they only needed for serious injuries or as a matter of course?
> What is Bobby's blood type?
> Can we start a blood bank for him?
> What other remedies are there?
> How debilitating is it?
> What other effects besides bleeding?
> Do tourniquets help?
> What about other children?
> What about my sisters?
> Is it ever fatal?

In time, over the years, the answers would come. So far, we had only the questions. So far, except for the hematoma and the trouble with circumcision at birth, the bruise on his arm and the oozing toe, nothing had happened.

Chapter 3

We did not know it then, but a great adventure was beginning.
It was an adventure that would lead us through terrible dark regions
of despair and up to the heights of joy. It was to plunge us into
struggle and lead us to creation. It was a journey of many thousand
days that began with the first faltering steps of our child. We,
along with him, were to learn to crawl and kneel, to stand and,
finally, to walk.

In those first days, bewildered and ignorant, our eyes were
closed to everything but the cataclysm. How could we interpret its
meaning? How were we to learn? Who would teach us?

My first reaction was to ignore it entirely. One only had to
look at Bobby, rosy and beautiful, to know that he was *perfectly*
well. Somehow, they had made a terrible mistake, those doctors.
Everybody knows that they don't know everything. After all, the
diagnosis was only a piece of paper . . . a series of blood tests. I
almost convinced myself that the few days in the hospital were
only a bad dream, that they had never happened.

But they had happened. It was no dream. Seven days after the
diagnosis, I went back to see the pediatrician. As I came into his
office, he was looking intently down at a paper, playing with his
pencil with great concentration. In the dark room, there was only
a single desk light that shadowed his face and eyes. He did not lift
his head for several moments; perhaps he did not want to meet my
questioning, still hopeful eyes. His silence continued, unbroken.
I tried to assume a normal voice, matter-of-fact, even cheerful.
"Tell me, Doctor, what can I expect?" I asked, pencil poised over
my notebook to take down his recommendations. "What shall
I do?"

There was only silence, only the scratch of his pencil doodling on the paper. Finally, with a sort of flat, hopeless voice that struck fear into my heart, he answered. "I don't know."

"But," I went on, speaking faster, "how will I know something is happening?"

"Watch for bruises," he said.

Then, although I knew already that it was useless, questions came tumbling out:

"Does it hurt?"

"It can."

"How does it start?"

"I don't know. Later, he may have trouble with his joints."

"But when?"

"Perhaps at the age of six." (At least that was something. Six was years away. Maybe it would be different then.)

"But how does it start?"

"I don't know. I have never treated a case. I have only seen a few cases in hospitals during my training."

"How often will he need a transfusion?"

"I don't know."

"What will happen if he does?"

"Well, we could do it at White Plains Hospital."

"You mean he has to be admitted to the hospital for a transfusion?"

"Yes."

"But can't you tell me anything?"

"No. I'm sorry. I don't know what to tell you to expect."

I was deeply shaken by this conversation. If the doctor didn't know, how could I? The doctor always knows. Every mother is sure of this. She calls the pediatrician, and he, like God, tells her when to feed and when to stop, when to add and when to take away. If the baby sneezes or wheezes, the doctor is the one who tells you, calmly and professionally, that it is nothing to worry about. If the pediatrician cannot tell you, then what? This essential rock of knowledge, this firm defense against a mother's unreasoning fear, where was it now? In front of me sat a troubled and hesitant man who knew little more than I. "What can I do?" I said, repeating in panic the meaningless question.

"Nothing. Wait and see what develops. Perhaps you should get in touch with the Hemophilia Foundation."

I went home.

Following his advice, I searched the telephone book and finally found the "Metropolitan Hemophilia Foundation." I called. Foundation was a grand name for an understaffed, struggling little group of parents who had only a volunteer to answer the phone. They had little time for babes in the woods like us. "Send in your money," said the voice. "We'll send you our bulletin. Come to our meetings."

One night I went. In a bare hall a small group was gathered. Almost all those present were parents of hemophiliacs, who, in addition to whatever time they could give to the foundation, were also bearing the emotional and physical burdens of their sons' illnesses. They were consumed in a tense discussion of new ways to raise blood donors. There was no time or energy left to think about raising money for research or for writing and publishing information. It seemed that the need for blood, and the difficulty of obtaining it, were so overwhelming that they were the only considerations.

But this didn't help me much. (And anyway, I told myself, *we* might never need blood. These intense, worried people were not *us*. It was only later that we too were to learn how much time and emotion is exhausted in this blood struggle.) What I desperately needed to know then was how to live with the knowledge of the disease.

Later that evening, over coffee, I timidly approached a group of mothers. They were talking feverishly about their own Johnny or Timmy, trading horror stories. I listened and heard things in those early conversations that I could not permit myself to repeat aloud to anyone, not even Bob, for years. There were stories of boys who had bled in their spines and become paraplegics (in teen age, I was told, very common), of bleeding into the kidneys and liver; the perplexing, terrifying terms, hematuria, hematoma; I heard how bleeding in the throat can be fatal, of boys rushed to the hospitals choking to death, of tracheotomies that did or did not succeed. As they talked, the full weight of the terror began to descend. Yes, of course, one could bleed *anywhere*. But how could anyone remain that vigilant? The women almost seemed to be reveling in this horror, trying to outdo one another with terrifying experiences in a sort of nightmarish *mano a mano*. Now I realize that probably it was only their way of releasing pent-up anxiety. But then I knew that if I listened to any more, I would go mad. I fled and never returned to those meetings. I regretted that I had gone at all, for the stories I heard in those early days lay at the bottom of my consciousness like a poisonous sediment, rising in the night to haunt me.

Instead, I wrapped myself in a cocoon and tried to *believe* that none of those things would happen to Bobby. I asked no more questions of the doctor. He, interpreting my silence as calm, noted in his records a month after our first interview: "Parents have adjusted to the hemophilia diagnosis and met several families who have hemophiliac sons and are getting along well." The truth was otherwise. I had not adjusted; I was simply frozen in fear.

During those early months I watched Bobby constantly. I checked him every hour, all over—sometimes many times during a single hour. I woke up at night and listened for his breathing. But no matter how hard I tried, the bruises began to appear, dark and blue, then turning into an ugly green and yellow, relentless, merciless stigmata confirming that "the piece of paper" had been totally correct.

First, he was bumping in his crib. Then he was trying to stand up, one hand on the play pen sides. A tottering step—down he went. Hard. Then he began to do more; in his tiny overalls and sneakers, he unsteadily trotted around the apartment. I tried to sew pads into his overalls, but the pads slipped or weren't in the right place. And in any case, it was a losing battle. Somehow the bruises always appeared somewhere else. You couldn't pad the entire child.

In the safe, benign environment of our little apartment everything suddenly became a hazard: the corners of chairs, doorknobs. I padded the edge of our coffee table. In this new world every common ordinary object had to be re-examined as a potentially dangerous instrument. Is there a slippery rug in the bathroom? Throw it out. The toothbrush: examine it carefully for hard bristles. "Strict care," warned the Hemophilia Foundation Bulletin, "should be taken not to give the child glass or hard plastic objects which, when broken, can be harmful." All right. Only soft toys and cloth books.

I did no housework when he was up, only when he napped. Or at night. I grew to have a love for the peaceful night when I at last could breathe a little, read a little. Until the night itself became dangerous, when we learned that, inexplicably, bleeding often grows worse in the dark hours just before dawn.

I began to develop a sixth sense, covertly watching, judging potentially dangerous situations before they became hazardous, staying alert without seeming to be, ready to let him move, but ready also to leap forward to catch him as he tripped. But it wasn't enough; even when his movements were still simple, there was always something I could not anticipate. Down he went, with my arms outstretched to reach him, too late.

Even very early, we were aware that there were varying periods of severity in the rhythm of the mysterious disease. "Bobby seemed to bruise more easily than previously," noted the doctor in his records. On May 15: "another episode of easy bruising. It was preceded by one day when he seemed unusually pale without being ill." We noticed that when he had a cold, or a slight temperature, the bruising increased noticeably. I grew afraid of every sneeze.

At first, following the doctor's advice, I tried to keep a journal of his bruises. On June 16, 1957, I was noting meticulously:

Sunday, June 16: He had an ear and eye infection. At this time, a bruise on the right side of his chest swelled noticeably. The protrusion was about an inch and a half. It was purple and blue colored. He had a temperature of 101°.

Monday, June 17: Bruise swelled.

Tuesday, June 18: A new bruise on the underside of the left arm, red and purple in color. By evening, it had swelled to 2 inches wide, 2 inches long, 1-inch protrusion. Wrapped with an Ace bandage.

Wednesday, June 19: Bruise on chest: bleeding stopped. Color starting to fade. Yellow-green on outside of bruise.

Thursday, June 20, morning: Bruise on left side of chest looks stopped. Color fading rapidly. Right upper arm, bleeding did not spread further. Swelling down. But back of right knee has streaks of blue, not real bruise; right calf swelled slightly, rather taut. Bobby still uses leg freely, with no signs of discomfort, but cannot straighten leg.

Thursday, June 20, evening: Arm has not spread. Color seems to be fading a little in center. But right leg swollen from knee to ankle, hot skin, taut; calf measures 8″ (left 7″), even foot looks swollen; seems to be causing him discomfort.

Friday, June 21: Chest fading. Arm fading on upper part toward shoulder; lower part still purple, but has not spread. Swelling gone. Leg (morning) measures 7½″, more flexible, foot less swelled, still discolored on back of knee, upper thigh, green, yellow, still taut. Evening: Arm O.K., still wrapped. Chest O.K. Leg seems a little worse, measures 7¾″, foot swelled, color same, skin taut but not hot, kept tightly wrapped.

Soon I gave up, because there was no way to record them all.

Indoors, at least, I had the illusion of being able to protect Bobby. Outdoors, it was a different story. The Spanish royal family, I once read, had padded the trees in their royal park to protect their little hemophiliac sons. I tried to assess everything in the path of mine. Holes in the ground: steer him away or fill them in. There were so many other things: swings and tricycles, fences and benches, slides, other children who threw stones or snowballs, or hit each other with sticks. Sometimes I tried to watch from behind the curtains, so that he could play a little more normally. I tried to outguess the unexpected. I failed.

Very soon I realized with despair that there was no way to avoid all hazards. Whatever I did, the disease would find a way to strike—sometimes, just as it had in the beginning, spontaneously, with no visible cause whatsoever. The bruises simply appeared: on arms, legs, body, and face.

During those months I learned a great deal about bruising. I learned that bumps on the head take the longest to go down, because the blood reabsorbs so slowly. I learned that bleeding in the large muscles was likely to be prolonged and difficult to stop, because of the large area into which blood could seep. I learned the color of surface bruises, and deeper ones, and that the worst ones did not discolor at all, because they were too deep. But they hurt and impaired movement.

What I was desperately trying to avoid, of course, was A Transfusion. I simply did not think I could face it. I dreaded the moment: foreign hands tormenting my child, having to leave him with *strangers*. No! I could not, I would not, accept it.

By chance, one of my acquaintances had had her baby at the same time as another woman she remembered well, because this lady had just given birth to a second hemophiliac son. She suggested that I get in touch with her hospital roommate "because they seemed to know a lot about it." I grabbed at this chance for information and called Joyce Stone. Joyce was a warm and quietly dignified girl. The appearance of hemophilia in her sons had been spontaneous. Yes, she said, Randy was born at the same time as Bobby, and a second diagnosis of classical hemophilia had been confirmed. While we had dinner in her home in Connecticut, around us played the Stones' older son, Skipper, who was nearly three. He was already wrapped in Ace bandages. It was Joyce who first explained to me how to use the elastic bandages to slow down bleeding, to give support to painful muscles. She and her husband, George, a husky giant of a Texan, explained about using ice packs on areas swollen by bleeding.

In the months and the years that followed, I too became adept at rolling and rerolling those elastic bandages. I learned how to strap muscles down in every part of the body: not too tight so as to constrict; just tight enough to support and take away pain. I learned about measuring bruises and applying ice. (The worst part about ice was that it had to be put in some sort of flexible bag that could be contoured to fit on a limb and tied on with an elastic bandage. I used ordinary kitchen plastic bags but, as the ice melted, they leaked, and then water would slosh over everything, sheets and clothes. But there was nothing better.)

Joyce and George wore an alluring air of serenity and near normality, but Joyce was constantly using the word that terrified me: "transfuse." To me, it was as explosive as an obscenity. While they talked, I tried to absorb, to learn everything I could. But at the same time I prayed that just perhaps, just perhaps, it would never come to us. Perhaps she hadn't been vigilant enough. I would be more vigilant. Perhaps it would never be necessary for Bobby. But there was no way to push it aside. Inexorably, the moment came.

It was August 1957, just two weeks before Bobby's first birthday. In six months I had already grown so accustomed to his bruises that this one seemed just one more. How it happened, I did not know. He may simply have sat down too hard as he was learning to walk. It was a large bruise on the left buttock. But this one began to behave differently. It swelled rapidly and then spread to the left side of the scrotum, which also began to swell. Bobby was very uncomfortable and would not sleep. Worried, we called the doctor several times during the night. Finally, at 4 A.M. we took him to the hospital. (Dear Lord, why do things so often get worse at night?) We were cold with fear and trying to hold on to our courage. I cannot forget the empty streets along our way, lit coldly by the lonely street lights, the sense of hibernating humanity behind the shutters and lowered shades. They, fortunate ones, were safe in bed, their children calmly dreaming. When Bobby arrived, his hemoglobin was low, down to 7.5 (normal for a baby is 11–12), his tiny scrotum had swelled to nearly eight inches in circumference.

Because his hemoglobin was so low, the doctor decided to give him whole blood. He had to be pricked, his blood crossmatched. This took more time. Only when the dawn had come did the doctor start to transfuse him. Hours had passed. The strangers wheeled him away on a stretcher to an operating room. We were sent away. When I saw him again he was tied into his little crib. Although he couldn't move, high crib pads that obscured all vision had, according to the rules, been placed all around the bed. Part of his hair had been shaved away because his veins were so tiny the doctor had gone into the scalp vein. The visiting hours were strict. They would not let me stay with him at night. I lay in my bed sleepless, worrying about his tears and his loneliness. I rushed back to the hospital and haunted the doorway to the ward, trying to catch a glimpse of him and waiting for the sacred moment when they would unlock the doors and let me in to see him. They kept him two and a half days because the doctor was unsure and wanted to take no chances. When we finally took him home, it seemed as if a year had gone by. It was the first real taste of what life was to be.

I knew then that I would have to make a great effort of will. All my life I had been mortally afraid of hospitals. It had begun when I was a child of seven and had my tonsils removed. I had almost bled to death. My parents had left me there alone, after the operation. In the middle of the night I unexpectedly began to hemorrhage. A clot developed in my throat and I was taken away and operated on again at three in the morning. Vividly, I still see the circle of doctors' faces grouped around me, like ghouls under the bright operating-room light. I remember waking up alone, terrified, in the dark, and not knowing how to call for help. So frightened was I by this experience that had I been able to avoid it, I would never have chosen to have my baby in a hospital. I could not find the courage to visit people in hospitals. I would even cross the street to avoid passing by their doors.

Now I had to face reality—that I would be spending a lot of time in them. I knew that, somehow, I had to overcome my fear, so that I did not pass it on to my son. If he was doomed to a series of hospital stays, he must not develop my unreasoning fears, for how much would they increase his suffering? I forced myself to be cheerful with him. I determined that he would never have to submit to that terrible fear of the small child, the disappearance of his parents. My instincts warned me that if this happened to him early in life, before he could reason or understand, it might leave him with lifelong scars. So I fought all hospital rules and strict nurses to stay with him for all his early transfusions. Although the needles might hurt, he would never feel abandoned.

In almost all hospitals, the rules were against such familiarity. In defiance of all reasonableness and humanity, parents were often treated as pariahs; or, at best, as annoying hindrances. I had to learn to stand my ground against a series of cold-eyed nurses, residents, and even doctors. I was often terrified of them, but I stayed with Bobby. And, although it is painful to say this, I was forced to conclude that there was a conscious cruelty in some of them. It was as if, in the soul of some of those who choose to work with the sick, there lies, side by side with the desire to heal and help, another darker emotion, more akin to the desire for power of the prison camp guard.

For his early transfusions I had to hold him down. But I did it, not a stranger. It strangled me with pain. I would look down at his pleading eyes while he screamed, but I would soothe him and tell him it would soon be over. Later, I brought books. I began to read him a story while the doctor prepared his needles and bottles, before they tried to get into a vein. Only for the few moments that were necessary for the puncture would I stop, and then I would resume the story as if nothing had happened. Wonderful Ludwig Bemelmans! "Poor Madeline would now be dead, but for a dog that kept its head"; and Pepito, and Miss Clavel, who woke up in the middle of the night and said, "Something is not right." We read them over and over. Soon he would be calm, his arm at rest while the plasma flowed. His faithful Teddy and his blanket came with us on every hospital visit, no matter what the hour. With Teddy propped up beside him, his blanket to stroke, and a story, very soon transfusions began to lose their terror.

Even before the age of four, Bobby no longer cried at all when they stuck him, although he often had to be stuck several times before they could find his small child's veins. As for me, no matter how many years have passed, I have never gotten used to it. Even now, when the moment comes to puncture the skin, to find and skewer the slippery vein, I draw in my breath sharply and hold it. I pray. When the needle pierces, I flinch. Only when the blood runs back, bright red, can I relax. It is a strange thing, but even when blood has to be taken from my arm, I think of him, and the puncture hurts far more than it should.

It was a blessing that it all started so slowly. Had I known what was to come, I do not believe that I could have accepted the burden. Would I have run away? I often wonder. Mercifully, we only have to learn to walk one step at a time.

After those August days, when we were home again, together, when it was all over, when there had been time to recover, things did not seem so insurmountable. I remembered that Joyce had said her son had transfusions "every few months." Well, I thought, if it is only to be every few months, I can just about do it.

Yet only a month later, in September, Bobby was in the hospital again, because of swelling bruises on the face and throat. Again in October. Always there was the same dehumanizing routine at the hospital: the high, obscuring crib pads (I removed them as soon as I was allowed to see him. As soon as I left, they were up again), the forced constriction of movement. (Rigid hospital rules decreed that all hemophiliacs must be tied to their cribs to prevent them from bumping themselves accidentally. This rule was absolute, no matter what the actual situation or the child's personality dictated. They untied him when I came. Otherwise, no one wanted to take a compassionate step that might result in bureaucratic problems later.)

While our fearful pediatrician committed Bobby to this hospital constriction for every transfusion, all our normal life stopped. I drove back and forth to the hospital as often as the short visiting hours would permit. Despite all my brave resolutions, each hospital visit drained me emotionally. For we, the healthy, think this way: we must wait until it gets better before we start to relax, to live. But what if it doesn't get better? Are we, is he, to wait forever? Is he to wait for his childhood?

Surely there had to be a better way, a more human way, to treat our sunny child. Through the hemophilia grapevine I heard that somewhere in Westchester there was a doctor who gave transfusions *at home*—a doctor with two hemophiliac boys of his own.

The waiting room of the modest little office in Mount Vernon, New York, was crowded. The phone was constantly ringing. But there was one fresh welcoming sign: there was no starched formality about the nurse. For the first time since our family had been set apart, Bobby and I were not met with hushed tones and strange, sidelong glances. Instead, we were met with a broad, welcoming smile, a cheerful, "Hi, Bobby! Would you like a candy?" (Could it be they didn't *know?*)

When our turn came, we were ushered into the cluttered office of Dr. Mario T. Bisordi. (Right away he said, "Nobody calls me Mario; everybody calls me Bill.") He was a handsome man, with the dark, dashing good looks of the film star Gilbert Roland, the same black sparkling eyes, the black mustache. As Bill talked to us, a wide smile often crossed his face and illuminated it. From some deep source it radiated simplicity and the expansive faith in life that is a treasure of the Italian soul. It was the sunny warmth of that smile, more than any explanations, that began to thaw the ice of fear around my heart.

He was the busiest doctor I have ever known; the real thing, an old-fashioned GP. (He quickly explained to me that first day, "No, no! I'm not an Internist. I'm a GP.") He was caring for all the needs of a wide and varied practice. He was delivering babies (he has delivered over a thousand). He was making twenty to twenty-five house calls a day. When we met, his fame in one particular specialty had grown to such a point that he was personally caring for all the transfusion needs and complications of sixteen of the twenty-six known hemophiliacs in Westchester County. Two of these were his own sons.

Bill is the kind of doctor everybody always wishes they had: realistic yet cheerful, with a kind, reassuring word and a healing presence.

Forgotten, apparently, were the crowded waiting room and the busy telephone. Bill seemed to have all the time in the world. Attentively, he listened to my hesitant descriptions of Bobby's diagnosis, of his few early problems. These things were still painfully difficult for me to talk about; never mind, he overcame my shyness. (Now I realize how very small and insignificant Bobby's problems must have seemed compared to the torment his own boys were in at that moment. But Bill showed no sign of this, made no mention.) The wonderful thing was, *he knew*. He talked about hemophilia almost as if it were as ordinary as a cold . . . there was no mystery, no need to use veiled phrases. After he had examined Bobby, he said, "He's a cute little fellow. Don't you worry. I can see that you're going to get along fine. There's no need to admit him into the hospital for a transfusion. I can't come all the way to you, but, well, how far are you from Cross County Hospital? ("Twenty-five minutes," I said.) O.K. Well, you bring him down there and I'll transfuse him as an outpatient whenever I can. You can keep the stuff there, or even at home, if you want."

I went home elated. Bobby was to be treated as an outpatient!

No more hospital stays! I could go with him, stay with him, and he would come home with me. There was hope, after all.

That was how we started going to Cross County Hospital. I would bring Bobby, lying on a blanket in the back of the station wagon, and carry him up in the elevator. Bill would give transfusions in the emergency room on the eighth floor, overlooking the miles of asphalt of the New York Thruway. He never missed a vein. Sometimes there would be two or three other boys waiting there too. Bobby remembers that he was impressed to see these big hemophiliac boys who gave him the bed to lie on, while they got their transfusions sitting up.

I might be worried, but when Bill came in, smiling, in charge, I felt immediately calmer. Sometimes he would be very much delayed. I would fret. It was only much later that I understood how sick his own two boys were all during that time, how strained he was giving so much to so many others.

While the plasma thawed in the sink, we had a lot of time to talk. I learned that Bill was the youngest of eleven children of an Italian immigrant family.

He had always wanted to be a doctor. "I was always talking about medicine, and then one day, when I was twelve, I found an old dictionary. In the back was a diagram of a skeleton. I studied the skeleton and learned all the parts. Then I looked up everything else I could find in the dictionary. I remember I once found a book on medicine by Logan Clendening and read it over and over." Bill had to work hard. He played the trumpet and the bass with local dance bands to pay his way through school. He did his pre-med at Manhattan College and went to medical school at St. Louis University.

In St. Louis, Bill met Nina; and with her, his fate. She was the tall, blond daughter of a German Swiss Bernese family of farmers who lived on a farm a hundred miles out of St. Louis. Hemophilia was in her family. Two brothers and two uncles had died of it. She remembers only that "I didn't know much about it; they were so much older. I just remember the funerals. It was just this strange thing that was in our family."

Bill knew. "I had read about it in my medical books. I had

never treated a hemophiliac, but it didn't frighten me. Anyway, I loved her."

Nina and Bill were married. They had a daughter, then two sons with hemophilia; later they had two more daughters and finally a healthy boy—six children in all.

It was during the years that we knew him best that Bill was treating most of the hemophiliacs in Westchester County. No one else knew as much as he did about the handling of the disease, and he could never find the heart to turn anyone down. The physical load was heavy, the emotional load beyond measuring. He was called out several times each night to make house calls and to give transfusions to other hemophiliacs. Often these were life-threatening situations. When finally, weary and exhausted, he would come home (and he *laughed* when he told me this), "Nina would say, 'Before you sit down to supper, you have to go and get plasma defrosted for the boys.'" His own boys' problems were severe and painful. His oldest boy was so proud that he never wanted to show his pain. Some nights Bill and Nina could hear him grinding his teeth all the way down the hall. Bill would rush in, anxious, and ask, "What's the matter?" and his son, tight with pain, would answer, "It's nothing, Dad, nothing."

Some days, when I would meet Bill at the hospital, his face, usually so merry and kind, would be clouded. I could see pain and torment in his eyes. But he would only say, "Billy Boy is having some trouble," or "Tommy is giving us some worry." Nothing more. The shadows would linger for only a moment. By the next sentence, he would be smiling again.

In addition to everything else, on top of his full practice, Bill was forced by his sons' disease to find time to hold down still another job. It was a civil service job for the State of New York: he was physician to the three hundred members of the State Public Works Department and their families. This meant about eight to ten extra house calls on an average day. But without the civil service job, he would not have been able to get medical insurance to cover his sons. He explained to me simply, "If I hadn't had that job, we couldn't have made it. We wouldn't have survived."

With inexhaustible energy and optimism, Bill pursued everything that could possibly help hemophilia. There were always piles of reading material on the subject on his office desk. After reading about Rasputin, he decided to take a medical course in hypnosis as a possible way of alleviating pain. When he finished and tried it on his boys, they just laughed at him. "Dad, you look so funny!" Instead, he used it successfully with women in childbirth, and on himself during a period of complicated bridgework because "I hate Novocain."

At the hospital, Bill would sometimes joke that he was getting "dishpan hands" from defrosting so many bottles of plasma in the sink. So he and a friend set to work developing an automatic plasma defroster. They devised a simple mechanism using a turntable made from a coffee can to rotate the bottle in front of an electric light bulb. The machine looked a bit eccentric, but it worked! No more dishpan hands! The trouble was that after months of effort, just as they perfected their invention, fresh-frozen plasma was switched from bottles to flat plastic bags. Back to the sink. Bill sighed, and then laughed and said, "It's the story of my life!"

Bill and Nina were forever organizing blood drives, to the point where, Bill says, "it even interfered with my practice, because I felt so indebted to people who gave blood for the boys that I felt terrible charging them for a visit. So I didn't." When a group of sanitation workers gave blood, Nina invited them home for steak dinners. She says, "Our whole life was hemophilia. Everything we did was because of it. Work and hemophilia. That was it."

Occasionally he would philosophize a little about medicine, although these times were rare, because Bill is not an articulate man and explanations of his philosophy don't come easily. He was too busy living it. Once he said, "The trouble with medicine these days is that it is losing contact with people. You know, medicine is not only called the 'science' but the 'art' of medicine. Science can do a lot, but you can't forget the art. A doctor has to be able to *feel* the patient's symptoms. Part of being a doctor is an interest in people." I half-jokingly asked him what his other interests were, besides medicine. He paused. Then that sunny smile crossed his face and he answered, "What am I interested in? Well . . . everything, I guess! I enjoy music. I enjoy my garden. I enjoy people. I enjoy living. I enjoy everything!" That was about as close as I ever came to getting him to describe the secret of the abundant energy in him, that joyous spark that gave him the gift of healing.

With Bill, we began to learn how to laugh again. He showed us that life had to go on, full and varied, despite everything. Bobby loved him because "he doesn't hurt me." I began to learn that the technical mysteries of transfusion were not so overwhelming. Bill taught me how to defrost plasma, how to handle the bags and the needles. This activity gave me a positive feeling of helping. My confidence grew.

It was lucky that we met Bill when we did, because during those first hard months, something else, something totally un-expected, had happened. I was pregnant again.

Chapter 4

Of course it was too soon. I had barely learned how to accept Bobby's illness. Emotionally, I was not prepared. Today I suppose that an immediate abortion would be the normal solution. But I did not even consider it. Perhaps I was too old-fashioned, or afraid. Anyway, it was illegal and we had no money.

Out of purest superstition I went to the gynecologist who had circumcised Bobby. He had not known or guessed that Bobby was a hemophiliac, yet he had succeeded. He had taken the time to visit me twice in the hospital after Bobby's birth. I had never forgotten him.

Dr. Callahan confirmed what I already knew. Cheerfully, he said, "You're quite right; you're well along." Only after my examination, when we talked in his office, did I tell him about Bobby. I could see how shocked he was, that he immediately remembered the circumcision. "Oh," he said, "I'm sorry"; but quickly, almost without a pause, he went on, "Well then, let's make this one a girl, so that you will have courage to go on and have others after!" That statement helped me through the months that followed.

There were some bad nights when I lay in bed awake wondering about the new life inside me. But Dr. Callahan was so unfailingly positive that he sustained my fragile confidence, nurtured my strength and my hope.

This was the easiest of my three births, and this time I was wide awake when the baby arrived. I heard the scream with my first rested breath. I asked, "Doctor, what is it, what is it?" "It's a girl!" he said happily. Anxiously I questioned, "Doctor, are you sure?" The doctor and the nurses all began to laugh as he answered,

"Yes, Mrs. Massie, I am sure." And I looked down and saw Susanna lying beside me, all beautiful and blond.

I had always wanted to have a baby in the spring, the 1st of May, I secretly hoped. In France, it is the day traditionally reserved for lovers and happiness, when everyone presents sprigs of lilies of the valley to those they love. And it was time for lilacs! More than any other flower, I love lilacs. I didn't quite make May 1—Susanna was born at five o'clock on April 30—but it was close enough.

How fortunate we were to have that surprise baby! Had I waited longer and chosen the time myself, I think I would have grown more and more afraid. Bobby had not yet begun his most fearful bouts with his disease. My hope and energy were still alive and fresh. I am grateful to Dr. Callahan for his understanding and his belief in the power of life and love which he put before his scientific knowledge.

I cannot imagine how our story would have continued had Susanna been a boy and a hemophiliac. I stand in awe before those who have lived with two or more hemophiliac boys and have gone on to have other children. I have heard of cases where there have been three, four; and in one family in North Carolina, seven hemophiliac boys. Sometimes there were sisters in between, sometimes only boys. What is so surprising to me is not only that these families have survived this terrible challenge, but that they have so often overcome it with their love and their strength. Such people are titans. I cannot be sure that I could have been so courageous. I gave thanks to God that He had been merciful and sent Susanna.

We almost got used to bruises. Cuts on the mouth were much more difficult.

Even when he was very small, Bobby was unusually curious. He stood early, he walked early, he wanted to explore everything. Perhaps because he was so active, he was constantly biting his tongue or scraping his lip. Even a tiny scrape took weeks to heal. Because the surfaces were wet, clots had difficulty forming. As soon as they formed, they were washed away by saliva, motion of the tongue, or any chewing of food. There was no way to apply pressure. There were a few surface clotting products that we would try, such as Topical Prothrombin, but mostly these just added to the mess by forming webby half clots that did not heal. Once he woke us up in the middle of the night and handed Bob a raisin-sized clot. I had to puree all his food. He went around with a diaper under his chin to absorb dripping blood which kept oozing slowly out of his mouth. His breath was horrible. I leave it to you to imagine what it meant to take him to the supermarket or the playground: the comments, the stares.

We learned not to panic at the sight of blood on a pillow, because we slowly came to understand that blood mixed with saliva looks worse than it is. Real, serious bleeding is thick and dark. It takes practice to tell. With difficulty we learned to keep calm, to measure, to watch before racing to the telephone.

Removing bloodstains became a peculiar household problem, but I became adept, thanks to one of the "Helpful Household Hints" that appeared in the Hemophilia Bulletin and advised cheerily:

> Soak the stains in lukewarm water, then rub out gently in succession of lukewarm waters. Hot water will set blood. Ammonia added to the water will help dissolve old stains. Javelle water may be used as a last resort for white cottons and linens. BLOOD ON BLANKETS may be removed by spreading the spot heavily with a paste made of raw starch and cold water. Let dry and brush off. Repeat until stain is gone.

Trying to guess the possible dangers was futile. Billy Bisordi once cut his tongue on a lollipop and bled for twenty-one days, needing twenty-one transfusions before it finally stopped. I tried to prevent Bobby from getting or finding lollipops as much as possible; people kept offering them. Occasionally I let him have one and prayed. One good thing, although we worried a lot about each one, his teeth all came in without problems.

The most frightening thing about these mouth cuts was that sometimes they would seem to be getting better and then suddenly, without any warning, often at night, they would begin hemorrhaging. There was no explanation. This was why, during any mouth bleeding, Bob and I took turns getting up every hour or half hour throughout the night to check his pillow for blood.

When Bill Bisordi could not transfuse Bobby at Cross County Hospital, we raced off, at strange hours of the night, to Mount Sinai Hospital, which was the only hospital to maintain a twenty-four-hour Emergency Transfusion Clinic for hemophiliacs. It took almost an hour each way for us to drive to New York, but we felt it was more than worth it to prevent his being committed to another hospital for several days.

One such night, at about 1:30 A.M., my voice tense with panic, I called Bill. We had to go to Mount Sinai. But Bill calmed me by saying, "Listen, Sue, for any normal family, a transfusion in the middle of the night is a catastrophe. For a hemophiliac, it is *routine*, and the more you can consider it that way, the easier it will be for you and for him." It was good advice, which we took to heart, and after that, whatever the hour, we would pretend to Bobby that there was nothing unusual about bundling him up and driving to New York at 2 or 3 A.M. Usually the sky would be pink with the first rays of dawn before we would finally be able to drive home and collapse into bed. Often Bob could sleep only an hour or two before having to get up and take the train back to New York and *Newsweek*.

There were bureaucratic problems at the clinic too. Hospital rules decreed that in case of hemophilia transfusions, the hematology resident was to be called. Very soon we learned that hematology residents had very little practice at getting into the tiny veins of a small child. Down would come some serious young man. He would try to get into Bobby's veins. He would fail. He would try again. Again he would fail. This sometimes went on five or six times, with me holding down Bobby, screams, and tears. Finally he would give up and call the pediatric resident, who most often was able to hit a vein the first time. Nothing we could say would convince the clinic that we could make everything easier by calling the pediatric resident immediately. This would never do. So each time Bobby was used as a pincushion.

Susy's very first outing was to the hospital. She had been born April 30. In mid-May Bobby had another severe mouth bleeding.

When I called Bill and he advised a transfusion at Mount Sinai, I said, "But, Bill, what shall I do with Susy? I can't leave her."

"How old is she?" asked Bill.

"Three weeks," I answered.

"When was she born, exactly?" asked Bill.

It was three weeks to the day. "All right," said Bill, "take her along."

We wrapped Susy in her blankets and bundled up Bobby. We tucked a diaper around his chin over his sweater to absorb the blood, and at 1 A.M. drove off to New York.

We were lucky. That night we got one of the hematology residents who quickly turned over his authority to the pediatric resident. (How I grew to love and respect those few who spared Bobby by not insisting on their bureaucratic privileges! They were so rare!)

There was a strange atmosphere in that night emergency room. Situated, as it was, on the fringe of the Upper East Side, it was common to have Bobby admitted at the same time as stab-wound victims and accident victims. A tough but pleasant night nurse, with flaming red hair and a Runyonesque gift of expression, ruled over this nocturnal domain. We loved it when she was on duty. That night, one of her admirers, a jolly cop on the beat, had come in to have a midnight chat and a cup of coffee. He put his cap on Bobby and gave him his nightstick to play with. Bobby cut quite a figure with his bloody diaper and his official regalia.

Wrapped in fluffy pink blankets on a neighboring bed where I had placed her, Susy, wearing her little lace cap, just lay there, her tiny hands clasped, looking wide-eyed at the lights in the ceiling. Finally, she went off to sleep.

Slowly, our family life was being precariously reconstructed. Sometimes it almost seemed normal again. I was beginning to relax a little, to lose some of the terror that had gripped me at first. This was a mistake. Hemophilia was to prove itself a more cunning, more surprising, more incomprehensible adversary than we could imagine.

It was Bob's birthday, January 5. Bobby was two and a half.

I had just finished baking a cake and I saw that I was late to meet Bob's train. There was always a neighbor with whom I could leave Susy, but in many small and some direct ways, these same neighbors had long ago made me feel that leaving Bobby with them, even for half an hour, was more of a responsibility than they cared to undertake. So I took him with me everywhere I went. As I did every night, I gathered Bobby in my arms and put him in his little padded car chair. Then, at a traffic light, it happened. I had to put the brake on suddenly because of a car in front of me. The whole chair, with Bobby in it, flew up into the air, and he hit the dashboard with a huge thump. My heart froze. Yet, although he screamed, he was quickly comforted. Shaken, I picked up Bob at the station. By the time we returned home, there was a huge swelling on Bobby's forehead. I called the doctor. Was Bobby sick to his stomach? No. Was he dazed? Had he lost consciousness? No. All right. Put ice on it and watch it. The bruise kept growing until the skin was stretched tight; then it stabilized. It took four weeks for the huge bump to go down. We breathed a sigh of relief. Everything was going to be all right after all.

Then, one morning, six weeks after the accident, I woke up to a strange, unnatural silence from Bobby's bedroom. I went in. He was lying in his bed. He did not recognize me; his eyes were strange and he could make no sound. "Bobby?" I said. No answer—only his eyes, looking at me unknowingly. I flew to the telephone. Thank God, I got Bill Bisordi right away. He said only one thing. "Sue, it could be the brain. You better get him down to the hospital as fast as you can. I'll be there." With desperate speed I called a neighbor . . . never mind that it was before eight in the morning. Could I leave Susy with her? I grabbed her from her bed, we bundled up Bobby, and careened off into the freezing winter air. I frantically rang the bell at our neighbor's house. It seemed a very long time before the door opened. When it finally did, I thrust Susy, still in her sleeping bag, at the person who answered, and we sped off. Only fifteen minutes later, when we got to the toll booth, Bobby began to froth at the mouth. Still no sound came. He is dying, I thought, here in my arms, on the New York Thruway. Bob was half-crazed; he drove the car faster and faster along the snowy road. It is a miracle that we did not have an accident. We screeched up to the hospital door, then had to wait . . . endlessly . . . for the elevator. In the familiar emergency room, Bill was waiting for us. He looked at Bobby and swiftly said, "It is the brain. You must get him to Mount Sinai as fast as possible. I have already called them. I have called the police. You will have to be brave. Get going. Good luck."

As through a mist, I remember the officer who suddenly materialized in his dark blue uniform and his boots. He was wrapped in a winter coat with a heavy black fur collar. He said nothing, but looked at us with compassion. We climbed into his police car, gently cradling Bobby, and from the Cross County Center, with lights flashing, we started down the Thruway to New York. I do not know the name of that policeman, but I will never forget his driving. Surely, steadily, with great skill, he drove at eighty miles an hour over roads covered with snow. He broke his silence only once to ask, "What is it?" I said, "He's bleeding in the brain." "Oh, my God," he said, and drove even faster. I remember noticing that even with his patrol car in full flashing light, many motorists did not stop, did not pull over, as the law requires. He had to slow down and start his siren to force them to make way for him. He radioed ahead to the New York City police for permission to come into New York with his sirens blowing. Permission granted. He flew up one-way streets the wrong way.

Normally, the trip from Cross County to New York takes at least thirty minutes. Thanks to his expert driving, we made it to Mount Sinai in less than fifteen. Before he vanished, I heard the policeman say softly, "I hope he'll be all right, lady."

There was no waiting that day. Six doctors were already waiting in a tight little group to examine him. Still stonily quiet, eyes simply staring ahead, Bobby had no reaction, seemed to hear no sound. He was gone, but into what world? "Transfusion," they said tersely. "We'll transfuse him first." Needles and bottles, already prepared, were rolled into place, and they poised to go into the vein. But then, as I held him down, he uttered one wonderful word, a connection with reality, the first sign of life. "No," he cried faintly. He had come back.

But what had caused it? What would be the effects? Would it happen again? What did it mean? They could not release him without looking, testing, and retesting. No one knew what had happened, or why. The chief of hematology at Mount Sinai came and pleaded with us to leave him in a ward, so that many doctors could examine him, so that he could be used as a subject for conference. We agreed, with one condition: that I be allowed to stay with him as much as I wanted. My mother came to look after Susy. Bobby and I began a new life in the hospital.

The first days were an ordeal. Batteries of tests were ordered. Some were awful to look at, but did not hurt, like the electrodes that were placed all over Bobby's soft blond head for encephalographs. Some I could not see and did not fear: the long series of X-rays. Some we were used to and we could sustain: pricks and blood analyses. Others were painful and terrifying. One evening, waiting in the hall, I saw Bobby being rolled away for a spinal tap. Could I be with him? No, was the answer, "but don't worry; he has been given a sedative." Unfortunately, with many small children, sedative drugs sometimes act not as a calmant, but as a stimulant. So it was with Bobby. Far from being asleep, he was wide awake. Impatient for their spinal tap, the residents went ahead anyway. The doors were slammed shut. I sat outside and listened to the sounds of struggle and terror behind the door. He was screaming —I wanted to beat the door down. But I could not. I felt as if the Gestapo had him.

They gave him transfusions around the clock. The chief of hematology himself had left orders that we could be with him during all transfusions. Nevertheless, one stubborn head nurse, probably feeling that this was altogether too *avant-garde*, had decided on her own to exclude me.

Transfusions had been ordered every six hours. It was very late at night. I was dozing in a chair down the hall in a dimly lit waiting room (there were no chairs in Bobby's cubicle) when I was jolted by familiar cries. I ran down the hall, burst into the room, and found a resident and two nurses huddled around Bobby's bed. A single bright light was shining directly into his eyes. They were preparing to hold him down and puncture his vein. He was screaming in terror. Only barely controlling a murderous rage, I asked, "Why didn't you call me?" Slightly chastened by my fiery glance, but nevertheless determined to justify her action, the head nurse said, "We thought it would be better if we just went ahead without you." My voice steely, I said, "The doctor has left strict orders that I should be there for all transfusions. I shall speak to him about this tomorrow." This invocation of supreme authority was enough. They allowed me to stay, to hold him, and the transfusion proceeded. I stayed with him afterward, until his cries subsided.

Those long nights in the hospital! At night, the corridors are so long, so empty; only the small light on the nurse's desk shines at the end of the lonely hall. In the night there are cries in those darkened, overheated wards, cries of children calling, "Mother, Mother, Mama, Mama." Cries, and not enough personnel to comfort them. As I had nowhere to sleep, I spent much of the night wandering among them, holding the hands and comforting the tears of these unknown children. Sometimes, during the day, I met their mothers: Puerto Rican women, black women, white women; sad-eyed mothers who came to visit their sick children, with the greatest difficulty snatching moments from their work. With rare exceptions, because of the strict visiting hours, fathers could come only on weekends.

I lived in the ward ten days. Bob came as often as he could get away from his work. I lost contact with the outside world. They gave me a white coat to wear, and because of it, the children thought I was a psychiatrist. I drew pictures with them, I played with them. What surprised me most was how quickly I simply no longer noticed their twisted bodies, their casts, and their wheelchairs. Instead, I became aware of and then overwhelmed by the strength and beauty of the spirit shining in their eyes.

I noticed, too, that those medical people who dealt most closely with these children were also somehow changed by it, made gentler and stronger, simply by the contact.

In one crib lay a dark-haired little girl named Stephanie. She was two years old. She had been born with a cleft lip, a cleft palate, and a hip defect. She was to undergo many operations to correct these deformities. Meanwhile, she had been encased in plaster up to her waist, with her legs spread-eagled. The smell of her was overpowering . . . but only at first. When one day my mother came to visit Bobby, she was shocked at the sight of Stephanie and whispered to Bob, "How can Sue hold her?" I was startled. I realized that at some time, a very long time ago it seemed, I had entirely ceased to notice her cast and her lip. I had simply grown to love her and to wonder at her accomplishments.

Bobby became the center of attention for the other children from the day a little Puerto Rican boy approached him, peered attentively at him, and then went off and whispered incredulously to another little boy in a wheelchair, "He has *blue* eyes!" Very soon, a little circle of children had rolled or limped their way to Bobby's bed, where they collectively confirmed in chorus the extraordinary fact. "Bobby has blue eyes! We've never seen anyone with blue eyes!"

The days passed while the doctors did and redid encephalographs, examined and re-examined Bobby's reflexes, peered again and again into his eyes with little electric beams. All the findings were inconclusive. In the spinal fluid, the doctors had found traces of old bleeding, but this finding was not definitive. It did not explain Bobby's convulsion. The chief of hematology was prepared to release him. He felt that nothing further could be learned, and that further complicated brain-testing might only harm him. But the chief of neurology, whom we had never seen, was so interested by the reports of his subordinates that he wanted to keep Bobby— indefinitely, it seemed—as a "case study," to keep on probing. We wanted to take him home, yet we were unsure and frightened by such authority. One day, two young doctors came down once again to tap his knees and elbows. Obliquely, they began to talk—in general, to be sure—about "the rights of parents," saying that "no one could be forced to stay in a hospital." We understood their veiled message. Bobby was about as well as he could be. They could do no more. It was time to defy the mysterious chief of neurology. We had to sign a frighteningly worded paper saying that we took *all* responsibility for our actions, and for *everything* that might happen to him because of our actions. We prepared to take him home. He was fine, if you overlooked a lot of needle marks and an infectious sore throat contracted in the hospital.

Bobby's new friends were sad when he left, and they asked wistfully, "Where is Bobby going?" I answered, "He is going home now, to play in his back yard." Their eyes opened wide, and one little girl said, unbelievingly, "Bobby has a back yard?" as if it were the most undreamed-of luxury. As we left, they crowded around the elevator, and even after the doors shut I could hear the children's voices echoing down the shaft, "Good-bye, Bobby, good-bye!"

We never did find out what had caused Bobby's mysterious convulsion. Bleeding as a result of the car accident? Again the doctors shook their heads and said, "We don't know, we can't predict." They prescribed an anticonvulsant dose of phenobarbital for six months. As for us, they said, we would just have to wait and see. There was one ray of hope, thin, but I clung to it. If it doesn't recur over the next six months, said the doctors, it probably won't recur again. We waited. It didn't. No one knew why.

(Later, many years later, I asked Bill Bisordi why he had had the foresight to call the police escort before we even arrived at the hospital. Then he told me. "There are two things in hemophilia that terrify me: the throat and the brain. I called the police right away because of our own experience. When Tommy was one and a half, he fell off a bench at a picnic. Nothing happened, and no one even noticed at the time. I was playing baseball. That night he was having convulsions every five minutes. His care was turned over to me, because no one knew what to do. Neither did I. I just had to watch him in his crib having convulsions every five minutes. I thought we were going to lose him that time. When I saw Bobby, I knew it was a neurological case. I knew we didn't have fresh-frozen plasma at Cross County then. Diagnosis in such cases is so difficult, but I had just proceeded on the premise that you have to treat it as if it was bleeding . . . and then see.")

That experience at Mount Sinai was a turning point for me. It taught me that if, compared to the healthy, we had cause to grieve, compared to others who were ill we had cause to be grateful. For the first time, I felt the relativity of our disaster. Not only were we fortunate to have only the problems that we had, but were *extraordinarily* fortunate to have had the preparation that we had. We had education, we could read, we could learn. We had energy . . . and, however modest, we had a back yard. How many did not have these comforts! For the first time since we had learned of Bobby's hemophilia, I began to turn outward. It was only dimly felt then; it was to grow stronger; but I began to sense that what had happened to us was a challenge, that we were meant to explore it, to learn from it. It was the first dawning in me of the determination to use what weapons we did have and to fight. It was the beginning of functioning on a new psychological level.

The brain episode was the worst of that period in our lives. Episodes such as the ones I have described earlier grew common. A few were uncommon enough to note. One Christmas, when Bobby was three, I was in the kitchen, finishing up, with a sigh of relief, the last of my Christmas cookies. I heard a funny tinkle in the living room. Bobby had taken a bite out of a glass "to see what it felt like, Mommy." Luckily, he hadn't swallowed any, but the bleeding went on for a month. Then there was the time that Bob was invited to give a lecture at Smith College. In the morning, a nursery-school classmate had pushed Bobby hard against a doorknob. As we were going up the Massachusetts Turnpike, his back began to swell very quickly. By the time we arrived at Northampton he was in considerable pain and could not sit up. We called the local hospital. After we had spent a time convincing them that yes, Bobby was a real hemophiliac, they assured us that yes, they knew all about it and had fresh-frozen plasma at the hospital. Bob gave his speech. Bobby grew steadily worse. In the middle of the night, Bob and I took Bobby to the neat little hospital. It turned out that there was no fresh-frozen plasma, after all; only regular plasma, useless for Bobby. Bob lay down on a table and gave his blood directly to Bobby. It was all finally over at 6:30 A.M.

Certainly by the time Bobby was five, we thought that we understood what hemophilia was about, that we were experienced. This was very far from the truth. The truth was that we just had completed our basic training; the real battles were about to begin.

Chapter 5

Since the farthest reaches of time, man has been fascinated and repelled by the sight of blood. Blood is sacred and all-powerful. A blood oath between men or a blood pact between savage tribes was the most binding of pledges; to break it meant death. Yet blood was also profane and demeaning: woman was strange, unclean, and inferior because, every month, she bled.

Blood was life, the vital force. But it was also the symbol of personality. It contained the essential elements of individual character; it was the person himself. The Christian Holy Communion is based on the dogma that wine represents (or, in the Catholic belief, becomes) blood, and that this blood is the life and person of Christ Himself ("This is my blood, which is shed for thee. Drink this in remembrance of me. . . .").

For most of recorded time, man had no true knowledge of what blood was or how it circulated in the body. Galen, the Greek physician of the Roman emperor Marcus Aurelius, decided that blood was laden with "vital spirits" which ebbed and flowed throughout the body like ocean tides. For fourteen hundred years Galen's view was regarded as inviolable, until in 1628 William Harvey proved that blood circulated over and over through the body as a result of the pumping action of the heart. Beyond this, over 95 per cent of what we know today about blood has been learned in the twentieth century.

Mysterious, powerful, vital, surging rhythmically beneath the surface, hidden except when it spurts dramatically forth, beautiful, crimson, terrifying, blood is one of the most spectacular of God's creations.

To the biochemist and the physician, the human body is a mechanism of 60 trillion living cells. These cells are linked together into tissue, and tissue is linked into complex organs. At the basis of each cell's structure and behavior is chemistry. The body lives, moves, observes, thinks, enjoys pleasure and suffers pain as a result of chemical reactions.

One essential chemical reaction is the nourishment and cleansing of each of the 60 trillion cells. This is the function of the blood. Blood, in constant flow, bathes every one of the 60 trillion cells, providing them with food and oxygen, while simultaneously washing them clean and carrying off their wastes. Blood is indispensable to every cell; no cell could exist without it. Ten pints in the average adult, pumped by a small, fist-sized muscle (the heart) through a circulatory system of arteries, capillaries, and veins which cover a distance of sixty thousand miles, the blood makes a complete circuit of the body more than a thousand times a day.

Essentially, what the blood is bringing to the cells is energy. Each cell needs food and oxygen to combine chemically to produce energy. Inhaled oxygen is picked up in the lungs by the blood and chained in a temporary chemical bond to the red blood cells to be carried throughout the body. Food passes through the stomach into the small intestine, where it is reduced to glucose, fats, and amino acid particles small enough to enter the blood stream and be carried throughout the body.

From birth to death, this endless cycle continues. Freshly oxygenated blood surges out of the heart through the aorta, the body's largest artery, flowing into subsidiary arteries and eventually into billions of microscopically small capillaries. By the time the blood reaches the capillaries, it is moving at a relatively slow rate, along channels so narrow that its own cells must slither through sideways. The walls of the capillaries are only one cell thick so that the nutrients are able, by osmosis and diffusion, to pass through the microscopically thin capillary wall into the cells. Inside the cell, food and oxygen are combined and converted into energy. Simultaneously, carbon dioxide, urea, and uric acids are passing the other way through the capillary walls into the blood stream to be carried away and expelled.

In yielding up oxygen and taking on carbon dioxide, the blood turns from a bright scarlet to a dull maroon. The entire cycle takes twenty seconds.

Blood, itself teeming with billions of cells, has four principal components. About 55 per cent of blood is made up of a noncellular fluid called plasma. The remaining 45 per cent is made up of three kinds of cells: red cells, white cells, and platelets. Floating in the plasma, the red cells carry oxygen, the white cells fight bacteria, and the platelets help to repair leaks.

Red cells outnumber white cells seven hundred to one. Their effectiveness in carrying oxygen throughout the body is due to their content of hemoglobin, a protein-and-iron compound which can pick up and carry more than half its own weight in oxygen, and which also gives blood its red color. It is the iron in hemoglobin that locks oxygen in a chemical embrace in the lungs, holding its grip until the destination is reached.

White cells are the body's roving guardians. Whenever invading bacteria enter the body, white cells rally in great numbers to attack, engulf, and destroy the intruders.

Platelets, tiny, flat, and platelike (hence the name), are the strangest of the blood's three cellular components. They have a strong tendency to stick to each other or to anything else they may touch, a characteristic that fits them admirably for the job of plugging holes and repairing leaks in the body's circulatory system.

Plasma, in which the cells float, is a yellowish solution, 90 per cent of which is water. The other 10 per cent is made up of a host of substances indispensable to life. Among these are the special plasma proteins like fibrinogen, albumin, and various globulins, which participate in the intricate series of chemical reactions known as coagulation.

It is in the plasma that Bobby's trouble lies. One of the plasma proteins necessary to persuade his blood to clot either is missing or is not functioning properly.

For all of us whose coagulation is normal, a small leak in the walls of our circulatory system is a minor concern. When we cut ourselves, our blood clots. That is, a clot forms, temporarily plugging the hole and forming a scaffold on which new tissue can form and reseal the wound.

Nature has provided at least three different overlapping, sequential systems that act to keep blood from flowing out of a torn blood vessel. The first is the action of the lining of the blood vessels, the second is the action of the platelets, and the third is the action of certain proteins and enzymes in the plasma that tend to promote the formation of a firm clot.

First, the blood vessel wall: When a blood vessel is injured, the muscular fibers in the wall immediately tighten and close around the injured area, tending by this retraction alone to limit the flow of blood out of the broken blood vessel.

Second, the platelets: Flowing through the capillary, they touch the roughened surface of the torn blood vessel, and, on touching it, stick to it. This temporary platelet plug further impedes the flow of blood out of the blood vessel.

But the platelets also do something else. When they touch the roughened surface they burst apart, activating a whole series of other plasma clotting factors, causing them to interact and catalyze a chemical process that eventually creates a clot and halts completely any flow of blood.

In every respect but one, Bobby's blood is exactly like that of the rest of us. His red cells are normal, his white cells are normal, his platelets are normal, and his plasma is normal except for a single protein called Anti-Hemophilic Factor or AHF. AHF is one of several plasma proteins that play an essential role in the first stage of coagulation. They have names, like Anti-Hemophilic Factor and Plasma Thromboplastin Component, but for ease in handling they have also been given numbers: AHF is Factor VIII, Plasma Thromboplastin Component (PTC) is Factor IX, and so on. In all, twelve factors, numbered in the order they were discovered, have so far been identified.

The sequence by which these protein factors chemically interact to start the clotting process sounds like a wondrous contraption by Rube Goldberg: Factor XII is converted to its active form, which activates Factor XI. Activated Factor XI converts Factor IX to its active form which, with Factor VIII, activates Factor X. Factor X, with Factor V, then converts prothrombin to the very active enzyme thrombin, which converts fibrinogen to fibrin. Fibrin finally makes up the substance of a blood clot.

Reading this, most laymen will appreciate what one hematologist told Sue: "Coagulation is one of the most intricate processes in the whole body. To me, it has always seemed a miracle that coagulation disorders aren't more common."

Bobby's deficiency is Factor VIII, or AHF. This coagulation disorder, called classical hemophilia, is the most common of the hemophilias; it occurs in 80 per cent of the cases of hemophilia. People who lack the functioning plasma protein Factor IX, Plasma Thromboplastin Component (PTC), have milder clinical symptoms; this deficiency is responsible for most of the remaining 20 per cent of hemophilia cases. There are other deficiencies: Factor XI, or PTA hemophilia, makes up about one per cent of all cases. And there is a bleeding disorder called von Willebrand's Disease caused by a combination of Factor VIII deficiency and a failure of platelet adhesion. Von Willebrand's Disease appears in women as well as men.

Most knowledge of these hemorrhagic disorders has come within Bobby's lifetime. When he was born, the difference between Factor VIII deficiency and Factor IX deficiency was known, but Factors X, XI, and XII had not yet been identified. Only as he has been growing up has the whole astonishing process been more precisely defined. And still there are huge gaps. A primary target of contemporary research is the structure of the AHF Factor VIII molecule. As yet, no one knows the chemical nature of this submicroscopic bit of protein.

Because it is absent or inactive in Bobby, his blood never clots properly. When he is hurt, he does not bleed harder or faster than normal; just longer. A soft and mushy semiclot forms, but it is rarely sufficient to plug the torn blood vessels firmly and effectively. Blood seeps around the clot, and it can be dislodged by even the slightest additional trauma.

The only way to remedy this situation is to activate his own blood-clotting mechanism by giving him AHF from somebody else. With someone else's AHF circulating in his body, then all the rest of his coagulation mechanism, which is normal, can be triggered into forming clots.

The only way to do this is by transfusion.

Transfusion, the transfer of human blood from one human being to another, was never performed or even dreamed of throughout most of man's history. Yet the procedure now is routine and one of the foundations of modern medical treatment.

It was not that earlier men were unaware of the healing power of another person's healthy blood. Indeed, they believed that blood held the life force, and they assumed that it contained the personal strength and other characteristics of its owner. The problem was that they didn't know how to acquire it—how to absorb another person's blood into their own bodies.

Some, like the ancient Egyptians, took baths in blood, hoping thus to soak up its useful properties. Others, like the Romans, drank it for rejuvenation. At the end of battle in the arena, the crowd rushed to try to drink the blood of the dying gladiators. In 1492, Pope Innocent VIII was in a coma. In an effort to save the elderly pontiff, the blood of three healthy young men was apparently poured down his throat. It was no use. He died immediately, and so did the donors.

Serious attempts to transfuse blood by opening a vein in the recipient began only after Harvey's discovery that the same blood circulated throughout the body. Thereafter, physicians began to experiment with the injection of various substances into the blood stream. Cups and bowls were used to collect the donor's blood and hollow goose quills or hollow silver tubes to infuse the blood into the recipient's vein. In the 1670's, Jean Baptiste Denis, physician to Louis XIV, revived an anemic boy by administering half a pint of lamb's blood (surprisingly, as mixing human and animal blood is usually fatal). Denis continued to transfuse patients until one of them, having gone directly to a tavern to celebrate his recovery, died. Denis was exonerated of a murder charge, but blood transfusions were banned in France. In England, transfusions were prohibited by Act of Parliament. For two more centuries, while millions of women bled to death in childbirth, blood transfusions did not take place.

It was not until 1900 that the most important single discovery in the history of blood transfusions occurred. This was the demonstration by Karl Landsteiner, an Austrian doctor who won a Nobel Prize for his work, that human blood could be divided into blood groups, depending on red-cell compatibility. Landsteiner typed these groups as A, B, O, and AB. Thereafter, donors were matched to recipients, and the chance of fatal or even harmful reaction to transfusion dramatically declined.

In the 1930's, the separation of blood into its major component parts, red cells and plasma, was achieved. During World War II, plasma, which can generally be given to anyone regardless of blood group, was widely used to combat shock in treating battlefield wounds, and thousands of lives were saved. Recently, the various protein fractions in the plasma, including the Anti-Hemophilic Factor (AHF), have been separated, purified, and concentrated so that now everyone who needs blood can receive the specific part of the blood he needs and no other. This advanced form of transfusion treatment is called component therapy.

But if the technique of safe blood transfusions is now perfected, the psychological reaction of many people to the idea of giving or receiving human blood often remains strangely primitive.

Not understanding that blood renews itself in the body, some people fear that to lose it is to give up some of one's own life force. "My blood is my strength," they say. Or, "I don't have enough to give away." Or, "I will be permanently weakened." Or, "I am afraid of damaging my own health." These fears are common.

Probably these fears also underlie the more prosaic excuses people are accustomed to offering. "I don't have time." "Nobody ever asked me." "I wouldn't mind giving once, but I don't want to be obligated to continue." "I'm afraid of the needle." "I can't stand the sight of my own blood flowing out through the tube." "I don't want to gain weight afterward." Frequently, all these reasons are wrapped into the statement, "I'm afraid." Some people are afraid and will not admit it, some are afraid and will admit it; often men are more afraid than women.

Hesitations still exist about *receiving* blood transfusions. Certain religious sects oppose blood transfusions as a matter of faith. They resist for themselves and their children even when the alternative is possible death. Some people still believe that blood carries personality, morality, and behavior. "I don't want the blood of a nervous person. I'm much too nervous myself already." Or, "I don't want the blood of a black"—only recently has blood been pooled in all parts of the United States without being separated or labeled according to race.

The fact is that so deep are the primeval taboos that most people are afraid to give blood until they have tried it once. And then most donors are willing, even eager, to continue. They discover what others have learned: that a donation of blood is one of the most meaningful gifts one human being can give to another. To the recipient, the gift may be everything, even life itself. To the giver, the physical loss is quickly replaced by the body and the spiritual gain can be overwhelming. Our friend Janet Dowling explained her feeling: "I get a profound emotional satisfaction because I am giving something of my own, something that is desperately needed. When I give blood, I feel that, no matter what else has happened that day, at least I've done one really good thing."

At the time Bobby had his first transfusion, AHF or Factor VIII had been identified, but it had not been isolated from the plasma it floated in. So, when he needed a transfusion, the doctors gave him plasma. But this plasma had to be specially prepared and preserved. AHF is highly unstable; once outside the donor's body, the AHF molecule apparently disintegrates or at least loses its capacity for useful activity unless it is stored at temperatures far below that of a room or even a refrigerator. Then the only way to preserve its activity was to deep-freeze it immediately after it was drawn from the donor's veins, and keep it that way until the time came to administer it to Bobby.

Our life, therefore, revolved around something called freshfrozen plasma, plasma that was taken directly from the centrifuge after the red cells had been separated and frozen rock-hard inside a closed, sterile plastic bag. Once Bobby began having transfusions either at home or at the doctor's office, we took the responsibility for keeping a supply on hand. Several times a month, we drove to the Blood Transfusion Association in Lower Manhattan or to the lab freezer at Cross County Hospital and picked up first two, then four, and later six, of the purse-sized bags with their lumps of yellow ice inside. We brought them home packed in dry ice and kept them in our home freezer. Then, when Bobby needed a transfusion, we called the doctor and, while he was coming, took a bag from the freezer and began to thaw it in a sink or bowl of lukewarm water. Normally, this took forty-five minutes. We could not hurry it, even in an emergency, because it was then believed that too much heat could destroy the AHF. Eventually, when the plasma was back in its liquid state, we hung the bag on a transfusion rack (or even a nail in the wall) and the transfusions began. Fresh-frozen plasma was not very efficient; Bobby was getting a large volume of plasma with only a small amount of AHF activity. What we needed was a higher concentrate of pure AHF. But that was for the future.

In those early years, one bag of fresh-frozen plasma cost $13.50. When Bobby was small, he had very few transfusions per year and he received only one bag of plasma in each transfusion. But as he got older, his usage increased and the bills got bigger. The Hemophilia Foundation, which made the plasma available and sent us the bills, asked for the payment either in money or blood. A typical bill read: "$553.50 or 41 blood donations." Naturally, they preferred that we pay in blood.

We began to give blood ourselves and to look for others who would help us. We discovered that many people will rally and give blood for one dramatic life-and-death crisis; our friends had reacted this way when they first heard about Bobby's disease. But when the need continues year after year, people forget. They have their own lives and their own problems. Nevertheless, the implacable notices kept arriving in our mail: You have used a large amount of blood. It is your obligation to repay it. Sternly, the Hemophilia Foundation warned all its members that if no effort was made to pay these bills, no further credit would be extended. That meant the child would get no plasma.

For most Americans who wish to participate, the Red Cross has worked out a simple, intelligent form of blood insurance: by giving a single donation during a year, the donor ensures that any blood he or his family may need that year will be freely supplied. Usually, these plans work through company blood banks. *Newsweek*, where I worked, had such a blood bank. But because of the enormous potential drain our family would create for this blood bank, I was excluded. The administrator of the *Newsweek* bank would not even permit my friends and fellow workers to donate blood for Bobby to a Red Cross mobile on *Newsweek*'s premises. "We're sorry, but this drive is for the *Newsweek* blood bank," they told me.

Thus in the autumn of 1960, feeling the weight of necessity and obligation, we agreed in conjunction with another Westchester hemophilia family to sponsor a neighborhood blood drive. Psychologically, it was a bruising experience. The Red Cross and Hemophilia Foundation organizers were professional and demanding. Nothing was left to chance, nor was there much room for shyness or sensitivity on the part of the sponsoring families. Obviously, some preliminary organization was necessary. The Red Cross could not simply drive up one day in a Bloodmobile, set up beds in a local meeting hall, tack up a sign, and expect that crowds of donors would swarm in off the street. When they decided to run a blood drive, they wanted to collect the maximum possible amount of blood. That meant putting a lot of pressure on somebody in the local community. And who, in the local community, was most susceptible to pressure, and most likely, if suitably prodded, to respond effectively? The family of The Victim!

In the weeks before the blood drive we were expected—and pressed—to do two things. First, to recruit donors. Our pleas, telephoned to every friend, carried door-to-door to every neighbor, tinged with the drama of personal tragedy and need, were counted on to provide a certain required minimum of pledged donors. Had we failed at this stage, the penalty would have been abrupt and automatic: our blood drive would have been canceled.

Beyond this, we were expected to cooperate in the effort to reach out beyond our friends and neighbors, and try to attract donors from the general public—in a word, to create, or at least submit to, publicity. Dramatize the need for blood, put a face on it—if possible, the face of a stricken child. It's easier for people to give if they know where their blood is going. Pity is a powerful motivation. Try your local newspapers. Don't neglect the local radio stations. Tell them how tough it is. Forget your dignity, your privacy, your pride.

All right. A smiling Bobby was photographed with a smiling Mayor of White Plains. (In the unbroken tradition of elected officials, great and small, who smilingly pose with sick children for newspaper photographers, the Mayor was absent when the time came to donate blood.) A reporter for a local newspaper came to see us. When her story appeared, Bobby, at four, fortunately was still too young to read it.

"Bobby Massie," she had written, "is doomed to a life of danger and constant threat of disaster. . . . He is a handsome little boy with an almost luminous personality and an astounding vocabulary. . . . Most victims of hemophilia do not die before the age of five, as victims did fifty years ago. They do, however, become hopeless cripples. . . . No single family can even begin to supply the blood requirements of a hemophiliac. The Massies are therefore wholly dependent on blood donations from friends, neighbors, and the generosity of the community-at-large."

When the blood drive took place, the "community-at-large" failed to appear. But most of our neighbors came—the Feidens, the Martinis, the Borgoses, the Deutsches, Janet Johnson, Julie Davidson, Barbara Rockefeller, Barbara Foley (more wives than husbands)—and many of them brought *their* friends, so that, in all, forty-five people came to the White Plains Armory to give blood for Bobby. We thought that this was wonderful; we never knew that there were forty-five people who cared that much, and we couldn't understand why the Red Cross attendants were grumbling that "only forty-five Massie donors showed up."

On the afternoon of the blood drive, a photographer took a picture of Sue and the other mother, and a few days later it appeared in the paper with the caption: "The grateful mothers were present to meet their friends and neighbors and to express sincere gratitude for those who gave their time and blood." I didn't like the wording, but the caption was true: we were grateful. Forty-five people had come, ten had been rejected for various reasons, but thirty-five had given blood. It had been painful for us, but that didn't matter. We had collected enough blood to last—in those days —a whole year.

Bobby's need continued to rise. In 1961, the year after our White Plains drive, he had 39 transfusions. In 1962, he had 54 transfusions, and in 1963, 67 transfusions. Then in 1964, when Bobby was eight and trouble with his knees, ankles, and elbows became chronic, the number soared to 103 transfusions. How do you get that much blood from your friends and neighbors? Does anybody have that many friends and neighbors?

By that time, we had moved from White Plains and were living in our crumbling Victorian house in Irvington. Bobby was in the third grade, speeding in his wheelchair down the hallways of Dow's Lane Elementary School. People still thought we were strange—two writers with a hemophiliac child, living without curtains or furniture in an old white elephant of a house—but somehow we felt more at ease and more secure. Partly this was because inside the thick walls of our big, old house, shielded by a wide lawn and ancient, giant trees, we felt protected from the outside world. But it was also because the small town of Irvington displayed toward us a generous spirit in a second, and much larger, blood drive.

This Irvington blood drive would never had occurred without the tactful understanding and practical Christianity of the minister of the local St. Barnabas Episcopal Church, David Matlack.

As part of his effort to involve his church in community problems, Dave arranged for the parish to sponsor a blood drive. A committee was organized, led by an active woman, Dorothy Stone, herself the mother of three schoolboys. *They* dealt with the Red Cross and the Hemophilia Foundation; *they* telephoned and pleaded for pledges in order to guarantee a sufficient number of donors. *They* put flyers in all the stores and in the post office, and announcements in church bulletins up and down the river villages. I helped in only one way: this time, keenly aware that Bobby himself would read most of the publicity, I wrote the stories, which the local newspaper printed without changing:

Except for a single, tiny protein substance in his blood stream, Bobby Massie lacks none of the ingredients that make up a normal eight-year-old boy. He reads *Superman* and *Robin Hood*, he watches *The Man from U.N.C.L.E.* and *Johnny Quest*, and when he grows up he wants to be a scientist or an inventor.

The drive was an overwhelming success. During three hours on an early June evening, 182 people came to the community center on Main Street. There were people I knew by name, people whose faces I recognized (including our village policeman), and people I didn't know at all. Bobby himself was there. At first, I thought he ought to say thank you, but it wasn't necessary. People seemed embarrassed, and we stopped after two or three.

The lines were long and, in the middle of the short donation period, the Bloodmobile personnel simply stopped taking blood and went out to supper. Many people, sitting on benches waiting to donate, gave up and went home. Dorothy Stone, watching it happen, was upset; when I heard about it the next day, I was upset. But there was nothing to do. For us, it was a community act. For the Bloodmobile, it was a job.

Despite these losses and the inevitable rejection of some donors for medical reasons, we collected 142 blood donations in those few hours. Again, we thought we had enough for another whole year.

Of course we were grateful to all the people who had given blood. Yet I had mixed feelings about these blood drives, the big, successful one in Irvington as well as the first, smaller one in White Plains. The problem was *having* to be grateful.

Before the first blood drive, the newspaper had declared, "The Massies are wholly dependent on blood donations from friends, neighbors, and the generosity of the community-at-large." It was true and we hated it. Nobody likes to be wholly dependent. Nobody likes to beg for charity. And begging for blood is just as hard, maybe harder, than begging for money. It destroys pride and independence. The people in our society who proclaim in booming voices that private charity is the answer to preserving pride and independence are always the donors, never the recipients.

Like most people who are dependent, I resented my dependence. I wanted to be myself and not always have to smile at every-body because I needed blood. Would it have been wrong for our society—say, in the form of the Red Cross—to supply us routinely with the blood we needed? Not because we had bowed to pressure to run a blood drive, begged our friends, extracted pledges from our neighbors, or even because the church, on our behalf, stirred up our town, but simply because we needed it? Wasn't this what the Red Cross was supposed to do? Isn't it what most Americans who regularly volunteer blood believe the Red Cross is doing?

The deplorable fact is that we Americans are afflicted with an appallingly inefficient national blood collection and distribution system. As a nation we are extraordinarily stingy in giving blood: In a country of over 200 million people, with more than 100 million qualified blood donors, only 3 per cent of the eligible donor popu-lation actually gives blood. Worse, we waste 28 per cent of the blood donated—one pint out of every four—by letting it become outdated. This unused blood is simply poured down the drain. There are appalling differences, from city to city, and from state to state, in the way blood is made available to people who need it. In some happy places, the community accepts total responsibility for replacement; in others, the individual user is required to replace what he uses, paying in either blood or money.

In every other advanced industrial nation—societies as diverse as Holland, Switzerland, Sweden, France, Britain, Australia, and Canada—some form of centralized national blood service collects and efficiently processes all blood. (In Sweden wastage is down to 3 per cent; in Britain, 2 per cent.) It is then distributed free to every citizen who needs it. Blood and blood products can be made available free because no one in these countries makes a profit on blood (as commercial blood banks and pharmaceutical houses do in America); because the state considers that its citizens need blood just as much as they need an army, or highways, or public schools, or judges, and therefore it pays the cost of collection, processing, and distribution; and most of all because all blood in those countries is voluntarily donated by socially responsible, public-spirited citizens, accepting this duty as one of the obligations of good citizenship.

Worst of all, in America, human blood often becomes a purely commercial commodity. The poor sell it—the majority of American donors are young unskilled male manual workers. The rich, the professional class, the upper middle class buy it, often substituting dollars for the time it takes to extend their arms and repay blood with blood. But this system is inadequate and on a local and national level as well as in countless, heartbreaking individual cases, America is short of blood. And so we have some bizarre and heart-rending stories appearing in our press about different methods Americans use or propose in trying to raise blood:

—A traffic judge in Lexington, Kentucky (where I was born), now gives speeders and red-light runners a choice between paying a $30 fine and donating a pint of blood. In the first week this policy went into effect, fifteen out of 190 defendants rolled up their sleeves at the local blood bank. (All right, let's make this practice nationwide and increase the fine. Then we'd have more blood or fewer traffic accidents. In either case, our country would be a better place.)

—Representative Edward Koch (Dem., N.Y.) has introduced a bill to give a tax credit of $25 for every pint of blood donated. (If we have to use money to persuade Americans to give blood, this is a better system than most. If three million taxpayers each gave only one additional pint of blood a year, it would cost the government a loss of $75 million. We could buy one less B-1 bomber a year.)

—In Miami, a black woman, Mrs. DeSola Brown, the mother of two hemophiliacs—Greg, seventeen, and Mark, nine—made twenty trips in 1973 onto Miami's skid row to coax alcoholics into trading their blood for drinks. "It's been almost impossible to find individual donors," she said. "We owe so much blood and have no way of paying it back. I had to find blood somewhere. I've been told I owe more than a thousand pints for Marky. Frankly, I've lost track on Greg." (There is nothing to say about this except that it is a national disgrace!)

As for the Massies, despite our blood drives, Bobby's needs continued to rise: 73 transfusions in 1965, 92 transfusions in 1966, 107 in 1967. And as he grew older and bigger, he began to need more plasma in each transfusion. We had assumed that the 142 blood donations collected in our Irvington blood drive would have paid for 142 transfusions. But in the fall of 1964, only a few months after the blood drive, the doctors calculated on the basis of Bobby's weight that he should start to receive two bags of fresh-frozen plasma with each transfusion. So our reserve was abruptly halved.

Nevertheless, we managed to pay back more or less what we owed. In part, we did this with cash, by making claims against the group major medical policies of our employers. The rest a few of us paid for by giving blood once a week, using an extraordinary new technique called plasmaphresis.

Normally, even the most faithful blood donor is permitted to give blood only once every eight weeks; it takes that long for the depleted red cells to rebuild to a safe level. But plasmaphresis does not deprive the donor of his red cells, only his plasma. In plasma-phresis, whole blood is drawn into a sterile bag. Then, while the donor remains on the couch, his plasma and red cells are separated in a nearby centrifuge, the red cells are brought back and reinfused through the same needle. The red cell and hemoglobin levels there-fore remain the same. Plasma protein levels return to normal rapidly—within two or three days. Thus, in theory, one could give plasma by plasmaphresis as often as twice a week. The ad-vantage for all hemophilia families is obvious: the amount of plasma available for extraction of Anti-Hemophilic Factor can be multiplied by many times.

Four of us were regulars in New York City's first plasma-phresis program at Mount Sinai Hospital: Sue's sister Jeannine, my brother Kim, Janet Dowling, and myself. Usually, we went to-gether into a pleasant hospital lounge. Here, we lay back on con-tour donor couches (much more comfortable than simply lying flat) and rolled up our sleeves, a nurse attached a tourniquet, and the needle went into the arm.

It was a warm, relaxing feeling, lying there, doing something important by doing absolutely nothing. While the nurses bustled about, attaching and clipping off plastic bags, we lay quietly, star-ing up at the bottles of saline water dripping slowly through the plastic tubing to keep the implanted needles free from clotting.

Lying side by side for an hour or so, we told stories, sometimes laughing so hard that the nurse had to calm us to protect the needles taped into our arms. I think we all felt that in those hours together we shared something special.

Sometimes other people came: our friends, Jeannine's friends, Kim's friends. Often, after these sessions, everybody who had given blood came home with me to dinner. Sue, who was pregnant, waited at home, never knowing exactly how many to expect. It was always a mixed group at these blood donors dinner parties, but because we all had something important in common, it was always fun.

Plasmaphresis was valuable to us. One plasmaphresis donation was worth four single blood credits or $54. Over the months, we gave a lot of plasma. But we never quite caught up and we were still behind, years later, when we moved to France, where blood is free.

Chapter 6

At the very first sign of joint swelling, ACT IMMEDIATELY! *Don't think it is of little consequence and will soon pass! Don't try to "get by with it" this time. A joint hemorrhage is a* SERIOUS *matter and unless treated immediately and properly can lead to permanent disability.*

> Home Care of the Hemophiliac Child,
> DOROTHY WHITE, R.N., B.S., M.H.A., 1962.

I remember waiting, always waiting for something. Be it to get better, or for a shot to end, or for school, and endless, endless clean white impersonal doctors' offices and clinics, where I sat and fidgeted among the worn magazines and plastic chairs.

> BOBBY MASSIE.

We should have known. *We should have known.* How many times I have told myself since then! Looking back now, it is so clear where we went wrong. But we did not know.

I love to dance, and I was happy that Bobby did, too. When he was five, I was teaching him the Scottish sword dance, using two broom handles on the floor. He was neat and agile, skipping over them. He loved to run, his sturdy little legs were always active.

It is true he was having recurrent bleedings in the muscle above his left knee, the one known as the quadriceps muscle, which controls and supports the movement of the knee joint. But neither we nor our doctor worried much about this. Occasionally, after such a bleeding, Bobby had a little trouble extending his leg, but we shrugged it off and said, "It's only a muscle." And we did nothing except wrap it up in Ace bandages. Our guard was down. We had been lulled into thinking we understood what had to be done.

One day it happened, quietly, without warning. The muscle

bleeding did not get better. Instead, it began getting worse. It began to hurt. I called the doctor. He was unconcerned; he thought I was overanxious. "Why don't we wait a little," he said, "before we give a transfusion. Let's wait and see what it does." We waited for one hour while steadily the knee began to swell and become increasingly painful. By the time Bobby finally had a transfusion his knee was swollen as large as a grapefruit. It was hot and, worse, it was bent. Bobby had begun to bleed into the knee joint itself.

Once started, it proved very difficult to stop. By the time we finally stabilized that first left knee bleeding, it was three months and thirty transfusions later. Bobby's knee was jackknifed rigid. That bleeding prevented him from walking for seven years. It unbalanced his body and was an important contributing cause of the hundreds of other destructive bleedings in both knees, in his hips, ankles, shoulders, and elbows that tortured him in the years that followed. It dominated his childhood, caused him a thousand nights of pain, locked him for years in casts and braces and, eventually, destroyed his left knee.

Joint bleeding is a viciously destructive form of internal bleeding. In severe hemophilia, it is inevitable. When a trauma occurs (and the cause of the trauma may be something as simple as walking), and when even a small amount of blood enters the confined space of a knee, ankle, or other joint, the result is devastating. The joint begins to hurt, then it swells. Seeking a more comfortable position, the arm or leg bends up, leaving the largest possible area in the joint socket for the expanding volume of fluid. When the joint cavity is filled but the hemorrhage continues, the increasing pressure on the nerves causes more and more intense pain. Even after such a hemorrhage is stopped, there is a delicate period which may last for weeks, when bleeding may easily start again in the wounded joint. Meanwhile, destruction is underway. It takes time for the injured joint to reabsorb the blood and to heal. Blood has a corrosive effect, and if it remains long in the cavity, or if hemorrhages recur frequently, the blood, like acid, eats away cartilage and bone. Eventually, there are bone malformations and changes. Motion in the joint is destroyed. The limb then remains permanently locked, frozen into the bent position. Well into our century this fate, in greater or lesser degree, was common for all hemophiliacs who did not die in childhood. Even up to the middle of the twentieth century, most severe hemophiliacs were in some way permanently crippled by the time they reached fourteen.

Joint bleeding (the medical term is *hemarthrosis*) is most severe during the growing years. This is because growth occurs in the joints. Bodies grow bigger and taller because bones are growing longer. This growth happens at the end of the bones—that is, in the joints. The process of ossification, when cartilage turns into bone, is nourished by blood. Because active growth is in progress, more blood circulates into a child's joints than into those of an adult. When growth is completed, less blood is needed in the joints. Then, as a rule, hemophiliacs have fewer joint hemorrhages. But if the joints have already been damaged, it is too late. The growing years, between six and eighteen, are crucial. It is then that the battle to save the joints must be waged.

The prevention of such joint bleeding and damage is a complicated hematological and orthopedic problem. In an attempt to stop repeated bleedings, the hematologist transfuses fresh-frozen plasma or, today, AHF concentrates. To rehabilitate damaged joints, the orthopedist and the therapist work gingerly with limbs, trying to find ways to restore movement and exercise without starting fresh bleeding. It is an exceedingly delicate balance. Often the best efforts meet only with failure.

Yes, it is easy to look back now and see what we all did wrong. But then, in 1962, when Bobby was five and a half years old, very little was known about the effective management of a bleeding joint. Among doctors, there was great disagreement on the best way to treat it. This disagreement continues to exist today. But one important thing has changed. Since 1962 much more has been learned about the most effective way of using transfusion to control joint bleeding.

Today, a joint bleeding is treated immediately and massively with AHF concentrates. In the days when Bobby was a small child, the emphasis was very different. Doctors worried more about the effects of frequent transfusions than the effects of joint damage. Today, as I write this, this statement sounds to me like the thinking of another century, yet it was only twelve years ago. Those who despair of our civilization need only to look at the startling progress in our knowledge of blood during these brief years.

In 1962 little was known about the Anti-Hemophilic Factor. The amount of AHF in each plasma bag was invisible, immeasurable. Transfusions of plasma met with very uneven results. In addition to this very practical problem, there were other severe complications associated with frequent transfusion. There was the fear of hepatitis. Doctors worried that the more transfusions received, the greater the danger of contamination and of contracting the hepatitis virus. And, in the still imperfectly purified fresh-frozen plasma, there were also other risks—risks of allergic reactions, hives, shortness of breath, and worse. Bobby experienced a few of these. Adrenalin was administered quickly and, mercifully, they passed. The most frightening specter was the fear that frequent transfusions would increase the risk of developing antibodies to the plasma itself. Then the child would no longer respond to plasma. It happened in a small percentage of cases, and this fear was more than enough to dictate reluctance in transfusion.

Today, because there have been so few cases among hemophiliacs, doctors tend to worry less about hepatitis. With more purified blood products, allergic reactions are now extremely rare. And the antibody reaction now appears to be a much more complex mechanism, one not necessarily linked to frequent transfusions. It is now recognized that the results of bleeding in the joints are much more terrible than the risks of treatment.

But then, fearful of the unknown and unproven dangers of the future, doctors decided to treat only tentatively and hesitantly the known and proved dangers of the present. They were thinking of the adult that *might* be, of the things that *might* happen, rather than of the child that was before them and the things that were happening. No one sufficiently pondered the Biblical injunction that "Sufficient unto the day is the Evil thereof." Plasma was administered sparingly, only after waiting to see if a joint would get better by itself. Very occasionally it did. This was enough to give false hope. Usually the joint did not get better; in fact, by not treating it, it got very much worse and thus, in the end, necessitated many more transfusions than if it had been treated immediately.

But how easy it is to see with hindsight! The fact was that the doctors were unsure. We were all unsure, and our fear of the future clouded our eyes to the present danger.

When Bobby began bleeding into his joints, there was only one place where we could seek advice: the Orthopedic Clinic for Hemophiliacs at Lenox Hill Hospital. Ruling this clinic with an iron hand was Dr. Henry Jordan, an autocratic Dane who had pioneered in orthopedic treatment for hemophiliacs. When we met him he was nearing seventy. He was world-famous. From this lofty position he brooked no controversy and no contradiction. His method was the one—the only one.

The Jordan treatment was immobilization, as total as possible, so that the joints would be protected from stress, from bleeding, and thus from damage. He believed in encasing the joints in various devices: first casts, then a series of stiff braces. It was his dream, he once said, to put a boy in braces from the age of five through the age of eighteen so that at eighteen he would emerge with his joints intact. He did not mention, or perhaps did not consider important, the effect on the boy's personality. Some of his devices, while benign, were so heavy and cumbersome that they looked like torture instruments of the Middle Ages. I have been told by others that Dr. Jordan was a very kind and humane man. Perhaps he was shy, but I know that I never heard from him a single soft or encouraging word in all the times that we saw him. In fact, I do not remember his speaking a single word to me directly, other than prescribing a cast or a brace.

At Lenox Hill they began to encase Bobby in plaster. His left leg was put in a cast. The casts itched, they hurt, sometimes bleeding went on inside them, and they became excruciating vises for the swelling joints. First it was legs, then arms. Then Bobby was put into a metal and leather splint. Still, the bleeding went on.

Faithfully, we reported to the Lenox Hill Clinic. In the main waiting room, there were long lines of wooden benches. We sat there, as if we were in court, waiting, waiting. It was obligatory to be there at 8 A.M., when the clinic opened. No appointments were made. You waited. Sometimes the doctors did not get around to you until the afternoon. I didn't object to this so much; I knew that Dr. Jordan was a very busy man and there were a lot of patients. But I did object to the heartlessness of the routine. You could not leave your place in line, because you never knew when you might be called. Mothers were so nervous about losing their places that they were afraid to leave for even a few moments to get a snack for their child. You brought what you needed or went without.

I read aloud until I was hoarse. Imagine yourself with a child in casts and braces, a child of six, seven, or eight. What would you find to amuse them sitting on the same bench for several hours? The time was endless. We all waited there, mothers of every race, tense and worried, with restless, bored children, reassuring in the same words: "It will be all right, dear; only a little while longer, dear. Try to be patient, dear; they will come and then you will get better."

Mothers were afraid even to ask "When will the doctor see us?" for fear that "Doctor" would get angry.

Whole days slipped away in this manner. But we went on waiting, for there was no other place to go. That was the problem. How well I came to know the sullen anger, the mutinous rage, that grows in the helpless. They say nothing. What can they say? But angry thoughts boiled in me.

When the moment finally came and it was our turn to move upstairs, another dehumanizing routine awaited us. Boys would be lined up in bare little cubicles with curtains. They sat there, alone in their underwear, apprehensive; sometimes another hour or so passed. Finally the curtain swished open. In crowded two or three doctors. They would pinch and manipulate joints, discussing among themselves what might be the trouble, rarely addressing the patient directly, as if, somehow, he had no feelings, no fears, no modesty. Then they would sweep out again imperiously. Outside, an anxious mother might venture to ask a nurse, "Will he have to have another brace?" (For her, this question was like asking what the sentence might be.) Brusquely, the answer would come back: "The doctor will decide that. You will have to wait to see what he says."

I remember one day especially. We had spent hours in the corridor waiting for the examining doctors. I was pacing the hall, feeling the rage boiling inside me, and finally I exclaimed out loud impatiently to no one in particular, "Where is that doctor? It's disgraceful the way they make us wait so long. We're human beings too!" Nearby stood another woman, who looked fearfully toward me and whispered, "Yes, yes, but what can we do? If they get mad at us maybe they won't see our children!" She was frail, small, with the fine, soft, blond hair of a child. Her skin was white, almost transparent. She looked very tired and I could see that she was really frightened, so I began gently to talk to her.

"When did you get here this morning?"

"We were here at eight," she answered. "From Long Island."

"What time did you have to get up to get here?"

"At five." Her husband was a truck driver. She had a seven-year-old hemophiliac son. He was in casts. The last time, they sawed through his cast and had cut his leg. His cast had to be removed and refitted again that day.

It was almost three o'clock in the afternoon. "Have you eaten?" I asked.

"No."

"Has your son eaten anything?"

"No."

Furious, I said, "Listen to me. You go now and take him to the cafeteria. Give him something to eat and have something to eat yourself. I'll keep your place; I'll wait for the doctor and I promise you that you won't miss him. He will see you." I finally convinced her and she went. I was still waiting when she got back, and the doctor still had not come.

That woman made a great impression on me. In her gentle and frightened eyes I saw inarticulate suffering. She was mute. I realized suddenly that we were not. I knew then that we would have to write.

The fearful gentle face of that unknown woman stayed with me, goaded me, even during our most discouraging moments. Throughout our work on *Nicholas and Alexandra*, she was the inspiration that sharpened my determination to persist, to succeed . . . for her, and for those like her, alone, afraid to speak, helpless.

Even after the doctor was seen and the prescription for new braces given, even then the waiting was not over. For then, Bobby and I were sent to wait in a dingy, dark brace-making shop on Third Avenue. The receptionist was rude. We often waited for two or more hours for no apparent reason. All this was for the privilege of ordering and then waiting six more weeks for a brace to be made. And then paying $300 for it, only to have it outgrown six months later and have to start the whole cycle over again.

During that hard time, two other things happened in our family. When Bobby could not walk and could not get somewhere in his wheelchair (up a flight of stairs, for example) I carried him. Once at Cross County Hospital when he was wearing casts on both legs I had to carry him up several flights of stairs. Then I carried him back to the car. When we got home, I carried him into the house, and then I went back to the car for several heavy bags of groceries. I was three and a half months pregnant. As I carried the last bag into the house, I felt something inside me snap. I began to bleed. The doctor ordered me to bed, but only a few hours later I was lying on a mattress in the back of our station wagon, hemorrhaging, as Bob rushed me to the hospital. With him in the front seat sat Bobby, with his casts and crutches. There was no one we could leave him with.

I remember the strong hands that reached out for me at the hospital door and gently put me on a stretcher. I remember the flood of attention, more than I had ever received before in my life, and how grateful I was, despite the pain. Before I lost consciousness, I remember musing on how wonderfully quickly hospitals can act when it is necessary. Then I was blissfully anesthetized. I lost the baby. Dr. Callahan was kind. He told me that it would probably have happened anyway. But this time, I did not believe him.

And Susy, our dear Susy! Her eyes had begun to cross when she was nineteen months old. Just before she was three, it was decided that she must be operated on. I was sick with worry that something malevolent had touched her too, and terrified that the operation would go wrong. I stayed with her in the hospital. For hours after the operation she was blind. I remember leading her in her little pink bathrobe to the window, and the glory of watching the new dawn with her, as she began, dimly, to see again. Bob had taken Bobby to Mount Sinai for a transfusion, and was waiting with him at Lenox Hill.

Months passed. There was no improvement. One day I looked

at Bobby, small and wan in his tiny wheelchair, his legs twisted, melting away before my eyes. I suddenly realized how much time had passed, and that there was no end in sight. One day one of the doctors said dryly, "He is a cripple. He will probably be crippled for life. He will never walk again." I tried to say to myself, "Face it, girl; it's true. You have a crippled son now. Accept it. Don't torture yourself with delusions." But somehow I could not accept it. Something didn't fit.

Bob had been doing research for a magazine article on hemophilia. Occasionally he heard talk that other methods were being tried. At a fledgling hemophilia center just begun at Los Angeles Orthopaedic Hospital, there was an idea of exercise. Bob wrote prophetically in his article, "Orthopaedic Hospital does not believe in immobilizing a joint, but in starting therapy immediately. Many people feel that the future lies in this technique." He interviewed a California orthopedic specialist who said, "In my view, the reason human beings are given joints is to move them. It is a well-known orthopedic principle that if you take any (injured) joint and hold it stiff over a long period of time, it fills up with scar and gets stiff and stays stiff."

Movement. To me, it made sense. I had studied ballet for ten years. In ballet it is a maxim that "it takes ten years to make a leg." Ten years of specialized training of muscles. If that were true, as I knew it was in ballet, then it was hard to believe that you could immobilize a leg for years and then expect it to work normally again—that no movement would result in movement.

I discovered a curious paradox in Dr. Jordan. The only other thing that commanded his interest as much as hemophilia was ballet. He loved it so much that he became the doctor specializing in the care of the dancers of the New York City Ballet. He worried over their professional injuries of tendons and muscles. He worked to help them move again. But for hemophiliacs he prescribed rigid iron braces.

That Dr. Jordan was a devoted man no one could doubt; that he had had some good results with his methods was also true. Yet when I met him, I had the feeling that he had somehow fallen in love with his own devices. And when it came to Bobby, I could not believe that this living entombment was the answer.

For although the theory was that total immobilization would prevent bleeding, in practice for us, it had not turned out that way. The joints inexplicably bled—spontaneously, for no reason at all, despite casts or immobilizing braces. Sometimes the braces themselves seemed to cause bleeding in the joint they were designed to protect, or in other limbs that had to strain to accommodate their heavy, unbalancing weight. We had to try to restore the leg to independent movement.

The idea of walking away, of saying no to Dr. Jordan, was a little like saying no to God. There was no one else who had as much experience in the field as he. Nevertheless, we decided to seek another opinion.

We could not afford to take Bobby to Orthopaedic Hospital in Los Angeles, so we took him instead to Dr. Robert Siffert, the chief orthopedic surgeon at Mount Sinai Hospital. He was not an expert on hemophilic joints and did not pretend to be, but he believed that joints should move. When I first took Bobby to Dr. Siffert, his left leg was jackknifed rigid. The muscles in his leg were so weak that he could not lift his foot at all when sitting on the edge of the doctor's table. The leg was misshapen, with a huge knobby formation on the outside of his knee joint.

The problem was to find the right balance between starting movement and starting new bleeding. In the years that followed, step by step, together we fumbled, learning by trial and error. If the right decision was made, it was more a lucky accident than anything else. We didn't know. The doctors didn't know. We all played our hunches and hoped. When things didn't work out, which was often, we gritted our teeth and started again. It took seven years of persistence and work before Bobby was able to straighten and use that leg again.

At first, Dr. Siffert decided on the bold course of putting Bobby in traction for several hours a day to begin pulling his leg straight. Traction! Terrified that the slightest movement would set off bleeding again, we rigged up pulleys and weights, and tied Bobby to his bed three or four hours a day. We did this throughout the summer. By the fall, although the leg was still bent severely, it had straightened enough so that we could think of putting a walking brace on him: a brace with a dial that we could adjust as the leg pulled straighter. At first, Bobby could not walk even with this brace, because his leg was too bent to touch the ground. He had to use crutches (and they could be used only sparingly because of the danger of starting bleeding in elbows and shoulders) or a wheelchair. Without the brace he could only skitter over the floor on his bottom like a crab.

I grew obsessed with knees. I seemed to be conscious of little boys' browned knees moving, bending in and out, everywhere I went. It was hard to look at little boys playing or running, unaware of their good fortune.

Gradually, very gradually, as the months stretched into years, Bobby's leg extended and he began to walk with the brace and no crutches. Some movement had been restored to the knee. The brace, with a flick of the dial, bent, so that he could at least sit down more or less normally at a desk or in a car. All this was already a miracle.

Braces taught a new way of life. I sewed long zippers in the inside of his pants, so that he could dress quickly in the morning. So that he would not have to wear special, "funny-looking" high shoes, I combed the stores for normal shoes with strong, thick rubber soles. We had a special heel put on these shoes, with holes to anchor the brace. For years one foot was much smaller than the other (we worried that one leg would end up shorter than the other), so I always had to buy two identical pairs of shoes of different sizes. I always kept hoping that I would locate another hemophiliac who would need the other one, because my Swiss soul rebelled at having to throw out two perfectly good shoes.

Then, after two years had passed, and we thought we were on the way to victory, the right leg, which had been supporting the weak, brace-ridden left leg, gave out and began to bleed repeatedly. Bobby was forced to wear another walking brace on the right leg. For two more years he had to wear two braces instead of one, and his stiff-legged gait gave the impression that he was walking on small, invisible stilts.

All during these years, bleeding was occurring unpredictably, maddeningly, from joint to joint. We would treat one; another would start the next day. Sometimes it happened even the same day: with plasma in him for one joint, another would start bleeding.

It would be the right elbow, then the left, then the left knee, right ankle, left ankle, right knee, left shoulder, left hip, or a combination of two or three.

The pain of these episodes was terrible. For all of Bobby's childhood, he lived with it and we lived with it. Doctors say that the pain of a bleeding joint is one of the worst known to medical science. Each of Bobby's joints behaved differently and had its own particular pattern of suffering. His right ankle caused him agonies, but it did not swell. His tortured left knee swelled until it seemed it would burst. Sometimes two joints bled at once. Bob constructed supports of cardboard and then wood to hold up the blankets at the bottom of the bed, so that their weight would not touch Bobby's excruciatingly painful joints. As the joint swelled and the pressure grew intense, he would try to curl up his leg. We fought to keep it straight, resting it on pillows, strapping it on splints. Sometimes we tried keeping his brace on for the night, knowing that the more the leg flexed, the longer it would take to straighten. Always, as the pain mounted, the leg would bend.

In the past, seeking to alleviate their agonies, hemophiliacs became drug addicts. Our doctor had seen such hemophilic addicts during his medical studies, and because of this we tried in every way to give drugs to Bobby as sparingly as possible. In any case, there is no drug that can completely alleviate the pain of bleeding joints. Besides, Bobby was very sensitive to any drug. They tended to excite, rather than soothe, him. We tried Darvon. We tried codeine, but codeine only made his eyes grow wild, blurred his vision, and did not take away the pain, only somehow made it pound through a haze of half-consciousness. Under its influence he would sometimes grow hysterical and violent, and scream, over and over, "No! No more pain! No more pain!" Sometimes when, for no reason we knew, transfusions did not help or only slowed the bleeding, the pain would go on for days and nights.

Through those sleepless nights, I sat by Bobby's bed. I soothed his forehead. I held his hand while he moaned, asking him to tighten his hold on my hand so as to forget the pain, as we were taught to do in childbirth. He would do this and, although he was a child, his grip would nearly crack the bones in my hand.

A terrible story I had read kept intruding into my mind. In

South America a child had fallen into a vat of boiling sugar and he died, slowly, in agony, with his mother watching by his side. Was it like this? I wondered. No, I thought, no; it must have been worse. How could she stand it, this unknown woman? If she could, then I must, for on that scale we were still among the fortunate ones. Yet tears that felt like liquid fire burned their way down my cheeks. Impotence, helplessness, choked my throat. I sat there numbly, hour after hour, as if the very act of witness would somehow help; but the pain continued implacably. And when he would finally fall asleep for a short while, exhausted, his eyes swollen with tears and struggle, I would simply lie on the floor beside his bed, listening to his breath, reaching for his hand, hoping, praying that the pain would stop.

When I am deeply upset, I cannot sleep. Blessedly, Bob has the capacity to shut out everything. During those long nights, he slept . . . and this was essential. We were soldiers in a battle. The struggle to keep us afloat financially depended on his energy. Without sleep, he could not write, and what would have happened to us if he had lost his job? One of us had to be rested enough to face the world.

For me it was late movies. How they helped! How many nights, when I was too tense and too worried to sleep, I would watch them through the night. *The Late Show. The Late Late Show. The Early Bird Show.* How many times I cried over *Casablanca*! I grew to love, as never before, those famous faces who were filling my lonely nights.

There were many nights when Bobby could neither lie down nor sit up in his bed because it was too painful, so I would move him in with me before the TV set, propping and supporting his pain-wracked limbs with an army of pillows. Wonderful Jerry Lewis! He actually made Bobby laugh in the middle of one of his worst knee episodes. Exhausted, and half asleep beside him in the middle of the night, I heard that laugh. It is still the greatest triumph of an actor that I have ever witnessed. When the magic medicine of movies worked, we would wake in the morning curled up side by side in blankets and pillows with the TV set still on. But the night always came again.

After three such nights, all life became a blur, and there was no reality but The Pain. Each of these episodes was like a siege during which we tried to hold our fortress against an invisible enemy that battered and battered. There was nothing to do but just take the blows and wait for the enemy to withdraw as inexplicably as it had attacked.

After these storms were over, there was such weariness, such exhaustion, as if we had been tossed, gasping, onto a deserted shore. Bobby recovered more easily than I did. I always wondered at his resilience. Somehow, as soon as things were better again, he would be as cheerful and active as before. For me, it took many days, and as I grew older and more tired, many weeks, to recover from this helpless watching of these terrible nighttime tortures of my son.

Chapter 7

SM

*What do I remember? I remember arm splints for shots, having
my arm tied down so the needle wouldn't move. I remember
staring at the light in Dr. Engel's office, feeling drowsy from the
Benadril, a stinging feeling through my whole body as I watched
the plasma as it hung from the light above my head. Slowly the
plasma would drip, drip, drip, drip, and I would be lulled into a
semihypnotic, sleepy state as I lay on my back—drip, drip, lulling
me into a daze.*

BOBBY MASSIE.

It was one of those lucky coincidences. Just before Bobby's
first knee bleeding we met the doctor who was to become a constant presence in our home for all the hard years of the bleeding
joints. In December of 1961, we were still running back and forth,
thirty miles each way, from Westchester to Mount Sinai at odd
hours of the night, when we happened to see Dr. Martin Rosenthal,
a senior hematologist. Shaking his head, he said, "I don't know why
you have to keep doing this. There's no reason he couldn't get his
transfusions at home. There must be a lot of our trained guys near
you. We have to find you somebody." He gave us the name of a
young hematologist whom we had met as a resident in one of our
nighttime excursions. He was just starting in practice in White
Plains, where we had just moved to a tiny two-bedroom house. He
agreed to come to our house when he was needed, and one night
a few weeks later we called him. But things did not go well. He
tried to get into Bobby's veins and missed. He tried again and again.
Six tries later, he still couldn't skewer Bobby's small vein. He did
something then for which I have always respected him. He gave
up. He said, "I can't do it. It's not fair to him for me to try any-

more. I'm going to try and get Lee Engel." Dr. Leroy Engel was a pediatrician, also just starting in practice, whom he had known during his residency at Mount Sinai. A short time later, Dr. Engel arrived. Calmly, he punctured the vein on his first try.

Only two weeks after that night, Bobby began to bleed in the joints, and in the six years that followed, from January 11, 1962, through May 23, 1968, when Bob took over from him, Lee gave Bobby 496 transfusions. I know he must have, once or twice, but I can't remember his ever missing a vein.

Lee Engel is a matter-of-fact man. He calls himself "old stone-face," but apologetically, a little shyly, as if begging you to understand that that isn't the real man, and if you would only persevere, underneath you would find the soft artist that he is at heart.

His eyes are his most distinctive feature: bright, searching, dark-brown eyes that take in everything, every detail of a child's condition, and relay the findings to a clear, decisive brain. He wears glasses, clear at the bottom with black rims on top, accent marks for those intelligent eyes under their bushy eyebrows. Lee remembers details. In college, his photographic memory could imprint and retain a page's contents in a few moments.

In all the years we saw each other, no matter what the hour of the night, Lee always arrived impeccably dressed: fresh shirt, tie, neatly pressed suit, hat and coat, driving his powerful convertible— the only outward contradiction of an otherwise totally unfrivolous spirit. (And when I teased him about being so dressed up in the middle of the night when we were running around distracted in our nightgowns and bathrobes, he always answered very seriously, "Sue, I never know where I might have to go to next.") He is always prepared. His doctor's case is precisely arranged with its neat rows of medicines and needles. But his notes are hit-or-miss, quickly scribbled in an illegible scrawl. He remembers.

On the phone his voice is always calm, low, matter-of-fact to the point of dryness. There is no bedside manner, but mothers trust him because they know that he is *good*, a superb diagnostician, and that he doesn't flinch during the hard moments. He is unsentimental, and that helps getting into a vein. His emotions never get in the way. Some doctors felt so sorry for Bobby that they found it difficult to stick him decisively. Lee is sure, and because of this sureness everything he does, the children say, "hurts less": shots, taking specks from eyes and beans out of noses, fixing scrapes, and removing splinters. As he himself always advised us, "If you have to do something painful, don't hesitate. Go in surely. It hurts less that way."

During those searing years, we needed that sureness, that dry approach, those cool and imperturbable nerves. There was rarely a day, excepting vacations, when we did not talk on the phone. Sometimes we went to him—to his office or to his house, where Bobby grew to know his three sons, their pet rabbits, gerbils, and turtles. But many more times Lee came to us—at least once a week, and during crises once and sometimes twice a day. Sometimes these crises lasted for weeks.

The routine was always the same. Lee would arrive, toss his coat and black fedora over the banister and, taking the stairs two steps at a time, go up to Bobby's room. With scarcely a word, he would methodically go about his business, setting out his needles and equipment. (Bob remembers that this routine always helped to calm him.) One of us would be thawing the bags of plasma in the bathroom sink. Then *ping!* he was into a vein and the plasma would start dripping. As soon as the transfusion was started, without fail Lee would call his service and say, "I'm at the Massies'; call you when I'm through." The whole process usually took about an hour, start to finish, and while the plasma dripped into Bobby's veins we talked or watched TV. I remember Lee, rocking back and forth in our old rocker, smoking the big black cigars he loved. We talked about the book we were working on, and he diagnosed Empress Alexandra's symptoms from the descriptions in the accounts that Bob was reading.

When it was all over he'd call his service once more. "Any calls for me? . . . O.K. I'm going home now." Many years later, when I called about a problem of Elizabeth's, I was startled when the service operator suddenly asked, "How's your son?" When I asked her how she knew, she said, "I used to take all Dr. Engel's calls."

There was one thing about Lee, though, that scared me. He

was very gruff on the phone when we called him at night. It took a lot for me to muster the courage to wake him. By the time he got to us, the gruffness was gone; but nevertheless, I would chew my nails and pace the floor trying to pull myself together enough to dial the telephone. Quite a few times we tried to get through the night rather than risk waking him. This was very foolish.

Once, many years later, we were talking and I finally found the nerve to tell him how afraid I had been of his voice. It seemed to break some barrier at last. Almost shyly, he said, "I know. I frighten people. My wife tells me that I'm—what is the word she uses—'austere,' 'serious.' Even when I kid around, people don't know I'm doing it. I have to be careful now, I've learned." I asked him why be became a doctor, and he answered, "I just don't know. I can't explain it. It's just that I always wanted to do it, as far back as I can remember. Even when I was a kid, I read everything about it that I could understand. I remember one book I read over and over, about a medical missionary—*Burma Surgeon*."

Lee came from a hard-working family of Jewish emigrants from Austria-Hungary and Russia, who had settled in a small town in Pennsylvania and prospered. "I always had to work in our garment factory . . . my father believed in that. At the age of five I was set to cutting out the long rows of hooks and eyes for bras with big, heavy scissors. I got blisters all over my hands. But I didn't like business. I didn't like money. I wanted to be a doctor."

A dedicated and intense student, he excelled in his studies, went to Yale, made Phi Beta Kappa, and applied for Yale Medical School. "When I was filling out applications and they asked why I wanted to be a doctor, I had a hard time answering. It was strictly a gut feeling. And when they asked what I wanted as a second profession, I couldn't think of anything else . . . so I left it blank." He was graduated *summa cum laude* from medical school.

And why did he choose pediatrics? "I really do like kids." And he added a little wistfully, "In fact, I think I communicate better with kids than with their parents. The kids understand me better. I know mothers keep looking at my face while I'm examining a kid to see if they can read anything. Nobody can tell anything by looking at my face . . . but they don't know how often my heart goes pitter patter."

When we met, Lee had just started his practice. Bobby was his first private hemophiliac patient. "I had seen hemophilia as a pediatric resident at Sinai. I'll never forget how, once, when I was chief resident and I was off duty, the interns panicked. A kid came in who was bleeding a lot. They got overzealous and overtransfused him. He went into pulmonary edema. They didn't know what it was and it lasted all night. That was always my big worry: overloading Bobby's system. I just couldn't give him enough to bring up his bleeding time because there just wasn't enough AHF factor in what we were able to give.

"With Bobby, I was impressed by how what seemed like a little bleeding would turn into a big one a few days later. And most of the time how quickly the plasma seemed to help him. I never knew whether this was simply because he relaxed when he knew he was getting the stuff or whether it actually relieved his condition that quickly.

"I was impressed by how much pain, how much abominable pain, he was in . . . how hard everybody tried to take it, how hard he tried to take it. That was what was so impressive: how he took it all the time.

"He was only stopped by his bleeding temporarily. I shouldn't say that I never saw Bobby depressed. Sometimes after a long period he'd really had it; but then, when it was over, he was off again and no longer depressed. When he was depressed, he got much less out of his transfusions. In his older years, things didn't respond as well. But running in and out the way I did, you don't see everything. A lot goes on that the doctor can't see, and that you could see better."

Lee Engel, cerebral and reserved, worked from the head; Bill Bisordi, open and warm, from the heart. What seems wonderful to me in retrospect is that these two men, the most important doctors in Bobby's early life, so opposite in temperament and approach, came to us and to Bobby precisely when we needed their special talents most.

Ever since first Bob and then Bobby learned to give transfusions, we haven't seen as much of Lee. Susy has grown up, and our youngest, Elizabeth, is of course less demanding of his time than Bobby was. Certainly it is easier on his schedule. But for all

those years he was a member of our family, and we miss him.
Probably because of the excitement and stress, Bobby bled on every
holiday. For years, Lee shared every family event, every Easter,
every Christmas. After the transfusions Lee would stay a while
and chat, munching on fruitcake or a gingerbread man.

And I remember that when Elizabeth was born, and we had
just brought her back from the hospital, Lee came to examine her.
Puffing on his cigar, impeccable and serious as usual, he walked
into our bedroom. I was nursing Elizabeth. "*Mazel tov*," he said.
Then we all drank champagne.

Blythedale Children's Hospital was just up the road from our
little house in White Plains. I often passed it while driving on my
errands and used to wonder what went on behind the walls of the
old house with the low buildings clustered around it. It was Lee
Engel who told me that it was a center for children with long-term
illnesses. He was on the staff of Blythedale and each week devoted
his days off from his practice to the children there. "Hey," he
exclaimed one day, "*that's* where Bobby ought to go for therapy!"
It was an inspiration.

Blythedale is a private charity hospital, supported entirely by
a yearly grant from the Federation of Jewish Philanthropies in
New York. A condition of the yearly grant is that there be no
other public fund-raising. When there is a deficit (and there always
is) it is quietly made up by the forty members of the Board of
Trustees from their own pockets.

Children are referred to Blythedale from all over the world.
They are rich and poor, they are of every race and religion. They
come when other medical centers have done all they can, and
spend from three months to three years living at Blythedale. It is
up to the staff to teach them how to grow and live with their illnesses. The challenge is enormous. Children come to Blythedale
with the most severe and disabling medical problems: children with
curved spines; with Perthes disease, a congenital hip defect which
necessitates wearing a wide-spread leg cast for many years; children
with cerebral palsy; paraplegic and quadriplegic children; and
children with "brittle bone" disease (*osteogenesis imperfecta*).

This is a particularly fiendish genetic defect. A child with this disease is born lacking the ability to make the substance that hardens bones. The problem lasts until adolescence when, for mysterious reasons, it seems to correct itself. By that time, a child may have had seventy-five to ninety-five fractures: from having his diaper changed, from being hugged, from turning over in bed during his sleep. How can such children learn to go to school, to play games, to make friends, to be happy?

Blythedale's approach to these problems is unique. The emphasis is on movement and independence. Many of the children are confined to bed, but they are not confined to their rooms. When we first went to Blythedale, I was amazed to see nurses vigorously pushing beds outdoors into the sunshine, where children flew kites from their beds into the wind. Today Blythedale has developed an even more flexible device, an electrically movable bed which even severely disabled children can operate entirely by themselves. Nicknamed the "Blythemobile," it is only one of a series of ingenious adaptive devices developed at the hospital and, like most of the others, made on the spot.

At Blythedale, the usual rigid hospital rules do not apply. Parents can come anytime, brothers and sisters can visit, even rabbits, turtles, cats, and dogs can visit. The focus is on the *child*, not the *patient;* what he *can* do and not what he *cannot* do.

Despite everything, the atmosphere at Blythedale is positive. I cannot call it lighthearted because the problems to be faced are too great; rather it is a special happiness that comes from the contact with human courage and deep compassion. Robert Louis Stevenson, himself a victim of severe tuberculosis, once wrote that "life does not consist so much in having a good hand at cards, but of learning how to play a poor hand well." It is that absolute determination to help those children who have been dealt some of the worst cards possible to play their hand well that makes Blythedale an exciting, inspiring place. I have never gone there without feeling better and stronger for the contact.

Ordinarily, Blythedale did not accept outpatients. Lee went to ask the director of the hospital, Bob Stone, if they would make an exception for Bobby. Bob had taken over as director of Blythedale only two years before we met him. He is a tall, soft-spoken man, totally absorbed by his job, who turns fierce when he is talking about the needs and problems of children with long-term illness. During the past ten years under Bob's energetic direction, Blythedale has exploded with activity and purpose. Lee explained Bobby's special need. Would they let him come and work with Blythedale's therapists? Bob Stone's reaction was, "If we can help him, we'll do it." And help him they did. During the two years that followed, Bobby and I drove up the road to the big rambling house three times each week for therapy. He worked with three therapists, one a girl who had had polio in her own childhood. Mostly he worked with the chief therapist, a remarkable Irish lady named Miss Margaret O'Neill. Miss O'Neill had a husky body with the strong arms and shoulders of a football player, developed over a lifetime of working to straighten and strengthen the limbs of hundreds of children. Her hair, once black, now was gray. When she worked actively with Bobby, a wisp or two would stray from her tight bun onto her cheek. She was always concentrating so hard that she never seemed to notice. She made Bobby work hard. She permitted no nonsense. He had to concentrate every minute he was with her. Yet there was something about her so warm and compassionate, so deeply encouraging, that I saw Bobby strain to try harder and harder each time as she would say, "Now, press down with your leg on my hand, Bobby. That's pretty good; now a little more, a little harder. Now, that's not so bad! All right, now once again. Count to ten this time while you push down as hard as you can." Over and over, her strong, experienced hands gently but firmly held Bobby's bent leg in a line while he tried to tighten his weak muscles in isometric exercises. She put Bobby in whirlpool baths, she made him lift weights. At first, the weight was only the weight of his own leg. Sitting on the edge of a table, he would try with great difficulty to lift his leg out in front of him. As his legs grew slowly stronger, she attached heavier and heavier weights to his ankle as he tried to lift his leg up. At home, following Miss O'Neill's instructions, I made weights, sewing little cotton bags which I filled with sand. Every day, I tried to do Bobby's exercises with him. It was a battle. Bobby would balk, get bored, refuse to work hard. I would scream at him in frustration, "Don't you know, Bobby, it's *your* leg!" I lacked Miss O'Neill's quiet authority. With her, he never did anything but try harder and harder.

Bobby would bring in his favorite things to show Miss O'Neill. He brought his precious lobster trap from Maine and put it next to him on the therapy table. He brought his butterfly net, and one day, when Bob Stone stuck his head into the therapy room, Bobby gave him a long lecture on insects, butterflies, and moths.

While Bobby worked with Miss O'Neill, Susy and I read books aloud together or chatted with the other children. We grew to know and love several of them. There was Annie with a curved spine, encased in plaster to her neck. And Christopher, who suffered from hydrocephalus. Bobby's best friend was a seven-year-old girl. Her eyes, black and warm as ripe olives, looked merrily out at the world from under the football helmet she had to wear to protect her head in case she lost her balance and fell. Marina had cerebral palsy. While they waited their turn for therapy, Bobby and Marina careened around the halls in their wheelchairs. Marina had a mischievous sense of humor, but she had trouble enunciating her words clearly. No matter; Bobby understood her perfectly, and I would happily watch them in a corner, chattering and laughing at secret jokes.

Once a month, up from Columbia Medical Center in New York would come Mr. Ernest Traber, the brace maker, to check on everybody's braces and casts, and to design and adapt new ones. A slight, balding man with a kindly smile, he had come to America from Austria-Hungary many years before. Mr. Traber died a few years ago, and with him, says Bob Stone, "a whole craft has died. We thought he was the best."

I often reflect how fortunate we were to have met Ernest Traber when we did, for it was he who designed the braces that helped Bobby to walk again. Practical and humane, Mr. Traber thought about one problem that few people considered: the financial burden on the parents of expensive braces. Mr. Traber designed braces so ingeniously that for the first time we could extend them as Bobby grew, which meant that they lasted at least a year and sometimes two. And, although they were beautifully handcrafted of steel and leather and took him weeks to make, he charged less than anyone else. One day, looking at a new, beautifully made brace he had just finished for Bobby, I said, "Mr. Traber! What if Bobby should walk in the mud?" He just smiled and said, "That's exactly why I make them—so he *can* walk in the mud!"

Thanks to the support of Mr. Traber's braces, thanks to the persistence of Miss O'Neill, thanks to hours, days, months of Bobby's work, slowly, very slowly, half a centimeter at a time, we managed to straighten Bobby's bent left leg, and to keep his right knee joint flexible. There was one six-month period when all improvement seemed to stop. We had extended the left leg almost straight, but not straight enough to walk. Miss O'Neill refused to give up, and the miraculous day finally did come when Bobby was able to discard his braces at last. "I remember marveling," he told me, "how easy it was to get dressed without a brace. Why, just put your pants and your shoes on, and you're off! Unbelievable!"

But the psychological and physical wounds of the long struggle are deep. Bobby's left knee was irretrievably damaged. I have covered over my scars more or less successfully. I thought I no longer remembered those days. But one day, many years after, when we returned from France, I went up to the attic and in a dusty corner I saw a pile of braces. I recoiled as if I had seen a skeleton. There they were, the tiny crutches, the tiny shoes, then larger and larger, with their worn-down heels, the worn leather knee covers, one brace after another piled like bones. Why had I kept them? Perhaps because they represented so many hours of waiting, such a great deal of effort and skill, so much money, so many things given up. I stood there in the attic and tears rolled down my cheeks before that mute testimonial.

Chapter 8

The first day at school is a milestone that every mother remembers. There before her, scrubbed clean, eyes shining, armed with a new schoolbag, is her precious child; scared, excited, *defenseless*, going into the big world at last. After the door of the school bus closes, that first morning, or after the familiar little back disappears into an unknown classroom, every mother frets, paces the floor, and gazes at the clock.

I was no different. It was only the degree of my worry that was different. I spent that day trying vainly to control the waves of fear that rolled over me when I permitted myself to remember that Bobby was out of my hands and entrusted to others. Did they understand? Would they watch? Perhaps, forgetful one moment with so many charges under their care, an accident would happen . . . and then the phone would ring. Would I be prepared? Should I leave the house during the school hours or simply wait to do my errands until he was back in my sight again—because what if I should be out when the awful moment came and at the school they panicked? Most of all, I worried about something else. Would somebody someday say something that would hurt him irrevocably, something so cruel that I could not smooth it over? I knew, of course, that I could do nothing but wait.

At home, we had already made the decision that Bobby was going to be treated normally. The long-range medical prognosis was that Bobby, depending on luck and circumstances, could have a normal life span. That could apply to any of us. The disease was most dangerous and destructive in childhood, but, we were told, after eighteen, when a boy has passed puberty and completed his physical growth, it seemed to be less active. Not that he would escape all problems thereafter, but they were likely to be less frequent. To reach that physical goal of adulthood in the best possible health was one of our two objectives for Bobby. The other, just as important and maybe even more important, was that he reach adulthood in good psychological health. Bobby was a curious, inquiring, outgoing boy with a happy nature. It was our job to protect these God-given qualities and never permit them to be crushed. It was we who had to help him fulfill the promise of his luminous personality, and bring him to that distant plateau as a vigorous, outgoing adult. If, at the end of the struggle, he was to emerge and live in a normal world, Bobby had to be taught to accept and understand prejudice, then to fight it, and finally to be strong enough to ignore it. He had to grow up thinking of himself as a boy who happened to have a problem, and not a problem who happened to be a boy.

At home, we could create an illusion of normality, however carefully disciplined and circumscribed. We could control the boundaries, we could gently push them out farther and farther, so that Bobby need never feel the invisible frontier that separated him from others. When children are small, all of them need a lot of watching. I could sit, unnoticed, and watch him play with other children. Bobby was not so different from the others, then. . . . But, if we wanted to continue the illusion of normality, we had to let Bobby become more active and independent. All parents feel the risk when they begin to let their children cross the street, go to somebody else's house, disappear down the block. The only difference for us was that we had a heightened understanding of these risks. We simply had to learn to accept them, and to live with a constant raw awareness of danger. This was the challenge. Every stage of growth meant new decisions. How far should we let him go? When? Could he be left alone with Sammy, who likes to whack his playmates over the head with a shovel? Should he climb trees? Could he sled? What about tricycles? bicycles?

There was no way to be sure. It was not enough simply to say Don't do this and Don't do that, because sometimes, whether he "did" anything or not, he would bleed. Other times, when he was more active than usual, inexplicably *nothing happened.* One day, walking around the house was enough to cause bleeding; the next day he could fall down a flight of stairs and there would hardly be a bruise. So we often guessed wrong, and when we did there was no one to blame but ourselves. Why couldn't we have foreseen? Why did we permit that? And who was to absolve me from the sense of guilt and failure? No one. Simply, it was necessary to begin again, to risk again, to try again to roll the boulder up the hill.

Yes, we worried when Bobby played with other children, but we wanted him to have friends. Yet fewer and fewer mothers permitted their children to play with him. Oh, it wasn't a mean, overt cutting off. Simply, they were "busy" or Tommy had other plans —unfortunately. "So sorry, maybe tomorrow." Occasionally, I would run into one of the neighborhood mothers at the super-market and she would say, "Oh, you know we'd love to have Bobby, but I would be afraid my little Johnny might hit him or something." I kept hoping they would ask, "Is there a chance he might come? Is there something I should know if he does come over?" But they didn't. It was easier just to cut him out, and then to add, "Really, I think you're so wonderful. I just don't know how you do it."

It was in search of companionship for Bobby that I swallowed hard and enrolled him in nursery school. At that young age the difference between Bobby and his classmates was scarcely notice-able. He remembers now that he was "never allowed to climb any-thing" but he marvels that in nursery school "I was still able to *run!*" Hemophilia had not yet touched Bobby's joints. He still looked like other children, the gulf could still be smoothed over. Like every other child his age, he loved ice cream, watched Captain Kangaroo, Tom Terrific and Mighty Manfred, was a loyal fan of the Mickey Mouse Club, and idolized Roy Rogers.

It was not until he began to bleed in the joints at age six that Bob and I understood that the biggest problem might be, after all, not what the disease did to his body, but what the world was pre-paring to do to his soul. For just as the time came when other children were growing more independent and could be ever freer, Bobby's frontiers became glaringly visible. At home we tried to treat his growing physical infirmities matter-of-factly . . . as some-thing annoying. About one thing we were very strict. No self-pity. Even if his legs were being twisted, there was no reason that his soul should be. We kept insisting that he think of himself not as an invalid but as someone temporarily out of commission, *only temporarily*. Keep the attitude positive; tomorrow will be better. But outside, no one would let him forget for a moment that he was "different" and "ill."

People mean well, but do they realize what happens when over and over again, on the street, in the supermarket, on trains, in school, they confront a charming little boy who happens to be on crutches or have his arm bandaged, and say, "Oh, poor little boy, what happened to you?" Totally ignoring the fact that the little boy had ears and understanding, people asked over and over, "What's the matter with his leg?" Insidiously, this repetition, accompanied by pitying looks and downcast eyes (and why do people so often lower their voices too, as if there were something shameful?), threatened everything that we tried to teach at home.

It was difficult to answer these curious, prying questions. If I said matter-of-factly, "He has hemophilia," there was a sharp intake of breath. "Oh, I'm so sorry," they would say as they hurried, frightened, away. Or, insistently, sometimes they would continue, still in front of Bobby, "But I always thought that meant they could bleed to death. I don't see what that has to do with a leg!" I would often see the happy smile on Bobby's face fade into bewilderment. He thought he was doing well. Why can't curious people realize how difficult it is for a parent, how wounding for a child, to have to explain over and over to strangers the thing that is causing him pain?

Over the years, we worried a great deal about the effects these constant, unthinking questions would have on him. And we continually searched to counteract this by looking for situations in which he would be treated by others as matter-of-factly as we treated him, in which he would be accepted and loved for what he had, and not pitied for what he did not have—perfect health. They grew harder and harder to find.

I keenly felt the ostracism of the outside world. How well I grew to know, and how hard I have fought, the sterility of bitterness! How much I wanted to shield Bobby from such wounds! Somehow, *he* had to make contact with life, real life, and remain hopeful. Yet no matter what we did, there was a limit to how much we could shield Bobby. To live and grow, a child needs more than parents. His image of himself comes from the way others treat him —his teachers, his peers, even the way that total strangers look at him. None of these could I control.

When he was very little, he hardly noticed. But even during his first days at nursery school he was pursued by these questions and they upset him. He did not know how to deal with them, and would come home confused and unhappy. Once, when he was five, he came home very distressed from a series of especially nagging questions from some children. So I said to him finally, "Look, Bobby, don't try to explain to the children. They are too little and they can't understand. Just tell them that a dragon bit your arm while you were fighting it in your back yard yesterday." Bobby was gleeful over this idea and for a while it ended the children's questions. But still these questions gnawed at him, and I knew it.

How well I remember the day when Bobby entered public school kindergarten. He had missed the first two weeks because of bleeding in the knee. He was on crutches. It was a totally new environment and the children, none of whom he knew, were already established in it. Not only was he new and different . . . he was late. As we entered the school door, I saw him hesitate, but I swept him along cheerfully. There was a long hall. And, as he traveled along on his crutches down the long hall, I saw his face begin to grow pale. By the time he reached the classroom, it was white. When we entered the room, all talking and noise stopped. The children stared at him. The teacher was elaborately kind.

I left, worried. Bobby made it through that day, but that night he came home and bled for three weeks.

Painful as it was, there was no other way but to keep trying. If Bobby were to grow up normally, that meant normal school, despite the fact that normal schools were neither equipped nor disposed to make concessions to his problem. The fact was, they did not want him at all. By law, public schools had to accept him, but it was made very clear to me that they would have preferred it otherwise. Principals were afraid, so afraid . . . of responsibility, of accident reports, of lawsuits, and God knows what else. He was

specifically excluded from all school accident insurance, and we
had to sign papers that we would never sue because of anything
that happened to him on the school grounds, no matter who was
responsible.

Happily, his first teacher in kindergarten was a kindly, experienced, older woman who took Bobby's condition rather more
calmly than did the administration. But at recess, Bobby was sent
to sit in the principal's office, alone.

Yet whether the school administrators were well-meaning or
not, whether they wanted to understand or not, after we had made
our best efforts to bridge the gap and explain, we had to entrust
Bobby to them, we had to expose him to physical hazards and to
psychological injuries that could wound forever. We had no choice.

Before Bobby entered each new school, my routine was the
same. First, I went over the physical layout as minutely as any
Secret Service man checking over a presidential route. Carefully
noting hazard points, I counted the stairs, checking their steepness,
their banisters, calculating the flow up and down at peak hours.
Next, the floors. Would crutches slip? I scrutinized the material
they were made of, the kind of wax used, under both wet and dry
conditions. Then I bought shoes with soles adapted to grip that
kind of floor. I went over Bobby's daily route. How many stairs to
the library? To the lunchroom? I checked the playground. Concrete under the swings was especially frightening. The slides? How
tall, and what was at the bottom? Who would watch him if a
swing hit him in the head or he fell off the slide? Later, when he
was at school, I had to fight to control my vivid imagination.

Physical layout made all the difference to Bobby's being able
to attend any given school. A school with a long, wide hall and
few stairs was the best. Then, with luck and understanding on the
teacher's part, Bobby could go in his wheelchair. But of course
most schools are constructed for healthy children only. No archi-
tect includes the possibility of illness in his designs: doors are not
made wide enough to accommodate a wheelchair, doors to toilets
are difficult to push open. There are no elevators. Generally he
could not eat lunch in the lunchroom because no one would bring
him a tray. In one grade—and I still bless her for it—a teacher
arranged for someone to carry his tray for him and that meant he

could eat with everybody else. Of course, when he was in a wheelchair it was impossible, because he could not get down the stairs . . . so I came to pick him up or he ate alone.

After I had checked the physical layout, I went to see the principal, then the teacher, the librarian, and the physical education teacher. It was very hard for people to understand a problem they could not exactly see—one that could be very serious one day and not serious at all the next—one to which flexibility was the key. They could not cope with a child who had such a variety of problems: one day an arm, the next day a leg, then two legs or two arms, or something else, totally unpredictable. In trying to explain the disease to them, the problem was always the same: How to tell them enough to educate them to possible danger signals, without making them overfearful; how to disarm fear just enough to give confidence, not too much to create overconfidence. It was almost impossible.

Usually, teachers were terribly afraid and overprotective. What was vital was to get them over their initial "Oh, poor little boy" attitude and persuade them to treat him like the others, to punish him when he misbehaved. I tried to emphasize that *nothing* frightening was likely to happen in a normal classroom situation. I tried to suggest to them that they not single Bobby out from the other children, but let him adjust normally to the class. Yet even after these talks I found that, no doubt meaning well, they would still stand in front of the class and make little speeches about "not hitting Bobby," embarrassing him horribly and making it harder for him to make friends. Or, even after I had explained that bleeding to death from a single scratch was a myth and that the real danger was joint bleeding, Bobby would come home to tell me that he had been forbidden to use blunt scissors to cut out and paste with the other children. But he had been turned out onto a cement schoolyard to play unsupervised.

Later, when they got to know him better and saw that he was really just a little boy and was not going to expire suddenly in a pool of blood in front of their eyes, teachers relaxed. But sometimes the damage had already been done.

Every day when he came home from school I would anxiously scan his face for changes; each day I found him slightly different from the way I had left him in the morning. More and more I saw a sad, serious, and thoughtful look coming into his eyes. Alone, he was traversing areas in his soul that I could neither touch nor comfort. And, I wondered, once he had crossed them, how would he emerge? Would he be shy and bitter? Would he be filled with fears?

I still remember vividly one day when I was most troubled by these thoughts. Bobby was seven. Two little neighborhood boys had stopped over. As they came in the front door, suddenly on the other side of the room they saw Bobby in a wheelchair. A look of shock and horror crossed their faces. Bobby noticed it. I saw the change come into his eyes, and he hesitated—but only for a moment. Then as they stood frozen by the door, he cranked up his wheels and rolled across the room at top speed. "Hi, fellas," he said confidently, "what do you guys want to do?" I was terribly proud of him. He had understood, but he was not afraid.

Bobby bled in his joints throughout his early school years; these crucial years of adaptation, of learning to read and write. We fought doggedly to maintain continuity and discipline in his education, but it was extremely difficult. There was never a status quo. He was absent a few days, then in school a few days. He would drop out for a week or two, then abruptly reappear for the next few weeks. In first grade he missed one half of the school year; thereafter he missed at least a third of each school year . . . but never consecutively. Because of these frequent and erratic absences, teachers found it hard to incorporate him into classwork and discussion, and he found it difficult, after weeks at home, to emerge from his own private world and swing into the routine of classroom and classmates.

We had no idea how to deal with these new problems. Perhaps a tutor? We had learned that in our school district the Board of Education regulations entitled a sick child to home teaching. Happily, I hurried to the school to make arrangements, only to find that we were not eligible after all because, on closer examination, the Board of Education regulations rigidly stipulated that a child had to be absent for thirty *consecutive* days. No exceptions. Discouraged but persistent, Bob wrote letter after letter, explaining Bobby's special need. Higher and higher up the ladder of the Board of Education superintendents he went. I followed up with politely nagging phone calls. Weeks passed. We persisted until the bureaucratic red tape was unsnarled—the district would pay for home teaching in our case, after all. But our victory was short-lived. Home teachers could not work out a sustained *home* program because Bobby was in and out of *school*. If they agreed to come every Monday, Wednesday, and Friday, what were they supposed to do when they found that Bobby had gotten well and was back in school on Friday? They wanted a steady job. The result was that we had a series of different teachers, none of them really connecting home and school. When Bobby missed the first months of first grade, he worked with an excellent teacher who taught him to read in two months. But then, when he went back to school, he found himself far ahead of all the other children. So he just sat in class with nothing to do.

(At that, Bobby was very lucky. Because of the erratic nature of their disease, most hemophiliacs in the early school years fall at least a year behind other children their age. They learn to read much later—and sometimes never are able to catch up academically.)

One reason we were so happy when we moved to Irvington was that the public school was next door to our house. There were no streets to cross; Bobby had only to cross a field to get to the school. I could even wheel him there. The halls were wide, the stairs were few. Perfect. But, as it happened, Bobby had another problem besides hemophilia. He was very bright. At that time, this too was a handicap which our public school system had difficulty handling. Slow learners, perhaps. But fast learners? Basically, the entire school program was geared to the "normal" child (whoever he or she may be) of the education manuals. Scattered efforts were made. Bobby was given harder books to read—alone. When in the third grade, he was put in a sixth-grade science class. But there was never any homework. The emphasis was on "group" teaching and classroom activity . . . and he was absent. Today he remembers: "People were well-meaning, but in school I was usually bored in class. I made careless mistakes because I was so bored. I had all this energy and nothing to do with it. I always wanted to learn new things that I didn't understand. I wanted to get on with it, to do something else." At home he was cranky. To my dismay, he sat, wooden, in front of the television set hour after hour. In fourth grade, his handwriting was illegible. He would be excited and happy about a group class project, only to miss it and find that the class was onto something else by the time he got back and his enthusiasm was useless. So he stopped caring. Watching him, I felt desperate and totally ineffective.

Where did he belong? I wondered. Perhaps we were wrong to press him into competing with normal children. The weeks were stretching on; he was becoming more and more handicapped. Were we right to keep exposing him to the disorientation, to the bruising sense of being very different? At Blythedale, where we went several times a week for therapy, Bobby had some friends. And the hospital had a school for its children. Perhaps Blythedale? We tried it for two or three days. Immediately, I saw Bobby's consternation. We had taught him that he was not sick. Now he was being sent to a school where all the children were bedridden. Many years later he confessed to me that "the idea of going to Blythedale scared me. I was lost and disoriented—afraid. It was not my world. It was too dependent, shut away from the outside. I remember how relieved I was when I saw Dr. Engel walking down the hall." But at that time, when he was eight, he could not express in words the apprehension and confusion he felt. He told us in another way—he immediately began to bleed spontaneously in his joints. I thanked the understanding director of Blythedale, and I removed Bobby.

But what was he? Handicapped or normal? Sick or well? He fitted no category. I had studied in France. I knew that the emphasis in French education was on intellect. Somebody told me there was a Lycée Français in New York City. Joy! On a cold bright winter's day I dressed Bobby in his best blue coat and leggings and we went to 95th Street and Fifth Avenue. When we arrived, my practiced eye took in the interior. Steep stairs, but there *was* an elevator. I noticed that the children were highly disciplined and supervised, I could well believe that the work was challenging. I needn't have bothered to consider these matters. When I went to see the director of the school, he agreed with me that Bobby was an exceptionally bright and capable child, but then said coldly: "Madame, no school and no teacher will ever willingly accept your child. And why should we, when we have so many healthy ones on the waiting list?" Mortified, cheeks stinging with embarrassment, we went home.

Would any private school take him? Distance was a problem. The only private school anywhere near us was a boys' school which, at that time, emphasized sports. It was spread over the crest of a high hill. The terrain was uneven and steep. In the Lower School building there were five full flights of stairs. The boys went up and down them constantly for each different class. The lunchroom was across in another building. Nevertheless, I went to talk to the director of admissions, Phil Havens. Phil's wife, Lee, worked as a therapist at Blythedale and, through her, he knew Bobby. Apprehensively, I waited for his reaction to our enrolling Bobby in the fifth grade. He smiled and said, "Bobby is a very bright boy and we want bright boys like him at Hackley." To spare his elbows we bought double sets of books—one to leave at school, one for home. Transportation was a problem—the school was four miles away. Bobby couldn't take the regular school bus and we couldn't drive him; we were both working then. So, straining financially, we hired a driver. Later, New York passed a bill that provides for transportation of handicapped children.

One of the important reasons we wanted Bobby to go to Hackley was that the school had an excellent pool. Doctors and therapists agreed that swimming is a wonderful activity for hemophiliacs, both psychologically helpful and of great benefit for joint rehabilitation. Up to that time, we had no access to a pool. When he took off his brace, Bobby limped badly. I was terrified that he would slip and fall on the slippery concrete around the pool. But it was a risk worth taking, for it allowed him, however irregularly, to exercise, to splash and play with other boys. His leg was bent and so weak that it seemed impossible to think that he would ever be able to swim normally. Yet there was that wisp of hope . . . and Bobby was very determined.

Hackley was a hard proving ground for Bobby. The boys were tightly organized into cliques. They constantly fought and tussled, as normal boys do. They called Bobby names ("Old

Leather Legs" was a favorite). One incident Bobby recalls vividly. "One day when I was away in Lower School assembly the headmaster announced that 'any kid who touches Bobby Massie will get three hours' (punishment classes on Saturday). When I heard that the next day I was livid. The kids used to taunt me, 'We're not allowed to touch you.' Then I would jump on them and beat them up. I hated being different, being considered 'bright' but hands off."

Nevertheless, physically challenging as it was, the academic atmosphere was better. Bobby's handwriting began to improve. The teachers were strict in demanding disciplined work. He had homework that began to absorb his hours and his energy. He began to *care* about being in school—and worry about his absences. There was still the same problem: He would work hard for a test only to miss it. He would spend weeks on a project, and then not be able to hand it in and tell about it. At ten, he was getting too heavy for me to manage and lift in his wheelchair. Bob, who was working at home by then, took over. So that Bobby would not miss exams, Bob would drive him to school and stay there all day, reading and working in the teachers' lounge, jumping up to push him around and to help him up the stairs from class to class. But during long stretches of bleeding, he would still be out of contact. He would get depressed. I would get gloomy.

One day, I saw a telephone company advertisement in a magazine. It extolled the public-spirited phone company which had brought *school* to *home* for one sick child through the miracle of an intercom. Galvanized, I sprang to the telephone. I was passed from one voice to another. No, they all said. The intercom was only for children who were "sick" all the time, or home for a long consecutive period. I insisted. To get rid of me, the anonymous voices finally transferred my call to a higher executive. He was sympathetic. He would see what could be done. The initial charge was high, stretched taut financially as we were, and there was a $44 monthly charge in addition. We would find the money somehow. To me, it seemed like the greatest bargain in the world. An intercom!

Once the decision was made, a team of telephone company repairmen worked with devotion. Technically it was difficult to install such a system at Hackley School. Bobby's classes met in five different classrooms. Patiently, the repairmen worked for weeks, unraveling and sorting out the phone lines to establish a direct communication to our house four miles down the road. (Sometime later, when the system was established and in perfect working order, vandals tore down and cut the intercom at the school. To reconnect them, the repairmen came back and worked all day in a drenching downpour.) Bobby's classmates took turns carrying the intercom from class to class. The teacher would plug it in and presto! not only could Bobby listen to all his classes, but simply by pressing a button he could answer questions!

Thereafter, whenever he was bedridden, he would call the school and ask them to plug in. Then, lying in bed, Bobby attended all his classes, even joining in the horseplay and jokes that went on before classes began.

Chapter 9

In the early years, well-meaning people, hoping to cheer me up, would tell me confidently, "Don't worry, Bob. Science is moving so fast these days that it won't be long before they find something for hemophilia." "Well, maybe so," I used to say; "I hope you're right."

Time passed and hope dwindled. We kept dreaming that "science" would at least come up with something less traumatic than transfusions. The easiest approach, if only it had worked, was through diet and vitamins. From the beginning, we got a lot of advice about what Bobby should eat. A Swiss doctor wrote to Sue's father: "The child needs calcium and potassium and various amino acids in rather strong doses. He should eat cheeses, butter, and wheat germ." Someone recommended bone meal. "Bone meal contains a lot of calcium, and calcium is important to clotting." I found an old medical paper titled "Hemophilia," published in 1932, which stressed a high protein, low carbohydrate diet: "It is definitely established," the author said, "that the absorption of protein food from the intestine is accompanied by an increased coagulability of the blood, so that the clotting time is usually shortened by 30 to 40 per cent for one to four hours after each meal containing protein." Hemophiliacs were urged to eat protein with every meal—to drink "milk, cocoa, or eggnog between meals and at least once during the night."

We were told that vitamins were important, especially Vitamin C and Vitamin K. Vitamin C has an effect on the strength of the capillary walls, and Vitamin K on the liver. Bobby took both. They may have helped, but the number of his bleeding episodes continued to rise.

In time—and not very much time, once his bleeding episodes

became serious and painful—we were ripe for more radical solutions. From time to time, reports of a miraculous new treatment or a spectacular medical breakthrough would race along the hemophilia grapevine. Some seemed to make sense, some were medieval.

One proposal, an injection of cobra venom, we never tried. Egg whites were highly thought of for a while: In England, a hemophiliac treated himself successfully by swallowing egg whites. He told his doctors, who ignored him, so he told his M.P., who stood up in the House of Commons to ask why British medicine had ignored this miracle. Subsequently, egg whites were tested at the hemophilia laboratory at Oxford and found to be valueless.

One hemophiliac was helped by bee stings. In Florida, a fourteen-year-old boy was bleeding in his kidneys. His doctor summoned a beekeeper, who plucked a bee up by its wings and pressed it against the boy's arm. The bee, naturally, stung the boy, and then was pulled away, leaving its stinger buried in the boy's arm. The procedure was repeated fourteen or fifteen times until the boy's arms and legs were studded with imbedded stingers. The next day, according to a now-yellowed newspaper clipping from the *St. Petersburg Times* dated May 19, 1957, the boy's bleeding stopped.

The folder in which this clipping reposes is filled with others:

—Under a headline titled "Fatty Diet Linked to Blood Clotting," *The New York Times* (March 26, 1960) announced that dogs at the Sloan-Kettering Institute fed on high fat diets had more difficulty dissolving blood clots than normal dogs on normal diets. (The motive of this research was to find ways to *prevent* blood clotting, the opposite side of the coin from hemophilia. Doctors interested in trying to prevent heart attacks caused by thrombosis were working to prevent rather than to cause blood coagulation. But everything was grist for my files.)

—Another *Times* clipping, dated May 11, 1964, announces "Tests Find Smoking Quickens Clotting." Here too clotting was the villain, not the hero. The announcement was made by the American Cancer Society, which hoped to discourage smoking; they suspected it led to thrombosis. Nevertheless, I was interested in their test, in which eighteen students inhaled cigarette smoke deeply for five minutes. Immediately afterward blood samples were taken and it was found that their platelet stickiness was 84.4 per cent higher than before they began to puff.

—Finally, there is a clipping that has no direct bearing on hemophilia, but which I kept because it backs up my belief that modern medicine is only scratching the surface. It is a story from *Time* (June 6, 1960), titled "Blood and the Moon." It reported the findings of a doctor in Florida that his patients bled more severely when the moon was full. . . .

Before we scoffingly dismiss all "miracle treatments" as hopelessly unscientific, let me add an opinion given me twelve years ago by Dr. Clarence Merskey, a hematologist then at Albert Einstein Hospital in the Bronx.

"The interesting thing," Dr. Merskey said, "is that every bizarre cure works for the man who invented it. I begin to believe they work *because* these men have faith in them. One Friday night one of my patients called me excitedly and said that he had found a cure for hemophilia: eating molasses. I discouraged him, saying that many other people had come up with private 'cures' and that all of them had eventually been found wanting, but that if he insisted, he could come in on Monday morning and I would run a test. Naturally, he came in on Saturday night with a very badly swollen knee. I am convinced that he bled because I had destroyed his faith."

There was one "miracle treatment" that we did try, and so did most of the other hemophilia families we know. Exactly why it worked in some cases and not in others is still unknown.

The cure was peanuts.

I was sitting in my office at *Newsweek* one Sunday morning in 1959, helping to close the magazine, when I picked up the Sunday *New York Times*. On the front page, leaping up at me, was a three-column headline: "Peanut Said to Cure Hemophilia." My head began to spin. This was not the hemophilia grapevine; this was *The New York Times*. I began to read. "The lowly peanut," the story began, "may become the conqueror of the disease of kings." The story went on to describe the experience of Dr. H. Bruce Boudreaux, a zoologist at Louisiana State University, who happened to be a Factor IX hemophiliac. Dr. Boudreaux had awakened one morning to discover that his knee, which had been swelling up when he went to bed the night before, was now much better; for some reason, while he slept, the bleeding had stopped. Very surprised—this kind of thing had never happened before—he tried to recollect the previous evening. He remembered that he had eaten an abnormally large number of roasted peanuts.

Thereafter, whenever he felt himself starting to bleed, Dr. Boudreaux ate peanuts. Up to the time the *Times* story appeared, he had been eating peanuts for two years and he had been giving a peanut extract flour which he had made to other hemophiliacs. One of his volunteers, a man bleeding from the kidneys, had gone right on bleeding through twelve transfusions. Then he took some of Dr. Boudreaux's peanut extract and his bleeding stopped. Dr. Boudreaux emphasized that he had no laboratory evidence that peanuts had this effect; he was simply reporting results.

I was excited. It seemed ridiculous: the peanut. But why not? Who knew what the eventual solution would be?

For days, the Hemophilia Foundation was besieged by telephone calls from hemophilia families. What kind of peanuts should they eat? How many? At what times of day? Trying to restore order, the foundation issued a statement that emphasized that only a very small number of hemophiliacs had been involved, that laboratory data was lacking, and that, as they put it, "much further work is necessary. . . ."

Nevertheless, like everyone else, we set about trying to lay hands on whatever it was that Dr. Boudreaux was eating. We telephoned him and he gave us his formula for preparing peanut extract flour. Sue's father took the formula to a friend who had a chemical factory in Philadelphia (he made ink). The friend declined, citing the food and drug laws, which prohibited unlicensed production of food or drug products for individual consumption. We looked for peanut flour in specialty food stores and diet shops. The trail led to the Brookhaven National Laboratory, to the Department of Nutrition at Cornell, to Tuskegee Institute.

Eventually, I learned that UNICEF was exporting American peanut flour as a protein source for undernourished children overseas. I wrote to UNICEF and it was arranged that I could purchase a fifty-pound bag from their regular supplier in Georgia. Whether it contained what Boudreaux's extract contained we had no idea. I hefted the sack into the garage, scooped out a pound or two, and brought it into the kitchen. Sue and I both regarded it with distaste.

But our distaste was nothing compared to Bobby's. He refused to swallow it. We tried blending it with all kinds of flavors. Sue made peanut cakes and peanut milkshakes. Bobby, who was three years old, closed his little mouth like an iron gate. What little he did manage to get down, didn't stay. It wasn't worth it; we gave up.

That was the end of the peanut story for us, but not for everyone. Naturally, along with everything else he was doing, Dr. Bill Bisordi got involved. Wanting to see for himself how peanuts worked, he tried them out on five of his hemophiliacs: his two sons, two other teen-agers, and a six-year-old. The problem with all the boys, as it was with Bobby, was getting the stuff down. The six-year-old, for his weight, needed two heaping tablespoonfuls a day; somehow he managed to swallow this. But the bigger boys needed half a pound. "They tried it in everything," Bill laughed. "Cakes, milkshakes, you name it. They couldn't take it. They said they'd rather have hemophilia."

Bill refused to give up. He persuaded a New Jersey drug firm to compress peanut flour into pills, which were easier to swallow, and then he persuaded the boys to eat seventy-five of these pills a day, twenty-five with each meal. Grumbling, the boys persevered for three months, and at the end both they and Bill were convinced that the pills had helped. But not enough to continue. Although Bill published the results in the British medical journal *Lancet*, neither he nor his patients had the will power to keep going. Except the six-year-old. "Jimmy had been having a bad time," Bill remembered. "On peanut flour, things got a lot better. He passed seven or eight months at a time without a transfusion. His parents needed all the help they could get; Jimmy's only sister was a severe diabetic. But they moved away and I've lost track of what happened."

Last summer, cleaning out his office, Bill found a large, round, unmarked cardboard drum. Opening it, he found that it was peanut flour which had been sitting there for more than ten years. He began to wonder if there wasn't some way he could use it. Perhaps as a breakfast cereal. . . . "You know, the stuff is 63 per cent protein. . . ."

When Bobby started going to school, we began to notice that every year there were certain months when he would bleed more often than other months. One of these bad periods was late April–early May, another was September. We had no idea what caused them (was it the weather or the change of season?), but as the pattern continued, year after year, we came to expect them and to call them "cycles."

We also noticed that there were specific periods and places in which Bobby did *not* bleed. He didn't bleed often in July and August; this was when we were in Maine. Again, we had no idea why this was so. We thought it might be the fresh sea air, the pine trees, the iodine in the seaweed that covered our rocks.

As time passed, we began to realize that we could make even finer distinctions in the timing of Bobby's problems. He tended to bleed when he was emotionally upset, angry, or frustrated. And he often bled when he was impatiently, and perhaps apprehensively, awaiting an important event: something that he feared, like an exam; or something that he wanted passionately to do, like a rare outing or a vacation trip. Whenever possible, we learned to keep things like this secret from him until the last moment.

Finally, we realized that we (Sue, especially) could tell in advance when Bobby was going to bleed. He would become pale, dark circles would shadow his eyes, and he would become cranky, irritable, and whiny. The next day, he would begin to bleed.

Eventually, trying to make sense out of what we were witnessing, knowing nothing about the possible physiological explanations, we reached some tentative, pragmatic conclusions: Bobby bled more often when he was anxious and unhappy. He did not bleed as much when he was happy. This would explain his troubles in September. School was starting. He had a new teacher to confront and convince about himself and his disease, new classmates, a whole new adjustment to make. In effect, he had to find his way all over again. In April and May, exams were coming; so was the summer with its trips and excitement—if he was well enough to go. Once in Maine in July and August, however, he was with his friends, who accepted him despite his braces, despite his days in bed. And although he was far more active in Maine, hopping from rock to rock, tussling with his friend Davey, he bled far less often.

But was this medically possible? Were there links of this kind between mind and body? Could Bobby's state of mind, his mood, actually affect the number and severity of his bleedings?

No one doubts that mental distress can cause physical symptoms; headaches, ulcers, and heart attacks are all around us. But what fascinated researchers from both a hematological and psychiatric viewpoint, and what was only dimly understood ten years ago, was the nature of the relationship between how a hemophiliac looked out at the world and how often and badly he bled.

At least three major factors are involved in bleeding. The first is the blood itself; the second is the blood vessel through which the blood is flowing (or, when torn, from which the blood is escaping); the third is the blood pressure, created by the heart, which keeps the fluid in circulation.

It is fairly certain that what happens in the mind does not affect the nature or composition of the blood itself. We made numerous tests on Bobby's blood at all parts of his cycles: when he was in a period of bad bleeding and when he seemed to have a period of remission; when he was happy and when he was sad. The results were negative. No one could find any evidence of change in levels of his AHF which related to his mood.

There was evidence, however, that what is happening in the mind, or to the mind, can affect both blood pressure and the strength of blood vessel walls. Anger, anxiety, resentment, and embarrassment cause an increase in blood pressure, forcing an increased blood flow through the smallest blood vessels. In addition, there is evidence that overwrought emotions can adversely affect the strength and integrity of the capillary walls. As these tend to become more fragile and break down under stress, while at the same time they are attempting to handle an increased flow of blood, the likelihood of bleeding becomes greater.

There is an opposite side to this proposition: a decrease in emotional stress has a beneficial effect on bleeding. As calm and a sense of well-being return to a patient, his capillary blood flow will decline and the strength of his vascular wall increase.

Now, ten years later, there is no longer any doubt of the existence of this mind-body relationship in hemophilia. The deeper causes and mechanisms are still unknown, but research in this area is intensive. The results, when they come, will certainly have implications reaching far beyond hemophilia. All of us would like to know why it is that happy people are usually healthier people.

The most famous case of the treatment of hemophilia through the power of the mind is the story of Gregory Rasputin and the young Russian Tsarevich Alexis. I have told this story before in *Nicholas and Alexandra*, where my emphasis was on its significance in the history of the fall of the Russian monarchy. I am retelling it here in outline because it is also an important medical story, suggesting what is possible in this shadowy area of mind and body.

About the Tsarevich, the facts are clear. Born in 1904, the only son of Tsar Nicholas II, Alexis inherited his hemophilia from his mother, the German Princess Alix of Hesse, who at her marriage became the Empress Alexandra. Tracing backward, Alexandra inherited the defective gene from her mother, Princess Alice of England, who, in turn, had inherited it from *her* mother, Queen Victoria.

Alexis' hemophilia first revealed itself at the age of six weeks, when he began to bleed from a still-unhealed wound at the navel. As a toddler, learning to stand and walk, tumbling and falling, he had the usual hemophiliac swellings and blue bruises. At three and a half, he stumbled and hit his forehead, causing a huge swelling that closed both eyes. He grew into a handsome, active boy, wanting to ride a pony and a bicycle and to play with other boys. His family tried to protect him; two sailors were assigned to watch him constantly to keep him away from physical danger.

Relatively speaking, Alexis was a mild hemophiliac. His hemophilia was much less severe than Bobby's, for example, and he had strikingly fewer bleeding episodes. The difference was that once the Tsarevich began to bleed, nothing could stop the hemorrhage. The best doctors in Russia and Europe could prescribe nothing except rest, ice, and immobilization.

A devout convert to the Russian Orthodox Church, Alexandra placed her hope in prayer. Alone on her knees for hours, she begged from God the miracle that medicine denied. It was at this moment, seemingly as an answer to the help she had implored, that Gregory Rasputin appeared.

The facts about Rasputin are far from clear, but this is the silhouette:

He was born about 1872 in a Siberian village. He grew to manhood there, chased—and caught—peasant girls, married, fathered three children, and became a farmer. One day, while plowing, he saw a vision and set out to walk the two thousand miles to the monastery of Mount Athos in Greece. At the end of two years, when he returned to his village, he carried an aura of mystery and holiness.

He became a healer. He began to pray at the beds of sick people, larding his language heavily with biblical quotes and old Russian proverbs. Peasants came to him, bringing not only their sick wives and children but their sick horses and cows as well.

When Rasputin began to travel again, his reputation preceded him. It was said that he was a holy man, a sinner who had repented and had thereby been blessed with powers of healing. He arrived in St. Petersburg and was brought before a curious group of bishops and priests.

Struck by his burning eyes and fluent tongue, and the apparent fervor of his faith, they gave Rasputin their endorsement. They thought him a *starets*, a peasant holy man, whom the church could use. For his part, Rasputin took his acceptance as no more than normal; he refused to humble himself and treated the dignitaries with spontaneous good humor.

It was the same when he moved into society drawing rooms. And when he was first called to the Alexander Palace to meet the Tsar and the Empress. From the beginning, Rasputin's manner was wholly self-confident; this, along with the power of his eyes, was crucial to his later success. But to Alexandra, the mother of a hemophiliac, Rasputin was the answer to her prayers, a man from God.

When Alexis was bleeding, the Empress sent a carriage or a motorcar to bring Rasputin to the palace. He would come up the back stairs to avoid attention. Entering Alexis' second-floor bedroom, he would take the white-faced Empress by the hand and murmur encouraging words. Then, waving the anguished parents and worried doctors to the other side of the room, he would approach the bed.

What was it, exactly, that Rasputin did for Alexis? The legend is that Rasputin used his extraordinary eyes to hypnotize the Tsarevich and then, with the boy in a hypnotic trance, suggested that the bleeding would stop. Medically, it could not have been that simple; hypnosis alone could not suddenly stop a severe hemorrhage. Nevertheless, we now know that hypnosis, properly used, can play a part in controlling hemophilic bleeding.

But if it is medically possible that Rasputin could have helped the Tsarevich by using hypnosis, inducing the contraction of the blood vessels and thus slowing the boy's bleeding, it is far from historically certain that he did so. There is evidence from that period to suggest that Rasputin did not even know the technique of classic hypnosis. Rasputin's daughter, Maria, who is still living today, vehemently denies that her father ever practiced hypnosis.

Nevertheless, in the light of what we now know about the relationship of mind and body, the question of whether or not Rasputin actually hypnotized the Tsarevich becomes a matter of degree. If, technically, it was not actual hypnosis that he practiced, it was nevertheless a strong power of suggestion. When Rasputin used this power on Alexis, distracting him, weaving stories, filling a darkened room with his commanding voice, he did in effect cast a spell over a boy overwhelmed with pain. The calm and well-being produced by the powerful flow of reassuring language must have produced a dramatic emotional change in the Tsarevich. And the change affected his body. As the pain receded from the center of his consciousness, the exhausted child dropped off to sleep, the bleeding slowed and eventually stopped.

The most extraordinary moment in the three-cornered relationship among Alexandra, Alexis, and Rasputin occurred when Rasputin helped to save Alexis' life although he and the boy were a thousand miles apart. This happened at Spala, the Imperial hunting lodge in the forest of eastern Poland in the autumn of 1912. Jumping into a rowboat, Alexis had fallen against an oarlock and injured his groin. After two weeks of apparently successful convalescence, he began to bleed. The doctors could do nothing and the bleeding grew worse. For eleven days, the boy lay huddled on his side, semi-conscious, screaming in pain. Alexandra never left him; she slept in a chair beside his bed.

When death seemed near and the last sacrament had been given, the Empress telegraphed Rasputin in his village beyond the Urals. Rasputin immediately cabled back: "God has seen your tears and heard your prayers. Do not grieve. The Little One will not die. Do not allow the doctors to bother him too much."

The next morning, Alexandra came downstairs smiling. "The doctors notice no improvement yet," she said to her husband, "but I am not a bit anxious myself now. During the night I received a telegram from Father Gregory and he has reassured me completely."

A day later, the hemorrhage stopped.

Although Alexis' doctor declared that "the recovery is wholly inexplicable from a medical point of view," and Alexandra was convinced that God, through Rasputin, had given her a miracle, there are several possible medical explanations of what happened. After a greatly prolonged period of time, hemophiliac bleeding may stop of its own accord. The great mass of blood itself crowding into the surrounding tissue may cause a back pressure on the injured blood vessel which will cause the wound to close. Similarly, the loss of a substantial amount of blood from the circulatory system can produce shock and fainting, accompanied by a general loss of blood pressure and a consequent slowing of the hemorrhage. After eleven days of bleeding without death, both of these factors may have played a part.

In addition, if his advice was followed, Rasputin's telegram must have had one beneficial effect on Alexis. The command "Do not allow the doctors to bother him too much" was excellent medical advice. It was Lee Engel who pointed this out to me one night in Irvington. He was giving Bobby a transfusion and together he and Sue and I were puzzling over the mystery of Spala. "Listen, Bob," he said, "if the boy had four doctors hovering anxiously over his bed, taking his temperature, probing his leg and groin, that was the worst possible thing for him. Even if a clot did form, it would have been very fragile, and one of these doctors' examinations could easily have dislodged it. If Rasputin's telegram gave Alexandra courage to tell the doctors to leave the boy alone, the effect could only have been good."

Finally, there is another possibility, directly related to Rasputin's telegram. If the hemophiliac patient bleeds more profusely under a condition of emotional stress, then anything that decreases that stress should have an effect on the bleeding. When Rasputin's telegram arrived at Spala, Alexandra was the only person with whom the semiconscious Alexis had any emotional communication. She, quite naturally, after eleven days of torment, was in a state of exhaustion and hysteria. To the extent that he had any contact with the outside world, Alexis must have felt and been adversely affected by her frantic terror. If so, then the sudden overwhelming change in his mother's emotional state produced by Rasputin's telegram must also have affected Alexis. Alone, the new aura of calm probably could not have stopped the hemorrhage. But together with the lowered blood pressure in the veins, back pressure on the wound, and the slow formation of clots, it must have helped.

Even today, more than sixty years later, this is about as far as speculation can go. But as we learn more, we shall perhaps understand better this mysterious medical story that had such fateful historical implications.

Many have told and many have heard the story of Rasputin. But not many have heard it at a point so distant from Russia or have made the story so important in their own lives as a South American boy named Oscar Lucas.

Oscar was born in 1932 in the town of Resistencia, in northern Argentina. As a boy working in his father's butcher shop, he dreamed of becoming a doctor. But there came a day when his father said to him, "I am sorry, my son, but your sister also wants an education and there is only enough money to educate one. Without money, she will have too hard a time, so I am giving the money to her. But do not give up your ambition. You are a man and you can work to educate yourself."

And so, a man at the age of fourteen, Oscar left home to go to Buenos Aires, three hundred miles to the south, to get an education. It took twelve long years of work by day and school at night. He changed his goal somewhat; the years and the cost of becoming an M.D. were simply too much. But in 1958, at the age of twenty-six, he graduated with a degree in dentistry from the University of Buenos Aires.

His graduation, like his final examination, was held in bed. Three months earlier, Oscar had been riding on the back of a friend's motorcycle down a busy street. The motorcycle was caught between a car and a bus. The friend was unhurt, but Oscar's leg was so badly crushed that it had to be amputated. Today he walks many city blocks on his artificial leg, waving away friends who try to persuade him to ride. "I am in charge," he says. "Not the leg."

While he was in dental school Oscar became interested in hemorrhagic problems in dentistry. He went to see Dr. Alfredo Pavlovsky, director of the Hematological Center at the University of Buenos Aires, and the greatest expert on hemophilia in South America. Dr. Pavlovsky gave Oscar a book containing all the papers presented at a world hemophilia symposium in New York in 1956. It was in English and Oscar perfected his English in order to read it. He was especially intrigued by the book's last paragraph, in which Dr. Tocantins of Philadelphia (the friend of Sue's father who had diagnosed Bobby) declared that he would like to know more about the relationship between "emotional stress and clotting time. . . . We all remember what is almost folklore on this subject —that Rasputin was able to stop the bleeding in the Tsarevich by hypnotizing him. As far as I know, there is no scientific account of this matter."

On graduation, Oscar was awarded a scholarship from the University of Buenos Aires for study anywhere in the United States. Pavlovsky suggested that he go to Philadelphia to work in the hemophilia group gathered around Dr. Tocantins.

Oscar had been in Philadelphia only a few months when he found himself facing a crisis. "I had to do a very difficult tooth extraction in a hemophiliac patient. The man, who was forty, was very emotional. He had a tremendous amount of anxiety about bleeding. He didn't want us to do it. I went home very depressed. I was lying on my bed, wondering how we could make him more confident and more cooperative. All of a sudden, my mind flashed to what Dr. Tocantins had written about Rasputin and hypnosis. The next morning, I went to see Dr. Tocantins. 'Oscar,' he said, 'let's try it.' "

By 1962, Oscar had extracted forty-three teeth from hemophiliacs under hypnosis, without using a single transfusion of plasma or plasma fraction. His procedure, which involved careful surgical technique, a protective splint for the jaw, and packing the socket with an absorbable hemostatic material, was described in a paper published in November 1962 by the *Journal of Oral Surgery.*

One night in 1963 he came to New York to lecture at Mount Sinai Hospital on his technique. The room was crowded; fifty or sixty dentists, hematologists, residents, and nurses were there to watch and listen. The mood was deeply skeptical, and before the lecture little smiles and low chuckles cropped up around the room.

Oscar began to speak, using colored slides to illustrate every step. He began by describing and showing on the screen some examples of the generally poor state of the average hemophiliac's teeth. Afraid to brush them for fear of causing the gums to bleed, he neglects them. They decay, and inevitably they reach a state in which a normal dentist dealing with a normal patient would automatically recommend extraction. This terrifies the hemophiliac— and the dentist. Eventually, when something has to be done, a major operation is scheduled, with weeks in the hospital and dozens of units of plasma transfused before, during, and after the operation.

Oscar avoided all this trauma, cost, and time by using hypnosis. "An emotionally tranquil patient has less bleeding than one emotionally distressed," he declared. But Oscar did not induce hypnosis and extract teeth on a casual, production-line basis. "On the patient's first visit, I explain in detail the purpose of hypnosis," he said. "I explain how it will be induced, what will happen while he is under hypnosis, and how he will be awakened. We talk, I answer his questions and try to allay his fears. Sometimes it takes several of these sessions to make him calm and receptive."

On the day of the extraction, the patient is hypnotized—there on Oscar's slide was a man with his eyes closed and his mouth open —and then Oscar suggests that the mouth is free of saliva. A series of slides from different angles showed a dry mouth. Next, in an extraordinary manner, the chosen area is anesthetized and freed from pain. Using a sharp dental prong, Oscar touches the back of the patient's hand, telling him that each touch is an injection into the hand of a powerful anesthetic. The patient is then told that now the hand is numb. Then Oscar tells the patient to raise his "numb" hand to his face and to touch that part of the face where the extraction is to be performed—on the screen the man's hand was on his jaw. At this point, Oscar suggests that all the anesthesia is transferred from hand to face. Then, touching the affected area with his sharp probe, Oscar demonstrates to his hypnotized patient that he cannot feel anything there. With some patients, to suppress bleeding, Oscar suggests that the area from which the tooth is to be drawn is ice cold. In response, the blood vessels constrict—we could see on the screen that the jaw had blanched white. Sometimes, to suppress anxiety further, Oscar asks patients to recall pleasurable experiences. One patient enjoyed himself hugely during surgery by returning himself to a baseball park for the climactic inning of a crucial game.

The lecture was impressive; the mood had shifted from skepticism to interest and a kind of tentative respect. But then an antagonist, a leading Mount Sinai dentist, got up to protest. "There is nothing very remarkable about Dr. Lucas' work," he announced. "Here at Mount Sinai we do the same kind of work without all this hocus-pocus about hypnotism." The dentist had prepared his protest in advance, and at this point he dramatically wheeled in a hemophiliac patient from whom he had just extracted a tooth. We all craned forward to look at the man, whose head was wrapped in bandages and whose face was barely visible. "Now," said the dentist, "Mr. Smith here has just had a tooth extracted without *any* transfusions *and* without hypnosis. We are able to do this solely by careful surgical technique."

Suddenly, there was movement. The patient, sitting in his wheelchair, was trying through his swathe of bandages to speak. "No, no, Doctor," he mumbled. "I had three transfusions yesterday and two today and . . ."

With the patient removed from the room, Dr. Martin Rosenthal, the distinguished Mount Sinai hematologist and medical director of the Hemophilia Foundation, stood up and ended the meeting. "I think we at Mount Sinai should be doing what Dr. Lucas is doing," he said. "His way apparently works and ours obviously doesn't."

Still only forty-two, Oscar is no longer a maverick. Now he is a professor at the University of Oregon Dental School, and he is An Authority. He has published numerous papers, and no world hemophilia symposium is complete without his report on his latest work. He is still handsome, still charming—and this year, twenty-nine years after he left Resistencia and seventeen years after leaving Argentina, Oscar Lucas is going home.

"I do not want to wait until I am too old. I have bought a hundred and forty acres in the town where I was born. I will raise grapefruit and have horses—perhaps someday you will send Susanna to my farm to ride. Maybe I will marry because I love women and I love children. No, I will not give up dentistry completely. I want to take back what I have learned to be useful to my own people. But I will go slowly. I want to enjoy life now."

At home, Oscar will again be living near his sister. "She is a wonderful woman. She is married and has two children and has become a wonderful lawyer. She is an Argentine congresswoman and is the vice-president of the Chamber of Deputies of our state. I am very, very proud of her. *She* has done a wonderful thing with her life."

There was never doubt in our minds that Bobby's bleeding cycles and many of his specific bleeding episodes were related to his mood. Bobby's hematologist, Dr. Margaret Hilgartner of New York Hospital, agreed. Like many other doctors, she had observed the same seasonal patterns in other hemophiliacs—a peak in April and another rise during September. Significantly, she also found that preschool children did not have these peaks and valleys. Dr. Hilgartner had even pinpointed a day of the week—Tuesday— when hemophiliacs seemed most likely to bleed. She suggested that this was because boys have more physical activity on weekends and bleedings started on Sunday would be serious by Tuesday morning. But she also felt that the fact that Tuesday was clinic day at New

York Hospital was important: the patient's anxiety would rise, creating stress, and therefore, possibly, initiating bleeding.

Dr. Hilgartner's observations and all of our own random, unscientific conclusions drawn from Bobby's daily life were confirmed—for me, at least—during a visit to Cleveland in February 1966. I was there writing an article on Dr. Benjamin Spock. On the staff of Case Western Reserve Medical School, where Dr. Spock was a professor, there were two young psychiatrists, David Agle and Ake Mattson, who were fascinated by the question of the mind-body relationship in hemophilia. After keeping exhaustive records and doing extensive interviewing of their patients and the patients' families, they were about to publish the first of a series of important papers directly linking hemophilic bleeding to psychological and social factors.

As we talked, I kept saying, "Yes, yes, exactly. That's exactly what happened to us." They had amassed clinical evidence to show that spontaneous bleeding could be triggered by emotionally upsetting situations, either actual or anticipated. They found that a stable, self-confident hemophiliac usually bled less. In their view, the worst environment for a hemophiliac boy was being placed in the exclusive care of a dominant, overprotective mother, who would try to seal her son off from life and the world. Frustrated, wholly dependent both physically and emotionally, bitterly resentful of this dependency, this child was not only certain to become a psychological cripple—he was also likely to bleed more often.

For me, the most dramatic part of their research was their finding that if a hemophiliac could break free from dependency and change his outlook and pattern of life in the direction of more independence, his hemophilia was likely to improve. They gave me the example of a man, totally dominated by his mother, who had had five hundred transfusions before the age of fifteen. Then he left his family to live with his grandmother in another town. Here, very much on his own, he plunged into high school activities, had girl friends, and bought a motor scooter—and bled less often. He graduated with honors, went to college, married, has three children and an executive job.

David Agle and Ake Mattson still do not know the physiological reasons for this mysterious change. "We don't think the cause is in the blood," said David. "There is no significant change in AHF levels and we are fairly sure that emotional factors are not affecting the strength or permanence of clots once they are formed. No, we think it must be the blood vessels. Oscar Lucas' work shows that under hypnosis an impulse from the central nervous system can command specific blood vessels to retract. We think that this must be true also in a more general emotional context. Somehow, an angry, depressed, frustrated hemophiliac is related to a weakened, dilated capillary blood vessel structure. Through these weakened, dilated capillary walls, blood tends to leak. In a happy, brisk, confident individual, the capillary wall structure tends to be stronger, the blood is sealed in, and the patient does not bleed."

Watching me scribble notes as he talked, David Agle looked at me thoughtfully and said, "The truth is that no one has proven how this works. No one knows. There is still so much we don't know about the working of the human body."

The episode in Bobby's life involving the effect of the mind on the body that was most dramatic involved the folk singers Peter, Paul, and Mary, whom we had come to know. One night, they were with us in Irvington. Near midnight, Bobby woke up with a sore right knee. Sue went up to see him. It was so late that she hesitated to call Dr. Engel; perhaps Bobby could make it until morning.

Sue came downstairs, worried, trying to compose her face. The rest of us were talking and didn't notice, but Peter Yarrow approached and asked quietly, "How is he?" Mechanically she replied, "All right." He pressed her and learned that it wasn't really all right. "Do you have a guitar?" he asked.

Sitting in Bobby's wheelchair in the darkened bedroom, Peter began to play and sing his soft and lovely songs. He sang about the melancholy Freight Train, the unusual Stewball, the immortal Puff. Bobby fell asleep and Peter tiptoed out. Bobby slept through the night.

The next morning he rolled briskly into our room in his wheelchair. "I don't know what happened," he said. "I listened to him play and the pain went away and I went to sleep."

Chapter 10

I have been going to one island off the coast of Maine since I was nine years old. For twenty years I went there every summer. Deer Isle is tightly interwoven with my personality.

My father had found a remote corner of Deer Isle and fallen in love with it. The wild, unspoiled forests reminded him of his native Switzerland. When he bought our point of land, it was part of a large tract that belonged to the widow of a Maine sea captain. Buying it was difficult for him; we had very little money. It was strange for the island too; ours was the first piece of land in that part of the island to have changed hands in twenty-five years, the first ever to have been sold to a stranger.

The trip to Maine was very long before the days of super-highways. It used to take us three days on the road from Philadelphia. And when we got there, we lived in a log cabin that had been built fifty years before by Swedish lumberjacks who had lumbered the tall, straight spruce trees on our point. We were alone; the nearest village was eight miles away. We had no running water, no electricity. One of my jobs was to clean the chimneys of the kerosene lamps every day. We brought our water in large cans from a well ten miles away. We learned to appreciate water. When it rained we collected rain water in barrels. (Nothing is better for washing the hair.) The roof leaked badly. When it rained, we heard a musical concert of ping, pong, ping in the twenty-six kettles and pans we had placed strategically around the cabin to catch the leaks. But, curled up under four blankets beneath the low, sloping roof, listening to the rain, it was the most secure feeling I have ever known.

Morning and evening we brought in the wood. The old, black

wood-burning stove gave off a sort of comforting fragrance that made all the meals taste better than any I have ever had since. My sister and I had no other children to play with, so I packed lobsters, went sardining with the fishermen, learned to clean cod and flounder and keep my footing in a rocking lobster boat while we hauled traps. One summer I helped to pull in herring nets, and salted the slithery, silver bushels of fish in the hold all the way to Southwest Harbor.

In the comforting fogs and dark forests I roamed alone, picking wild flowers, gathering shells and starfish, making balsam needle pillows for my Christmas presents. We kept our stale bread and fed the seagulls who flew around us by the hundreds and learned to take the crusts from our hands.

It was one of the strict Swiss family rules in our house that we had to gather a quart of berries before we were free to play. I grew to love those moments of total solitude. Out on my own, deep in the forest, gingerly stepping on the piles of brush on which the wild raspberries grew, sometimes sinking through up to my waist, I would hang my berry bucket on a branch, pick with both hands, fill my mouth with small, savage, fragrant berries, and share the flowers and the sun with the bees that buzzed around me. The trees creaked in the wind like the masts of ships. Later, in the cabin, the sweet perfumed juice would drip, drip, into the jam kettles as we made jelly for the winter.

We made moss gardens, collected plants and driftwood. I would sit for hours in a makeshift tree house nestled in a great fir that was hoary with Spanish moss, contemplating the horizon, spinning dreams of pirates. Captain Kidd had sailed these waters, and year after year we went off digging, hoping to find his treasure. We ended up finding Indian clam heaps and an arrowhead or two, but the magic hope stayed with us.

In weeks of fog I would curl up in a corner of the cabin and read, hardly lifting my eyes except to eat. I devoured books, first fairy tales, then great sagas, then Dostoevsky and Tolstoy. Mysterious strangers on boats were often blown into our cove by winds and fog, and we would take them in, feed them, play cards and weave tales until the fog lifted and they sailed away.

I learned to know the forest's and the beach's most intimate changes. I knew where to find the best mussels, the juiciest clams. Like an Indian, I could read the signs of weather and wind, growth and death. I knew the seasons and secret places of blueberries, of raspberries, of the tiny lingonberries that grow under the firs; of the fat blackberries that ripen in the warm sun at the end of August, when the mornings are already sharp with the smell of autumn.

My father taught us as children the varieties of tasty mushrooms that sprouted like gold under the fir branches after the rain. Crawling on my stomach, rain dripping down my back, Swiss Army knife in hand, with a basket lined with moss, I would uncover the fertile spots and come back sometimes with two pounds of mushrooms in less than an hour. My mother would simmer these tasty morsels in butter and wine. If I was lucky, or the season was right, I would find the regal bolet, king of mushrooms, all toasty brown and white. My mother would cook these in butter and sour cream, Russian style, and then, warmed with wine, she would often be inspired to tell again the great tales of her years in Russia. We children never tired of these stories— ballerinas decked in diamonds, pulled in sleighs by dashing admirers who wore cloaks lined in sable!

At night, the sky blazed with stars. There were so many, and they were so bright! The Milky Way spread like a great river of diamonds, and I would lie for hours on the sand of the beach, the sky a huge perfect cup over me, and lose myself in finding the constellations. All summer there was nothing to do, and there was everything.

Perhaps I linger too long over these memories, but when I think back over all these years, I know that this intimate contact with nature was a reservoir from which I drew strength when times were most difficult. In later years, often desperate and sad, I used to go back to Maine, for however short a time, just to touch the earth. For I had faith in that place. In our family we believed that the very air, that air perfumed with the salt of the sea and the smell of the firs, had magical, curing properties. One of my sisters was fragile in childhood and often ill, with unexplained low fevers and aching joints. After a summer in Maine, she would come back strong and brown.

Grappling with the unknown mysteries of Bobby's disease, dismayed by the bewilderment and helplessness of doctors, secretly in my heart I believed that somehow Maine would help.

It was a great risk. The coast was jagged rocks; a fall on any one of them could have been very serious. On the island there was only a country doctor. The nearest small hospital was almost an hour away over country roads that were sometimes hazardous and closed by fog. There were no supplies of fresh-frozen plasma nearer than Boston, more than five hours away by car.

But we decided to risk it, and we went there every year of Bobby's childhood. And, mysteriously, he *was* better; no matter how sick he had been through the year, he had fewer transfusions there. Neither we nor Dr. Engel ever understood why.

Bobby and Susy loved it there (Susy called it "Happiness Land"). Every year, as the time approached to leave, they would count the days, the hours, the minutes. They would cheer as we crossed the final bridge that linked the mainland to the island.

Bobby had chores, even when he was very young. He stood on a stool and pumped water, he brought in wood, he helped uncover the ice all covered with sawdust in the icehouse. Then he and his sister would roll over and over in the soft shavings, giggling.

Providentially, during those summers in Maine, when Bobby was growing ever more aware of his handicaps, when he was struggling with the ravages of his disease and forming his self-image, God provided him with friends—strong men of courage and heart.

The rough fishermen, friends of my youth, were not over-sentimental. It was somehow not difficult to explain to them. They accepted Bobby's problem as another act of a capricious Nature— a Nature they lived with and whose power they did not question. What had struck Bobby was the bolt of lightning that singles out one tree and not another, the wind that suddenly comes up from no one knows where, or the calamity when one fisherman and not another accidentally falls off his boat and sinks to the bottom like a stone in his black rubber boots. (The lobster fishermen still venture far out to sea in the roughest weather although most of them cannot swim.) These things happened, and others, and life went on.

One fisherman said to me, "Sue, it's not *if* it happens, but who it is going to happen to next."

When Bobby was three years old I would take him to the lobster pound to watch the fishermen bring in their traps. Bobby was fascinated and longed to join them. One afternoon around four, an old lobster boat pulled in. At the wheel was a tall, strong man with friendly blue eyes. With him was a little boy, nine years old—his son, Alfred, who was already hauling with his father through the school-free months.

The fisherman saw Bobby standing there wistfully on the dock, trying to fish with a little bamboo pole. And a dream suddenly came true. Just as in a fairy story, the friendly man smiled and said, "Well, son, I don't think you'll be a-catching much there. Would you like to come aboard? We'll take you for a spin." Bobby's face glowed. We stepped aboard and took a spin around the bay, the water sloshing briskly under the bow. The fisherman had cookies left over from his dinner and he gave them to Bobby —found a Coke too, under the dashboard. The crusty traps were piled up in the stern and the smell of rotten herring bait rose up around them. We got acquainted.

His name was Jim Greenlaw, from Oceanville, on the other side of the island. By the time he delivered us back to the dock, Bobby had found a hero. Jim invited him to come back. "You just be here any time around four on Tuesdays and Thursdays, and we'll take another spin."

And that is how Bobby began a friendship that nourished and strengthened him all his young years. We got to know the family well. The Greenlaws lived in a rambling, ramshackle clapboard house set in the middle of a field of wild flowers. There was always scaffolding somewhere on the house; Jim was forever trying to shore it up. In an old apple tree there was a swing. The house always smelled of cookies and fresh baked bread, or chowder bubbling on the stove. Nellie, Jim's wife, baked wonderful lemon pies. There was a patch of garden flowers, an old car that was constantly breaking down, some chickens in a makeshift pen, a fine old mutt dog, and lots of cats. In the back, Jim had a workshop, cluttered and cozy, where he fixed his traps and painted his buoys.

There was something courtly and old-fashioned about Jim, a sort of perfect natural courtesy. His ways and manners were those of a prince—one of those gentle, kind, protective princes who live in fairy tales. And he always treated his wife, Nellie, as if she were a princess, rushing to help her lift her kettles, building her fires. His daughters were beautiful, one dark, with bright brown eyes, the other two with great clear blue eyes and blond hair flowing over their shoulders. All five of the children worked. One daughter who worked summers as a waitress walked more than six miles to get to work at 7:30 for the breakfast serving, and then walked back six miles at night after clearing up dinner.

Lobstering is a hard life, and there is not much money in it to feed seven, but the house was always gay and hospitable, and we had some feasts when Jim could spare a few lobsters for the family, or bring in, as he would say, "a mess of crabs." He loved his boat, and he used to tell me how much he enjoyed his walk "to the office," that is, down to the water three-quarters of a mile away, down a winding steep path that wound through forests (you had to slither over a cliff and skip on rocks over a little brook), and then —just when you wondered where the sea was—there would be a sharp incline and, there in front of you, a secret cove, rocks covered with seaweed, and the boat, bobbing and waiting.

How grateful I was to him! Through the years, Bobby would look forward to coming to Maine, to seeing Jim, who treated him not like a "poor little boy" but as a friend. I would try to thank Jim, to tell him how precious his strength and confidence were to Bobby. He'd always answer in his quiet, kind, Maine voice, "Aw, Sue, don't thank me. I'm really selfish. Little friends grow into big friends and Bobby's going to be my helper one day." And he would always introduce Bobby as "my future partner." Bobby would beam proudly. Not every boy had a lobsterman as a pal.

I remember one moment especially. It had been a terrible year; Bobby was seven and had had repeated bleedings into his knees all winter. A heavy brace weighed down his left leg. He had gotten very adept on crutches, careening around corners, balancing on one crutch, and he was proud of his skill. Back in New York people kept pitying him. He really couldn't understand this. But these people didn't really depress him. He knew that they couldn't skitter around on crutches the way he could.

Yet I knew that what Jim would say would matter a lot. The wrong word might shatter Bobby's fragile confidence. Inside, I worried and wondered what I could do to soften the blow. Naturally, as soon as we got to Deer Isle that summer, Bobby wanted to see Jim. As we walked toward his house, I grew more and more nervous. After all, they hadn't seen Bobby for a year, they had never seen him on crutches, and I hadn't had a chance to explain anything. Nellie was in the kitchen as usual and just as friendly, though she threw me a glance of sad concern. But she smiled at Bobby and said, "Well now, Bobby, it's sure good to see you. Jim's still down at the dock, but he'll be back soon." Bobby, impatient, set out to meet him. The grass in their field was very high, higher than Bobby's waist, but he started to push his way through on his crutches.

And then he saw Jim coming over the bluff in his high rubber boots. Bobby started to move through the grass as fast as his crutches would allow. I saw that even from a distance Jim had seen. I held my breath—how could he possibly know how much his first words would mean? And Bobby, suddenly overcome with shyness, realized too; he hesitated and stood suddenly still! in the middle of the field, like a bird poised to fly away. Jim kept advancing, and then I heard him boom out gaily, "Well, by gorry, Bobby, you sure do some good on them crutches!" A great broad grin broke over Bobby's face and he started running, yes, running, on his crutches, as fast as he could to meet Jim. When they met, Bobby dropped his crutches, fell into Jim's arms, and Jim swept him up in the air and whirled him around.

That summer, when Bobby could not manage to walk very far with his bent leg, much less swim, he went hauling with Jim and Alfred. Just the nearby cove traps to be sure, but still. . . . With Bobby's arms clasped tightly around his neck and Bobby's good leg tucked under his arm, Jim carried Bobby, brace, crutches and all, on his back down the rocky path under the trees, down the cliff, across the brook and down to the cove, a distance of nearly a mile. And then, when the tide was low, sure-footedly over the slippery, seaweed-covered rocks. I followed along, a little frightened. What if he should slip? But I trusted Jim. He would lift Bobby into the boat and off they would go. Bobby handled the winch and the hook, helped Alfred haul aboard, opened the traps, helped take out the lobsters. "Carefully now," advised Jim, "get 'em behind the ears." Bobby looked in wonder at the other sea creatures that came up in the traps—sea cucumbers and hermit crabs that skittered backward across the deck. Bobby would handle the ropes, would get the fresh wind in his face. And, as they sped over the sparkling blue waters, Jim would tell him stories about the surrounding islands, islands with wonderful names like Dumpling, Lazy Gut, Enchanted, and Phoebe.

Then, when things got worse and Bobby couldn't use his legs at all, Jim came to him and asked him to help him paint his boat. "We really could use you, Bobby, you know. We've fallen behind this winter and it would be a real favor." Jim gave him a job painting buoys and brought him a wooden fisherman's needle and taught him how to knot and weave trap bags. This work absorbed Bobby for days. Jim promised to make Bobby his own small lobster trap and send it to us in New York, "so you can keep your hand in through the winter and practice." I could not imagine how even Jim could manage to send a lobster trap through the mail. One winter day, a long flat package came. Bobby said, "It's the lobster trap." Seeing the shape, it seemed unlikely. But sure enough, it was. Jim had carefully numbered all the slats, and sent the screws to put it together. A miracle of Yankee ingenuity, it could be entirely reassembled into a perfect barrel-shaped trap. For Bobby, Jim had created the world's first entirely collapsible lobster trap. He sent a scaled-down buoy as well, which Bobby painted in Jim's colors, orange and white.

Over the years, the lobsters grew more scarce. Jim had to give up his beloved *Nellie G.*, the sparkling blue water, and the fanciful sea creatures that came up in his traps. For him, the time for fishing has passed. Now Jim is on land; he has become a carpenter. As for Alfred, the little blond boy who helped his father, and who was Bobby's friend, he has grown tall. Today, he is at the University of Maine, studying psychology. His plan is to work with handicapped children.

There were other friends, too—like the sheriff in Stonington who owned the finely crafted old brass and leather telescope that had once belonged to Captain Kidd's first mate. Back in England, the mate was hanged, but the telescope was found behind a false wall in a house that was being torn down on Petit Manan Island, north of us. The sheriff loaned Bobby the telescope, and Bobby happily sat on a hilltop and scanned Stonington harbor for alien sails.

Almost everybody on Deer Isle knew about boats and the sea. Stories of men who had sailed the seas, and the cheerful, rugged independence of those who told them, fed the children's imagination and nourished their dreams. One of our good friends in those years was a storybook character named Bert Dow. Bert was a man of the last century, but such was his tough Maine health, his sheer dog-gedness, that he had managed to live on through most of our own. His life encompassed the change from sail to the jet plane.

At the age of nine, Bert had run away from home and signed on as cabin boy on a great sailing ship. Under sail, he toured the world, following the wind. His ships carried barrel staves to the Caribbean and brought rum back. He sailed to Africa and around the Horn more times than he could count. "A-hauling mahogany, I spent seven years on the Gold River—I was a king down there," he'd muse. He sailed on three-masted schooners, four-masted schooners, and finally on the greatest of all, the *Thomas J. Conlin*, one of the only two seven-masted schooners ever built. During the First World War they carried explosives to England, and Bert was aboard. Some of these ships, partially converted to steam, went right on until World War II. "And when the sailing ships stopped, well," said Bert, "I did too."

So when we knew him, he was finishing his life where it be-gan, on Deer Isle. He lived with his brother, Frank, an old bachelor too, but a farmer who was as attached to the land as Bert had been to the sea. Frank unyieldingly refused ever to set foot on any boat. Bert worked the farm with his brother; long ago he had helped to build their house with his own hands. In the winter Bert would go off for days alone into the forest to log with his horse

Trigger. In the summer he gathered hay onto a rickety hay wagon. Our children would go find him in the fields and help him. Then Bert would bring them home, laughing and rolling around in the huge piles of hay, clippety-clop, clippety-clop. We have movies of Bobby lying in the hay wagon, front teeth missing, happily chewing a piece of hay—only the braces on his legs a sharp reminder that life was a struggle.

At seventy-five Bert was tall and straight as a spruce. He had huge, strong hands and arms, and sometimes I would go looking for him down at his dock and find him carrying logs the size of trees on his shoulders.

Whenever he could, Bert would steal away to the sea. Bob had a small sailboat, so leaky and old that it had a tendency to fill up and sink at the mooring. Bert would come down to the cove and help him fix it. He knew all about ropes and knots, and he would carefully splice and repair. And sometimes Bob would turn around and find him suddenly quiet, a sweet, musing smile on his face. "I just like to hear the wind in the sails," he'd say. And he would sit a long time, in the tiny boat in our small cove, sunk in happy reverie.

On an old launch, borrowed from the local doctor, with Bert as skipper, we spent many happy afternoons. From his childhood, Bert recalled without error sweet-water springs on every island, and all the best berry places, despite the fact that some of them were entirely hidden by years of tangled growth. We would land on some isolated shore, Bert would laconically mutter, "Follow me," and he would lead us through brush and tangle, and then with a wide, powerful fling of his arms, sweep open a thick wall of bushes. There would be a fairylike clearing, rich with a tangle of large, ripe raspberries. When had he found it? "When I was six," said he.

We loved to go fishing with him. We would go far out on the ocean and there might be six or seven boats around us also trying for cod. Bert would study the water attentively, turn the boat around a few times, stop the motor, let it drift, all the while scanning the surface and then cocking his head down low to the water. After a few moments he would grunt laconically, "Here." And he would start pulling up fish. All the while nobody around us would be catching anything. Astonished, we would ask, "But how do you *know?*" And he would answer mischievously, "It's easy. You just have to talk to the fish and ask them what they'd like for dinner."

Many times, on foggy days, we would just go and sit in his old kitchen with the wood stove. Bobby would bring Bert chewing tobacco and Bert would give him donuts and cookies. Then Bert would spread out newspapers for a tablecloth and we would eat donuts and sip strong coffee. Bert would sit there, with Bobby or Susy on his lap, the only man I ever saw could chew tobacco and suck a lollipop at the same time. Every so often he stopped talking to spit tobacco, always hitting the same dime-shaped spot, a feat that Bobby admired greatly.

And he would spin his tales. He would tell us about the time the rum barrels broke in the ship's exhaust system down in the Caribbean and all the sailors were drunk from the fumes and lying on the deck giggling, or about his St. Bernard who traveled with him on the world's oceans for sixteen years.

Then he would spread out his old pictures of all the ships he had sailed on, and of himself when he was young and handsome. His bright blue eyes were still the same, although they now teasingly looked out from a grizzled thatch of hair. "No, I never married," he said. "The life of the sailor is too hard for a lady."

At the end of one summer, when we came to say good-bye, great tears began rolling down those leathered cheeks. Bert hugged Bobby very hard. And during the winter, before the flowers of spring, he died. He is buried in the Deer Isle cemetery with an eloquent epitaph: BERT DOW, the graven stone reads, DEEP WATER MAN.

During those summers, God provided for Bobby not only heroes, but also the most precious and irreplaceable gift of all— children of his own age. Friends.

The loneliness and ostracism of the drab months of winter, the sharp pain of never being asked to birthday parties, of missing school outings, of forever being looked on as a curiosity—all these and more were made bearable, I think, because of the rich and full days of summer Bobby spent with his friends in Maine.

The only house anywhere near us had belonged to Daisy Conary, the Maine sea captain's wife who had sold our cabin to my father. Rambling and comfortable, it sat on a little bluff overlooking a wide field of grass that swept down to the sea. The house came to be owned jointly by three families, all young, with among them a total of twelve children who in those years ranged in age from infants to about twelve. If you add visiting cousins and friends, the total tribal count sometimes rose to twenty. Their names still sound in my ears like poetry—Roger, Holly and Gardy, Connie, Davey, Tom and Alexander, Hank, Maggie, Tiz, Martha and Kate. All now grown and scattered like petals across the land.

We called it the Red House. It always bustled with noise and activity, doors slamming as children went in and out, hammers banging in the tool shed, dogs (two Huskies and two Labradors) barking or chasing the three or four cats. The hammocks strung between the old apple trees in the field were always furiously, wildly swinging. The game was to swing as high as you could and then, at the peak, jump out and roll in the grass.

Making the lunch sandwiches was an assembly-line affair. Two giant loaves of bread were spread out neatly on a twelve-foot counter in the kitchen. One child would then methodically move along spreading peanut butter or tuna fish, while a second child followed along slapping the sandwich closed. Milk was bought in gallons—six every day. At dinner the children grouped around an enormous wooden table; whole turkeys were devoured at a sitting. (The adults, outnumbered and benumbed, ate later.) Then, with children wandering around in pajamas of many colors, stories were read or there was singing accompanied by an accordion.

Activities were myriad and complicated. Thanks to one of the talented mothers, the children were constantly inspired to make mobiles out of shells from the sea, to build looms and begin to weave, to make sea shell collections and leaf rubbings. They made their own pots from the clay of the cove, hauling the clay up from the sea flats and then firing the pots in the oven of the big kitchen stove. Groups and clubs formed and re-formed like clouds in the sky. They were generally classified as "The Littles" and "The Bigs," but within these general groupings there were middles and submiddles. The important thing was that everybody could find a friend to suit his mood of the moment.

There were boats. All the children learned to row, and later to use a motor and to sail. And they all splashed and swam in the icy Maine water as if it were the Caribbean. There were picnics and wienie roasts on the beach.

Every day there was usually some kind of gathering expedition. A group would set off for blueberries in the blueberry field (two measuring cups was considered a pretty good net yield, considering how good they taste sitting in a sunny field) or for raspberries on the ledge or wild flowers for dried bouquets. And with such a lot of manpower, there were very frequent expeditions for the clams that abounded on our shores.

One very foggy and rainy summer, the children formed "The Red House Players." They put on several unforgettable performances in the loft over the old barn. They strung up sheets for curtains and rummaged for old costumes. They wrote, directed, and produced entirely themselves, and put the smallest children to work making tickets which were sold to adults for five cents to finance future productions. Memorable productions included a play based on James Thurber's "Many Moons" and an entirely original play with incidental songs called *Mosquito Man*. The leading role was played by Roger, oldest and tallest of the group, with Susy, wearing a flowing pink strapless gown fished out of the attic, cast as the Maiden in Distress. Her entire role was to exclaim, after Mosquito Man had dispensed with Tomato Man (played by Bobby) and other dastardly villains, "My hero! Kiss me." At the very idea, the puritanical Mosquito Man promptly swooned. Curtain.

The total eclipse of the sun in August 1962 was a great scientific event at the Red House. The children read books on astronomy, followed all the newspaper accounts, and set to work making paper bags with small slits covered by film to protect their eyes. These of course quickly bloomed into gaily painted paper heads of animals and monsters. Then they all gathered in the living room and watched the eclipse's shadow being thrown up on a white wall. At the crucial moment, we rushed down to the shore.

As the sun was slowly being lost from sight, the cove grew strangely quiet, the birds stopped singing. Just before this magnificent natural wonder took place, as we were sweeping up children to go to the shore, Susy came running out of the house, shouting, "Mommy, Daddy, the most exciting thing is happening!" "Yes, yes," we said, "we know; it's the eclipse." "No," she cried, "I just learned to tie my shoe!"

Every summer the climactic social occasion was Bobby's birthday. There was no reason for this except that it happened to fall at the height of summer at a time when everyone was together. Over the years, traditions developed. For instance, Bobby's cake was always chocolate with whipped-cream icing, decorated with blueberries and raspberries. So lost in the ancient annals of Conary Cove lore is this that no one remembers how or when it first happened, but it lasted and is now immutable.

The children in the Red House sometimes worked for weeks concocting Bobby's present. It was A Project, demanding hours of consultation and decisions. Every child contributed, whatever his age. Triumphs included a large wooden car with wheels slightly askew, in which every child had driven at least one nail; a ferry boat decorated in bright colors and built of old pieces of a Victorian chest; and later, a complicated sailing game, the board carefully drawn from real charts of our waters, with obstacles and storms. Five tiny sailboats, whittled of balsa wood and fitted with different color sails, set off on this course, which had to be plotted with a compass.

And then, with everybody cleaned up for the occasion, the present would be ceremoniously brought to the party, which was held at our cabin. We organized treasure hunts, with clues graduated in difficulty for children from three to fourteen. The others ran from clue to clue; Bob carried Bobby on his back. There were sack races, potato races, egg races, blindfold games, and special tests of skill, like trying to extinguish a candle with a water pistol at twenty paces. Grownups enjoyed this. We made fresh ice cream, priming the father at the churn handle with cans of cold beer. After supper, we all gathered around our big fireplace and sang folk songs and toasted marshmallows on alder sticks.

For us, the wonderful, blessed thing was that there were so

many children. There was always someone to play with, somebody who wanted to come to the cabin to play cards or talk. One
summer, when Bobby was seven and we had begun the long road
back to straighten his rigid bent leg, he had to lie in traction for
three hours each day. His leg was tied to ropes and a pulley, and
he had to lie quite still, with a pillow supporting his knee. Every
morning a little visitor from the Red House would arrive on foot
and tap at the door. "Is Bobby home?"

Of all the Red House children, there was one who was Bobby's
best friend, his buddy, his pal, the recipient of his secrets. Davey
Gardner and Bobby met at the age of two. They began their first
important mud construction projects at three. Year after year they
went on to greater exploits.

When Davey was little, he was chunky, round-cheeked, very
blond, and had gray-brown eyes. He looked as if he were made of
some wonderful flavors of ice cream. Later he grew tough and
wiry. He was full of physical energy, constantly in motion, and
always had skinned knees. At first Bobby and Davey could run
together, but after the age of six, Bobby's joints were attacked. The
long months of enforced inactivity, the wheelchair, crutches, and
braces took him further and further away from his peers. In New
York, Bobby's friends came to our house more and more rarely;
finally they stopped coming altogether. But Davey somehow grew
along with Bobby. All summer, like Tom and Huck, they were
inseparable. When Bobby was in daily traction, Davey came every
morning to play knights with him. Restraining his own love of
running and playing ball must have been hard on Davey; sometimes he would disappear for a day or two, and I knew he just
wanted to race around with the others at the Red House and let
off steam. But he always came back. I marveled at his loyalty.
What an understanding of true friendship existed in the heart of
that child!

However handicapped Bobby was, he and Davey managed to
do most of the things that boys love.

"We were fascinated with knives," Bobby remembers, "and
this distressed everybody. We made swords out of poplar sticks.

We took walks, we fought a lot and beat each other up. I was stronger than he but he was more wiry. Davey loved Indians and snakes. He was very woods-minded and wanted to be tough.

"We would race over the ledges. I would use my brace to catapult myself onto the next ledge. I could move very fast over the rocks, and I liked it better than sand because my brace was so heavy I couldn't run through sand."

Davey shared that precious moment one summer when, after years mostly in a wheelchair, Bobby was able to walk with his brace all the way to our point. It was only a fifteen-minute hike through the woods, but it took five years of hope and work for Bobby to accomplish it.

During all those crucially important growing years, Davey's loyal friendship was a solid rock on which Bobby could lean. It is possible that in itself it made up for all the other slights, and gave Bobby the confidence and the joy to keep fighting. How can it be measured? How can a mother find a way to thank him?

Behind this idyllic existence, in the shadows always lurking, was worry. For our life in Maine, as everywhere, was only an illusion of normality. It took a constant, disciplined effort to push into the far corners of my mind all the terrible ifs. Every rock, every slippery ledge, was a hazard. The uneven terrain in the forest was full of hollows and hidden holes. There were fishhooks and knives. Not to speak of the consequences of falling off a boat—the braces on Bobby's legs were like heavy anchors.

Even the splendid isolation of the cabin, that source of calm, was a threat and danger. When occasionally we went out at night, I spent my evening suppressing panic. The cabin had no phone. The only lights were kerosene lamps. What if a lamp fell over? What if Bobby woke in pain and no one could reach us? As we drove home from these evenings, all the way along the road I prayed and held my breath until we arrived at the cabin. Then I would rush in, heart tight, to look at him as he slept. Only then could I, in retrospect, enjoy the party.

So we put in a telephone, the link that tied us to hospitals and doctors—and safety. And with the phone, down through the forest on hundreds of yards of expensive cables and poles, came electricity. Bobby was not aware, to be sure, that these measures were taken for his safety. He loved the cabin as it was, dark, primitive, and exciting. He complained bitterly when the oil lamps were converted and the hand water pump was removed. One day, when he was five years old, alone with his grandfather, he asked, "Grandpa, do you like what's going on?" My father agreed that he wished it didn't have to happen. "Oh, well," sighed Bobby, "you know, we men, we have to give in sometimes." But he swore that if the cabin were *his* he would have everything—electric lights, telephone, automatic pump, hot water, refrigerator—ripped out again.

The only fresh-frozen plasma available was what we brought with us. We stored our precious supply at the Red House in the freezing compartment of a refrigerator placed in an entry way, so that we could come at any hour without disturbing them. Many times in the small hours of the morning, I would sleepily extricate the vital bags from between the ice cream and the frozen juice. We used our supply with care, for when we had no more, we knew we would have to leave.

At first, to find a doctor who was able and willing to give transfusions, we had to go to a hospital in Ellsworth, an hour and a half away. Later we were able to find a young doctor in Blue Hill, a village only an hour away. We always had to find young doctors because older doctors generally knew nothing about hemophilia and were afraid to treat it.

We had phone numbers where the doctor could be reached at every moment in his day. We were umbilically tied to his family plans. When sometimes he was unreachable (he liked to go fishing), we had to swallow hard and hope that no emergency would happen just then.

Whenever we went for a transfusion, it meant an hour traveling each way and at least two hours at the hospital. Sometimes, if the doctor was definitely waiting for us at the hospital, we started thawing the plasma in the car, with warm water sloshing out of the saucepan I had brought along for the purpose. It was always the same wearying routine: the choking worry as we bounced over the country roads, with books and faithful Teddy to hold; and then again the waiting, this time in the neat bare wood halls of a country hospital, the forced words of cheer, repeated over and over, like a Buddhist chant, as if the monotonous repetition would bring relief. After it was over, we wearily drove back through the deserted countryside to the haven of the cabin, and sank into bed, temporarily eased. Sometimes the bleeding stopped and sometimes it didn't. We often had to go back the next day and the next, or night after night.

All those years, whenever we traveled, we had to travel with dry ice. Fresh-frozen plasma had to be kept deep-frozen all the way. If it thawed even slightly, it lost its potency and was useless. I don't imagine that dry ice intrudes much on the consciousness of most people. We had to think about it a lot and we became very knowledgeable on the subject. The only place dry ice was available was in ice cream factories or wholesale frozen-food depots. Anytime we wanted to go anywhere, we had to have some. Thus, even short trips were accomplished only with careful advance preparation. I had long ago given up hope that I would ever see my beloved Europe again.

We found a frozen-food depot in White Plains which agreed in advance to sell us dry ice the morning we were to leave. In those sweltering ninety-degree days of June and July, dry ice evaporated in twelve hours. And once the ice was gone, the plasma would thaw in twenty minutes. So our trip had to be geared to the hour of opening of the depot in White Plains. Bob would drive over early in the morning, pick up the dry ice, and then we had to drive directly to Maine. There could be no lingering on the road, no stopping overnight. Immediately on arrival, we rushed to the safe haven of a freezer. If we were lucky, and had a piece left over, the children were delighted. They quickly discovered that when dropped in the toilet, dry ice made glorious gurgles, and clouds of Hades-like mist rose mysteriously from the toilet bowl. There are always compensations for everything.

At the end of the summer the whole process had to be set in motion again for the trip home. We geared our departure to the twice-weekly arrival of the ice cream truck that came from Bangor to Stonington. As insurance, we located all the milk and ice cream companies on the route from Deer Isle to Boston. When there wasn't enough dry ice in Deer Isle, we called ahead and usually managed to get more in Bangor or Camden or Rockland. Then we would race for home.

As the years went by, dry ice became harder and harder to come by. Companies began to ship ice cream in refrigerated trucks. But fate was kind. For just as dry ice disappeared, we began to get the new concentrated AHF, which needed only normal refrigeration and could be kept on ice in a picnic cooler. It was a narrow escape: until then, without dry ice we could never have left the house for more than a few hours.

Robert Massie: At the end of one of these summers, as we were driving home for the beginning of school, the accident we had escaped on the isolated, rocky coast of Maine finally happened. It was early September, 1964. Bobby was eight, Susy was six, and Sue was three months pregnant with Elizabeth. We had been driving all day, and by late afternoon all of us, including the two cats in the back of the station wagon, were hot and thirsty. At a Howard Johnson's restaurant on the Massachusetts Turnpike, we halted for that all-purpose American procedure known as "the family rest stop."

Sue and Susy went in first. Just inside the entrance as they went in, Sue noticed a man mopping the floor. They came out and Bobby and I went in. The man and his mop had disappeared, but with my first steps, I noticed that the floor under my feet was wet and slippery. A danger signal flashed, and I started to turn to warn Bobby— Too late! Behind me I heard a thump and clatter as body and braces hit the floor.

Bobby had not had a chance. He was wearing his heavy brown shoes with special ridged rubber soles to grip when he jumped from rock to rock in Maine, but as soon as his feet touched the slick, soapy floor, he slipped. He lost his balance backward, overcorrected forward, and both feet went out from under him. Instinctively, he tried to protect his body by putting out his right arm. Sprawled on the floor, he began to scream. I turned him over and saw something horrible: his hand was hanging at a grotesque angle from his forearm. He had broken his right arm.

I was almost overcome with shock. The world around me

became unreal. My head was nine feet off the floor, my hands were at the end of six-foot arms, everything blurred except the crazily askew arm on the floor. I forgot the elementary first-aid rule, dutifully learned as a Boy Scout, that broken limbs must not be moved. The only thoughts in my head were hemophilia . . . hemorrhage . . . transfusion . . . hospital . . . doctor!

By good fortune or God's mercy there was someone in the restaurant who kept her head. A tall, gray-haired woman, a customer, had seen what had happened. She got up quickly from her chair and kneeled beside me next to Bobby. Seeing the arm, she quietly told a waitress to bring us a piece of heavy cardboard. From this she made a temporary splint. Then from the soda fountain she asked for crushed ice, which she packed into the cardboard around the arm. Thereafter, until the ambulance arrived, she sat quietly beside Bobby, making certain that his arm remained absolutely still. Later, we were told that what happened in the first minutes was of crucial importance. Ice and immobilization were exactly the treatment Bobby should have had. In the confusion, we never learned her name, but to this unknown woman we owe much.

As soon as Bobby was wearing his improvised splint, I rushed to the receptionist, a woman wearing glasses, staring in horror from behind the cash register. I explained to her that this was not a normal broken arm, that Bobby was "a bleeder" and that it was urgent that we get him to a hospital or a doctor immediately. She said that the nearest hospital was Harrington Memorial in Southbridge and that the fastest way to get there would be in a State Police ambulance. I begged her to telephone quickly.

While she dialed, I ran out the door to tell Sue. Only a few minutes had passed since she and Susy had come out of the restaurant. They were still in the car, arranging saucers of milk for the cats, waiting for us, unknowing. I was incapable of cushioning the blow. "Bobby has broken his arm!" I blurted. In Sue's face I saw a mirror of my own shock and terror. "No! Oh, no!" she cried and dashed ahead of me into the building. Susy, her little face awestricken, knowing as well as any of us the implications of what had happened, began to weep. "I didn't mean it, I didn't mean it," she sobbed. Later, when we had time to think about it, we realized what she meant: normally jealous of this older brother who routinely gathered so much interest and affection because of his disease, she had secretly wished his comeuppance. Now that massive disaster had struck him down, she was overcome with guilt.

For the next twenty minutes, the restaurant was in an uproar. Bobby, Sue, and Susy were crying. I was wild-eyed, rushing every thirty seconds to the cashier, demanding to know when the ambulance would come, insisting that she call again, shouting that she must understand that Bobby was in critical danger. Four or five times, while I danced in agony in front of her, she phoned the police.

Time seemed to stop. Every few seconds I looked at Bobby and the same sequence of desperate thoughts raced through my head. How much bleeding will there be? Suppose he has to lose the hand? How can we prevent it? What in God's name can we do? Where is the ambulance?

Nothing happened. Nobody came. The restaurant world swam crazily around us. Suddenly, frantic with worry, I decided to take him to the hospital myself. Of the sea of faces I demanded whether anyone knew the way. A waitress said she did but she couldn't go; she was on duty. With a cry, I leaped to drag her bodily into our car. At that moment, a Massachusetts State Police ambulance, pulsing with lights, screeched up to the door. The trooper and I put Bobby on a stretcher and loaded him through the back door of the ambulance. With Sue, Susy, and me perched inside, we set off at ninety miles an hour for the hospital.

We were met in the emergency room by a nurse who said that she had had two calls. One said that a boy with a broken arm was coming in, the second that a boy with hemophilia was coming. She was surprised to find they were the same boy. Despite this double alarm, no doctor was there. The doctor had preferred to wait at home until the nurse took a look at the case and phoned him her evaluation. While we waited for his routine to be observed, we ourselves thawed the fresh-frozen plasma. When the doctor arrived fifteen minutes later, I explained how the tubing and valves of the administration system worked, he put a needle into Bobby's other arm and, at long last, the transfusion began. With the bag of plasma inverted on a stand over Bobby's head,

and the yellow drops, precious now as liquid gold, falling rapidly
into the filter chamber, then sliding in a constant flow down into
Bobby's outstretched arm, Sue and I, for the first time, sat down
and began to breathe again.

While the needle was still in his arm and the plasma on a
portable stand, Bobby was wheeled into the X-ray room. With
the arm exposed for the camera, I saw it for the first time since the
moment of the break. It did not appear to be badly swollen, but
the X-rays showed a fracture of two bones, the ulna and the
radius. The local doctor suggested that we call our own doctor to
decide what to do next. We telephoned Lee Engel and he suggested
that we bring Bobby to him. Carefully, we resplinted the arm and
packed it again in fresh crushed ice.

It was dark outside when we left the hospital and were driven
back to the restaurant. Our abandoned car and cats were alone in
the parking lot. We set off for home. In the car, we were pleased
to see that Bobby's appetite remained: with his good hand he went
rapidly through a box of French fries. At midnight, we arrived at
White Plains Hospital. Dr. Engel was there, his familiar face
radiating normality, and he had brought with him an orthopedic
specialist. The two doctors worked simultaneously; while Lee gave
another transfusion, the arm was set into a cast. "What do you
think?" I asked, when they had finished. "I don't know," Lee said.
"We'll just have to wait and see."

For the next three days, Bobby had transfusions twice a day,
along with codeine, Darvon, and Demerol. In a week, with the
transfusions cut to one a day, he went back to school. Being unable to write or draw, he could only sit in the classroom and listen.
During the month that followed, Sue and I did little but drive the
car. Twice, then once, a day to the doctor for transfusions, four
times a day to school. (Bobby had to come home for lunch because
he couldn't carry a tray.)

Although the arm itself was useless to him, it gave Bobby
little trouble as long as it remained immobile in the cast. It was
once the bones had healed and the cast was discarded that his arm
problem began. During the long period of immobilization, the
muscles controlling the joints had atrophied and, when he began
to use the arm again, he began to bleed into both the elbow and

the wrist. This meant more pain, more codeine, and after a difficult decision, the arm was resplinted. Bobby's piano lessons were abandoned; the strain on the arm was too severe.

The months went by. In time, the muscles strengthened, and Bobby began to use the arm again, but he still was unable to straighten it completely. The accident had struck a permanent blow. Until it happened, the right arm was the single limb with which Bobby had never had a problem. Thereafter, his right elbow, along with his left knee, became his most severely affected joint.

The episode had two footnotes. Blue Cross refused to help with our expenses at White Plains Hospital because we had already made a previous claim for treatment of the same injury the same day at the hospital in Southbridge. No excuses, no exceptions.

The other footnote was happier. The Massachusetts state trooper who took us to the hospital was a silent, burly man named Officer Jerry Charette. Learning that I worked for *The Saturday Evening Post*, he asked, somewhat embarrassed, if I would do him a favor. Norman Rockwell, the illustrator, was one of the area's famous citizens. Could I, as a *Post* writer, get Norman Rockwell's signature for him?

I wrote immediately to Mr. Rockwell. He replied:

Dear Mr. Massie,

I sent the autograph to Officer Charette as you requested. It's always wise to keep on the right side of the police.

Sincerely,
Norman Rockwell

Chapter 11

How can time be measured for a *healthy* child who is immobilized in bed? For that was the trouble: Bobby was not really sick; he was caged. What to do when these long days stretch into months and years and become a way of life? During long sieges of bleeding Bobby was forgotten by the outside world, as if he had gone away on a long journey. Occasionally, there would be brief communiqués from the classroom. Sometimes the whole class would write letters and send pictures. Usually this happened only once. A few teachers did try to help Bobby keep up with the class by sending mimeographed sheets of classroom work. A small emissary would arrive at our back door bearing these papers, and after a few minutes of conversation with Bobby in his bedroom would disappear again. But this work was not nearly enough to occupy the hours.

How to fill that active, restless mind? Somehow I had to find ways to bring the world into his room. If only we had had our families or our cousins close by to spread the load and vary the stimulation for him, but they lived far away. Bob was working very hard to try to support the crushing financial burden of hemophilia. He worked all the time, days and nights, weekends. That left only me. I searched my mind for every idea, every resource my education had given me.

It was hardest when Bobby was very small. I scoured the stores for games. I kept him lavishly supplied with crayons and paper. I tried to read to him a lot, but I couldn't do this all day. (How much easier everything seemed when he could read to himself!) I started reading stories of knights who did Brave Deeds Against All Odds. In a toy store one day I discovered, to my joy, miniature knights, about three inches high, whose lances and tiny swords, sashes and ribbons all could be taken apart. They were expensive. We could not afford to buy more than one at a time. The first one, proudly mounted on a white horse, we called Sir Bobby. Some time later I was able to buy a Black Knight who became Sir Bobby's sworn enemy. We called him Sir Evil. He was *always* vanquished in the end. As his little army slowly grew, Bobby developed whole imaginary worlds around them. When, at the age of six, Bobby was in traction three or four hours every day, he would spread out his knights on the sturdy wooden bed table that Bob had built for him, and invent battles and jousts for his knights.

Not long ago, Bobby noted nostalgically in his diary: "Sir Bobby was the first knight I ever received, when I was four. In my childhood games he was the hero of all occasions—strong, handsome, gallant, good sport, articulate, excelling in all things. I quite unabashedly attributed all these qualities to myself by virtue of the fact that we were namesakes. As my collection grew, Sir Bobby assumed increasing importance among his men. Whenever Sir Bobby's sword was snapped, his crest cracked, or his lance topped off, his entourage was quick to replace the damaged item with one of theirs; but Sir Bobby's head, with its brown hair and little mustache, remained the same through each and every rejuvenation, as did his knightly color, purple. Sir Bobby could do anything, and for me, at that time, that must have been very important."

The collection and the stories grew. Finally, after four or five years of birthdays and Christmases, we were able to buy the castle. This castle and the armies that defended it from so many attacks continued to occupy Bobby hour after hour. They were so precious to him that in nine years not a soldier was lost.

There was one very strange thing that I noticed: immediately before the beginning of a bleeding, Bobby would often be irritable and difficult. Yet during one of his bouts of terrible pain, and immediately after, a kind of gentle sweetness would come over him. He never complained then . . . he just bore it bravely. It was beautiful, but disturbing, because it only happened when he was very ill.

As soon as he was better, yet still immobilized for a long period, he became, like all invalids, cranky and demanding. By nature he is stubborn. This is a blessing; it has helped him overcome great challenges. But when he was a child, it was not easy to live with.

No more than any other child did he want restrictions. Almost daily we fought and struggled about how much he was to do. Out of sheer rebellion, he would refuse to do his exercises with me. He wanted to push out, to do more. He got as tired of hearing "no" as I got tired of saying it. His strong will wore me down, pushed me to tears of rage and frustration.

It was hard not to be sorry for him. I had to fight myself not to make allowances for him, not to let him use his disease to get out of responsibilities. I didn't always succeed. Each step of the way I worried about how he would emerge.

He had two great natural advantages: a good sense of humor and enormous curiosity.

During all those years of Bobby's childhood, trying to help him overcome apathy and boredom, I put into action the principles for fighting depression that I had developed for myself. When legs cannot move, it is important that hands be kept busy. So I taught Bobby to sew buttons and to knit; later he learned to weave. Before he could read, I taught him how to cook. But not as a game . . . as a serious business, to teach him discipline and develop in him a sense of perfection in small tasks. This was important because with little or no challenge from the outside he had to learn in other ways to strive for excellence. I trained him as a kitchen helper and let him help me on the condition that he accomplish professionally the tasks I set him. There are many things in cooking that children can do very well. For instance, little fingers are better than big ones for rolling and crumbling bread crumbs. In ascending order of difficulty, I taught him to peel, chop, fold, and roll. Cooking is an especially gratifying activity, one that satisfies all the senses at once. Best of all, unlike all the other arts, when you are finished you can eat your creation.

Christmas was the apotheosis of our cooking activities. Over the years we developed and perfected an elaborate series of cakes and cookies. We started baking weeks before the holidays. We made gingerbread men for all our friends, dressing them and painting individual names on each one with colored sugar icing. This cookie making has become family tradition, and the gingerbread men have become so sophisticated that they are now given different ages, sexes, and personalities.

Music helps loneliness, too. Even when we were straining for money, I managed to save enough from our food money to enroll us both in the Little Orchestra Society series in New York. Here, not only was music played, but instruments were explained. I taught him about ballet, which I loved. When we could afford it, I took both Bobby and Susy to ballet performances. But as Bobby grew more handicapped, even these rare outings became impossible. Our cities are not prepared or designed to accept the physically handicapped. For Bobby to be able to attend any performance, he had to be accompanied by two adults. To get there we had to drive, because buses and trains are difficult to manage—too many stairs, long distances to reach the theaters. Yet the law did not permit parking the car close enough to any theater so that I alone could push him in his chair, and I couldn't deposit a six-year-old child in a wheelchair and leave him alone on a curb while I searched for a parking lot. Once we got to the theater, we couldn't climb a flight of stairs to the cheaper seats we could afford; and it was almost impossible for Bobby to squeeze past a row of seats. So we couldn't go. Nevertheless, even when he couldn't see performances for himself, Bobby could listen to his records and dream.

As he grew older, I turned his eyes to the sky, to stars and space. When his joints kept him confined to bed for many months, I hung above him a mobile of our solar system. Gently the air pushed the planets, which turned in orbit. On his seventh birthday, we gave him a telescope so he could gaze at the moon for himself.

I turned his interests toward science, to develop an inquiring, unsentimental approach. He needed to develop objectivity to face his own problems. Searching through catalogues of educational toys I came upon a series of musical science records. They were wonderful! Wittily, in music and song, they explained some of the basic scientific rules and phenomena. I heard him playing them over and over in his room. I did my housework to the lilting strains of:

> *Vibration. Vibration.*
> *Vibration is what causes sound.*

> *Vibration, vibration.*
> *Vibration causes sound.*

Or, to a calypso beat:

> *What do we mean by metamorphosis?*
> *Metamorphosis, metamorphosis.*
> *A certain kind of change is what it is.*
> *That's what we mean by metamorphosis.*

Then a serious voice would announce: "Every action causes an equal and opposite reaction." The powerful whine of a jet plane followed. Then, in rock beat, triumphantly:

> *And that's how a jet plane flies . . .*

You can see that these songs made a great impression on me. (It was from these records that I myself finally understood at last why a jet plane flies.) Sometimes I still find myself humming the tunes. Worn and rutted, we still have the records. Now Elizabeth listens to them.

From the very beginning, we explained to him the nature of his own disease so as to take away his fear and help him understand what was happening to him and why. At eight, he was peering through a microscope at slides of his own blood. Dr. Engel prepared the stains for him. I took him to visit the laboratory of the hospital. In fifth grade, as a project for the school science fair, he produced a scientific analysis of his own hemophilia, complete with graphs he had made of his own bleedings over several months.

Through his microscope he began looking inward and at the miracles of the world close around him: dust and feathers, salt and insect wings. I bought him a little ant colony which he carefully watched; I provided him with books on the weather and on insects.

Thanks to the healing summers in Maine, he grew to love and respect nature and to draw comfort, as I had, from its harmonies. Today Bobby is a crusader for the environment. But already, back in third grade, he grew so outraged at the proposed devastation of the Storm King Mountain in the Hudson Valley by a Con Edison electric plant that he wrote a letter to President Johnson, accom-

panied by "before" and "after" drawings. (*Before:* the sun is shining and smiling, birds are flying, colors are bright. *After:* the sun
is frowning, no birds, no trees, black and white.) The President responded with an autographed picture and urged Bobby to write
to his congressman.

These were the years of collections. First it was models of
dinosaurs (age four). Then (at six and seven) he collected insects.
He caught a praying mantis and examined it for several days before
releasing it. Ruefully, he found that "the bugs were always getting
loose, and they never ate what it said they should in the books.
They never did anything right, so I let them go."

In Maine he began a rock collection. His Grandfather Todd
(Bob's stepfather) helped him to start a penny collection. I would
bring home all the pennies I could, and he would spend a lot of time
examining each one with his magnifying glass, always hoping to
find the 1909S VDB worth $150—the treasure of his dreams. We
provided him with ship models to assemble. He began a stamp
collection.

A series of pets slithered and scampered through our house
during these years. There were two sleepy green turtles, a chame-
leon bought at the circus, who lived a reasonably long life in a jar
with Bobby feeding him flies. There were two dogs—both killed
by cars. There has been a series of prolific and durable cats, all of
them from Maine, all of them with good, sturdy, no-nonsense
characters. Finally, Bobby had a white mouse named Trixie, who
had an aggravating habit of exercising on the wheel of his (her?)
cage at 5 A.M., waking the whole house with creaks and squeaks.
Trixie came to a sad end. Left behind with friends when we went
to Maine one summer, Trixie refused to eat and died of a broken
heart and an empty stomach.

Of all the things that occupied Bobby, the most important, and
the greatest blessing, were books. Thanks to his home teacher, he
was reading freely at the age of five. He began to devour books.
Quickly he worked his way through all the fairy tales and children's classics. By the time he was ten he had swallowed the complete Sherlock Holmes, all twenty-nine volumes of Tarzan, the spy
stories of John Buchan, Dickens, Robert Louis Stevenson, and

Edgar Allan Poe. His favorites were adventure stories. I looked for stories of the lives of men who had begun in adversity and ended in glory: Abraham Lincoln, Teddy Roosevelt.

From the beginning, Bobby followed the NASA space program. He was fascinated by every detail about space exploration and spacemen. He read science fiction and started to develop and write his own adventures. At ten years old, over a period of several months when he was repeatedly in bed with knee hemorrhages, he invented a race of super space creatures, the Birdgonians.

For his Birdgonians he created an entire world and life style, complete with subterranean houses, school system, battles, legends, customs and caste systems, even insignia for the army patches. He drew hundreds of pictures of his world, created a new language and alphabet. This work occupied him for weeks, absorbing an enormous amount of creative energy.

There were times, especially when I had to go back to work, when there was nothing else for Bobby to do, nothing else to keep him company but the television set. Sometimes, during his long recuperative periods, Bobby would watch TV for most of the day. I was grateful when it would distract him and make his loneliness more bearable. And it served another important purpose—it kept him quiet and occupied, so that he would not move or disturb the fragile clotting in his joints.

Every week, Bobby counted the moments until his favorite programs, *Lost in Space* and *Star Trek*, came on. More and more he identified with the young boy and girl in *Lost in Space*. He wrote them fan letters.

His greatest dream was to write an episode for *Lost in Space* based on his Birdgonian space world. I tried to explain to him that opportunities for ten-year-old free-lance TV writers were likely to be rather slim, but undissuaded, he sent off an elaborate letter with story suggestions for several episodes to Irwin Allen, the producer of the show. Week after week went by, during which he eagerly and hopefully awaited the arrival of the mailman each day. Finally, he did get an answer from a public-relations man, along with some photographs of the cast. But to his great disappointment, no assignment.

With friends a man lives and thrives. Take them away, and a man is left with himself and soon he will crumple and die. A man truly needs friends, to live and be happy.

Bobby wrote this when he was ten.

Pets and stories, knights and telescopes, pennies and stamps—all of these were fine, but they didn't quite make up for that one thing: friends. Hemophilia Foundation information sheets warned of the dangers of a hemophiliac becoming too attached to his mother; this, they said darkly, could impair him for life. All right. I agreed. Anyway, he was *bored* being with his mother all the time. But what was I to do about it? The Hemophilia Foundation information sheets did not offer any suggestions.

In his early years, Bobby was never invited to birthday parties. Susy often was, and when she went, I tried to gloss it over. But my heart ached. He loved company so much. Even today, Bobby always sleeps with his door wide open and I wonder if it is not a reaction to all the closed doors of his childhood. By nature, he was more gregarious than Susy; he *needed* company. When the cycles of illness and isolation stretched on and on, he would grow depressed, and depression caused more bleeding. Happiness *is* the best medicine, but how to find it?

I tried to enroll him in the Cub Scouts, but they wouldn't accept him. We tried to send him to a day camp but "the responsibility," they said, "would be far too great for a junior counselor." Perhaps they were right. But what hurt was that nobody was willing to ask what was involved; the simple word "hemophilia" (and it could have been cystic fibrosis, epilepsy, or any chronic disease) was enough to make them say no.

I sent him to Sunday school hoping that there perhaps he might find friends. But it was the same problem as school—no continuity. His cousins lived far away. I tried to import Davey Gardner, but Davey lived first in Providence, then in Washington, three hundred miles away. Davey's mother worried when he traveled alone, and I didn't blame her. So at most, Davey could come only once or maybe twice a year. Even so, just the *possibility* of such a visit

could pull Bobby out of a long siege of bleeding. After one of these
visits, when Bobby was eight, he wrote:

May 18, 1965

Dear Davey:

Do you remember when you walked out of my classroom
with Tom? I was very sad for I knew that I would not see you
until I go to Maine, and I knew that I would miss you.

When I got home I missed you so much I called out "Davey!"
even though I knew that you weren't here. I decided I would write
you a letter. So this is it.

I am writing to you from my desk in my room at about 4:10
on May 18, 1965. There are a lot of noises in the house. Susy calls
downstairs to ask whether she can wear a bathing suit and Daddy
is saying "NO!" The baby [Elizabeth] is crying. A shriek of delight comes from Susy's room and I hear Susy calling, "Daddy may
I wear these shorts?" and Daddy says, "Yes!" Before I wrote this
letter I looked all over for this yellow paper and Daddy found it.
Mommy is in town and will be home later. I am tired and don't
have a lot to say, but please write to me and I hope you and your
family are well.

Your Best Friend,
Bobby Massie

P.S. I will send you your kit of squirts and things to you later.

When Bobby was five years old, for a while he had one wonderfully loyal friend, a beautiful dark-haired little girl who lived
across the street. Her name was Susan Price and she came over to
play every day when Bobby was sick—until she moved away.
(Since then, most girls that Bobby has liked have all looked a little
like her.)

Otherwise, there was almost no one. I asked—in a quiet way,
I begged—for children to come over. Very occasionally, pushed
by his parents, one would come on a sort of duty visit. When the
child was with him, Bobby's face was illuminated; he was gay and
happy. But soon, very soon, unaccustomed to having to play quietly
for long periods, the visitor would beat a retreat, to run and play
outdoors. I tried to be cheerful.

(But I can see his eyes fill with pain, and all I can do to reach
him in that lonely world is to bustle about busily plumping pillows,

overelaborately arranging the room—all the time sharply aware that these gestures are pitifully inadequate. Still, they help me. My body is aware of a thousand tiny signs of improvement or worsening. I read them silently, swiftly, like a farmer scanning the earth and sky for portents of the weather to come. The expression in the eyes—a dark large pupil is a bad sign. Color of skin—is he growing paler? My hands and fingertips like antennae lightly run over knees, trying to learn the extent of the turmoil. They support the leg—while I sneak a sidelong look to see how much it pained him. I try to move with confidence, quickly, but not abruptly, talking, talking positively all the while.

(I rage at the slights inflicted on him by giddy friends who promise things and then disappear for carefree afternoons and holidays, throwing back over their shoulders in silvery voices, "I'm so sorry, but you know I promised to go. . . ." He doesn't complain, but my heart is tight when he nonchalantly asks, "Any mail for me? Did anyone call?" At times, I'm ashamed to confess, I want to wish suffering on them—not much, to be sure—but enough to cure their youthful selfishness. I have to hold my tongue and repeat over and over to myself, "Why should they know? It's not their fault." But I remember. And those precious few who do take time, well, I have to keep myself from lavishing thanks on them, from showering gifts. For that would be just as wrong. No, this is one barrier against which all my energy and determination to overcome are powerless.)

A visit was such an important event to Bobby that each one is meticulously recorded in his diary: "Today is a good day, because Beth came over. We looked at the cats, played Memory and Sniff and just read. I am very glad I didn't have another shot today."

Tuesday, March 21, 1967
Dear Diary,

Today was a good day, not as boring as most. The reason for this is that I had Nick Benson over to my house. We had lots of fun.

First he came at 11:30 and we played. Then we went to the Irvington Pizza Shop, the food was absolutely delicious. Then we spent the rest of the afternoon playing.

During that time Nick and I wrestled on my bed to see who

was stronger. Nick is on the wrestling team at school. Yet he couldn't make me surrender or hold me down.

Accidentally, Nick hit my chin and I bit my lower lip. It didn't stop for about 3 hours, but right after it started again. Dad took me for 6 units of plasma. He told me that wrestling was not so bad.

Dr. Engel took all the stuff that Dad and Mom had put on off after the transfusion. We found to everyone's surprise it had stopped. That's the best example of clotting I've ever seen.

Well, sianara!

Sincerely,
Bobby Massie

P.S. I got a new *Mad*!

Thanks to this carefully kept diary, it is easy to list the visitors for September 1966–June 1967. They were: my parents, my sister Jeannine, my friends Janet Dowling and Liz Parks. Bob's brother Kim came twice. The mayor called once. The minister came twice. Beth Drill (an elementary-school classmate) came three times, Peter Kmetz and Nick Benson (Hackley classmates) came respectively three times and twice. Otherwise, Bobby spent his time with Mrs. Connors, the friendly babysitter who took care of Elizabeth while I was working; Dorothy Robinson, the cleaning woman, who came once every two weeks; and Dr. Engel and Dr. Newman (Dr. Engel's partner).

To this general exclusion there were two exceptions. At nine or ten, all the children in our neighborhood went to dancing classes. Bobby was wearing a brace on each leg. Nevertheless, Jane Drake, the neighbor who was in charge of the invitations, called me one day and said, "Look, I don't know if it's possible for Bobby to come, but we don't want to exclude him if he can." I was joyous for days afterward. Although Bobby did miss a lot of the classes, he went whenever he could, shoes shined, wearing a blue blazer, just like all the other boys. Thanks to this understanding neighbor, he attended each year until we left for Paris.

And then, there were the Russians.

Just north of Irvington—across the Tappan Zee Bridge, which spans the widest part of the majestic Hudson—is the small town of

Nyack. In Nyack there is a large Russian community, some three or four hundred families, who came to settle there in different waves of emigration. There are old émigré families who left at the time of the Revolution, there are others who managed to escape the wrath of Stalin during the upheavals of the Second World War, and there are new families who have arrived during the last ten years. Such is their sense of shared community responsibility that on holidays the gentlemen still observe the old Russian custom of calling on all the old ladies; and when the snow falls, the teen-age boys immediately go out to shovel the walks of all elderly people. Together, the Russians of Nyack raised the money for and with their own hands built a Russian church that stands high on a hill overlooking the Hudson. On the knife-sharp, biting cold, clear days of winter, sometimes we could just glimpse its golden cupola far away across the river.

My first Russian teacher, Svetlana Umrichin, lived in Nyack with her family. During the most difficult times I took comfort in her house, where the Umrichins—father, mother, son, daughter, and old grandmother—would enfold me in their friendship.

Svetlana called almost every day during times when Bobby was suffering a series of agonizing days and nights with bleeding joints. One day she asked, once again, "How is Bobby?" I answered, "Better now, thank God." She said only, "What time?" I answered that he had seemed better sometime in the afternoon. Svetlana exclaimed, "I knew it! I knew it!" The Russians had all prayed for him in church that morning.

The Umrichin family invited us to share their warm celebrations at Christmas and Easter. Our children were always delighted to find that when all the Christmas lights in our town had been extinguished, the streets of Nyack where the Russians lived were still blazing (Russian Christmas is celebrated on January 7).

Most of all we loved the Easter celebration, the most beautiful of all Russian holidays. Late at night, there was the mystery of the crowded church, smelling exotically of incense and ringing with the magnificent Easter music of the Russian church. Easter Day at the Umrichins was filled with celebration. There were gifts and food, talk and gaiety, and friends coming in and out to visit. These holidays were events of the year for Bobby and Susy.

It was one of those times when Bobby had missed school for weeks. It was spring, the weather was beautiful, but I could not notice the bursting buds or the daffodils. There was only one sight before my eyes—my son, with his pale, wan face sitting disconsolately in his wheelchair. He was desperately lonely. The phone rang. It was Svetlana calling about my lesson. I confessed to her the frustration I felt. The next morning, the phone rang again. "Suzanne," said Svetlana, "you know, there is a very nice couple in our community, Catherine and Peter. Peter is a carpenter and Catherine is a very good cook, a very motherly person. She is at home all the time. They have very nice children. Bobby met them at Christmas. They wonder if Bobby might come over and spend the day with them." Wonder if he might come over! My heart leaped. On a sunny spring Saturday I drove him to Nyack. He came back with his face transformed. His cheeks were rosy, he was chattering about Catherine making bread and giving them the most wonderful tea, about playing the piano with Irina, who was eleven, and card games with Serge, who was nine, and how Serge pushed him all around the yard in his wheelchair.

That night I was warm with hope. How could I thank them for what they had done? What could I *do!* The next morning the phone rang once more. Again it was Svetlana, arranging my next lesson, and oh, by the way, she added as if in afterthought, "Peter and Catherine wish me to thank you for sending them Bobby." (*Thank me!*)

The only child who was close to Bobby—his only real companion—was his sister Susanna, twenty months younger than he. From the time she was born, Susanna always had a faraway look in her blue eyes. In photographs of her as a little girl you can see her looking out at the world, surprised and a little wistful. A chronic disease is visited on the entire family; each member must learn to deal with it in his or her own way. The path of a middle child is always hard, but to be the younger sister of a brother with a mysterious disease is even harder—always to have to play second fiddle, always to have your own needs shadowed, molded, dictated by a dramatic disease. There is the fatigue of the parents, the drain on the family resources, the imbalance of having to pay more attention to one child than to another. Without even noticing it, without even meaning to, parents tend to think, *Thank goodness, she is healthy*—and to take this miracle for granted. And if parents forget, other people forget even more. Without realizing it, and in Susy's presence, people always asked first, "How is Bobby?" and only later, sometimes nudged by me, they remembered to add, "Oh, yes, and what about Susy?" This hurts. Maybe this was what was in Susanna's wistful glance when she was little.

Susy and Bobby pummeled their way together through childhood. During their early childhood years, in our tiny house in White Plains, they shared a first floor room. They devised a number of daring sports. They would leap off the top of their dresser and land with a whack on their beds. They fought so much that the two of them decided to divide their turf with a chalk line. Unfortunately, a clever Bobby had managed to include the door in his territory. During battles, Bobby would prohibit Susy from crossing his line and getting to the door. Rather than give in, when she had to go to the bathroom Susy would climb out the window, go around the house, come in the front door, and go to the bathroom. And when she was really aroused, she would run after him brandishing her shoe, which scared him. ("Susy," Bobby says, "when cornered, would let out a scream and it would always be my fault. She had the hardest heels I've ever felt.") But all this I learned only later. Such was their shared intimacy that all these escapades were kept as comradely secrets.

She has needed all that stubborn spirit. From the age of five, Susanna has loved horses. Where this passion comes from is as mysterious a genetic secret as her brother's hemophilia—perhaps from some distant, dashing Virginia ancestor. We saw it first when she was five. One summer, without fear, as if it were second nature to her, she mounted a huge horse. Her legs were so short that they almost stuck out straight over the broad back of the beast. We smiled. But she wasn't smiling. She was deadly serious and totally confident. That day, she won a blue ribbon—for walking. In our home movies, there we are, clustering about her, congratulating her with silly grins on our faces. Susy is calmly patting her mount, as if she had done it all her life.

From that moment, she has single-mindedly clung to her dream. Every Christmas, the requests have been the same: books about horses, miniatures of horses. Today, her shelves are crowded with horses in wood and porcelain, metal and straw, from Mexico, Greece, Russia, and China. Her shelves bulge with horse dictionaries. She has studied equine anatomy, memorized the names and victories of famous race horses and jumpers, studied the biographies of famous riders. Her letters, and even the good-night notes she leaves on our pillow, are signed with the carefully drawn head of a horse. It has been a lonely passion—but maybe it has sustained her.

We couldn't help her. We knew nothing about horses. For many years we couldn't even afford to pay for lessons. She has had to go her own way alone, sustained only by her vision. It has developed in her the discipline of the champion. You can see it. Her room is always neat, she is always well groomed. Quietly, she shuts herself up in her room for hours and when she comes out, her work is done. She gets straight A's in school. No one pushes her, whether she is learning a language, doing her eye exercises, or wearing her nighttime orthodontist's braces. No one has to remind her. She *knows* where she is going.

In a family of noisy temperaments, Susy is the quiet one. She grew used to sitting on the edge of conversations, looking, listening, noticing everything. She lets others exhaust themselves in talk, and then when she disagrees she just digs in her heels and doesn't budge. And when occasionally that fiery temper that awed Bobby suddenly explodes, the family—startled and chastened—has learned to back away and give her room.

Despite everything, she is overcoming all obstacles to become an excellent rider. Somehow, more and more often, we, who didn't know a Morgan from an Arabian, are finding ourselves cheering at Madison Square Garden or squinting and sweating in the sun at local horse shows. Slowly, her lampshades are blooming with ribbons she has won. She has ridden in England, in France, in Mexico. She is becoming her dream.

Not long ago, Susy and I sat and talked about her perceptions of those early years of Bobby's illness. She surprised me by the frankness and ease with which she spoke.

"It wasn't until I was seven or eight, I think," she said, "that I began to get a real awareness that something was different about him. But I got it from others. It had never occurred to me before that he was in any way ill. For me, he was absolutely normal—at home, everything was natural. He was just a brother, like any brother, whom you beat up and fight with. For me, transfusions were normal and routine . . . like washing behind your ears. I remember wishing I could take peanut pills, too. I liked standing on the back of the wheelchair and whirring around with him. I liked to jump around on his crutches. And when Dr. Engel came to give him transfusions, I had a game. I liked to jump from one end of the transfusion stand to the other. Everybody told me not to do it, but I liked it.

"But from the outside, I began to feel *something*. I would overhear things at school. I heard kids whispering, 'What's the matter with him?' when he was in a wheelchair or on crutches. You know, kids can be mean. They were always staring at him.

"Even later, when I heard the word 'hemophiliac,' I didn't associate it with him somehow. That was for somebody else. When I saw somebody else in a wheelchair it just didn't occur to me that my brother was that way.

"When we fought, I had a big advantage over him—I could run away. I used to slug him and then run away quickly. He depended on his wits to trap me. I was always under restrictions about hitting him, but I used to threaten that I'd hit him with my riding boots or my crop, and that really scared him.

"When he was really sick, I felt bad. I often felt responsible because although you didn't know, I used to slug him in private. I would taunt him and make him run, and when he was sick I used to think it was my fault. Then I was sad, and when everyone was running around taking care of him, I stood looking on. I felt like a shadowy figure and I couldn't do anything, so I would just go away in my room. I used to wish somebody would come and talk to me and tell me it wasn't my fault, but of course you didn't know I did these things. Then when he would get well and start to bug me again, rages would come over me and I'd go pull his hair. Sometimes I got so mad at him because he was so bossy and know-it-all that I wanted to take his crutches away . . . something really mean like that.

"One thing about Bobby: I remember that I knew very early never to show pity. Maybe it was because I sensed that if I did, he would try to take advantage of it. So, after a fight I'd say, 'Go and croak if you want to.'

"I remember a really nice thing he did. Once, when I was eight, I was sent to my room without supper by Granny because I had hit him a lot. It wasn't my fault, and he knew it. He came up secretly and brought me potato chips and a tomato.

"It's true, it was hard for me sometimes. He was always singled out. He was always so intelligent and witty and had something to say. I was shy; I wanted to say things so much. He would get all the attention. I was counted on to be a 'good girl.' I would get bitter and say to myself, 'One of these days I could just die and then they'll see. Then they'll cry.'

"I'm still very touchy about things I hear in school. In science, when they start talking about it, I turn red. There are hemophiliac jokes. Didn't you know? The kids tell them and say things like 'poor twerp hemophiliac,' not knowing about Bobby. And I say, 'My brother has hemophilia,' and they get embarrassed. Even now that he's grown up I don't accept the fact that he is that kind of 'hemophiliac.' To me it seems like a minor obstacle. Bobby is just like any other brother that you get really mad at and really love . . . and hemophilia is like having crossed eyes or split ends in your hair.

"I learned about carriers from an article Daddy wrote. I read it when I was eleven. I had never thought about it at all before, but in that article I read that some girls had trouble getting married. It seemed very strange to me, because I always thought that when you love somebody you take them whether or not there is something wrong with them. My first reaction when I thought about it was, 'Wow! You better get a rich husband!' And then, 'Boy! Am I glad Mom and Dad have been through it and I'll know where to turn for help and I won't have the rocky road that they had learning about it.' Sure, I'll tell my fiancé, so he knows the facts. I want to have a child or two. And now in Biology, when the kids say to me, 'Gee, you know you might be a carrier,' I say, 'So?' I know."

What does Bobby remember about all those school years? I asked him and this is what he answered:

"I remember how scary the brace was, because it was so heavy . . . and I remember books. I read so many. I remember I loved *The Good Master* just like you did when you were a child . . . and a book that Dad read me about a bear and the light. There was one about a runner, a world champion, who had his legs badly burned in a gas explosion and to recover he.ran every day, never walked. I was impressed that he had come from so far behind.

"I never had to tell the kids very much. The teachers had usually explained it. Then the kids were automatically disoriented and immediately prejudiced—they had *heard* about me before they met me. It would have been better if nobody explained.

"About sports—well, if I had thought about it, it might have upset me, so I didn't think about it. It was as if they never existed. It was as if somebody said, 'There are magic carpets, you can ride one.' Well, I didn't have any.

"When the world was in tune with what I wanted it to be, I was happy. When it wasn't, I didn't pay any attention to it. Really, I lived in my own bubble . . . like a spaceman. I was very out of it and totally involved in my own thoughts, in my own world that I had created for myself. I thought of myself as very advanced, very precocious. I liked your friends . . . I used to feel I could talk to them without any qualms, without any feeling that they were older.

"There was nothing at school that stimulated my imagination . . . only what I did at home. I was pretty much in a hurry to grow up. Growing up was the answer to get out of all that dumbness. I remember how amazing it was for me to find how much intellectual activity can distract the mind and alleviate pain.

"I had a whole series of psychological defense lines. I was alone a lot, so much in day-to-day circumstances. So I became independent.

"The marvelous thing was to find out that when you are different already, you can be entirely yourself. To be radically different is to have an enormous advantage. You can be exactly what you want. You can be in many groups at the same time."

But, I asked him, what was the one thing that he wanted to do most and couldn't? Then Bobby, who had been talking steadily, fell silent. Finally he answered, so quietly that I almost couldn't hear him. "Walk," he said.

It happened in the supermarket. Bobby was two, and had a black eye and bruises on his arm. These bruises were not serious; I knew this, and I had ceased to notice them. We were, in fact, very happy that day. But, waiting my turn in the line at the checkout counter, I suddenly became aware that people ahead of me were looking at me disapprovingly and casting sidelong glances at Bobby. I heard the woman ahead of me hiss at the clerk, so that I could hear, "I think people ought to *do* something about people who do things like that to children." I was startled; then in a flash, I understood: they thought I had been *beating* him. Somehow we got through the line and, as fast as I could, I wheeled my cart and Bobby out of the store. After that, I was afraid to go to the supermarket; I dreaded running that gauntlet. I wanted to leave Bobby at home, but I had no one to leave him with, so I tried to hide the bruises as best I could with long-sleeved shirts and big caps.

It was then that I first knew how much my life had changed, and realized that all my relationships with a world I thought I understood had irrevocably altered.

We had thought of ourselves as being just the same, except that this problem had happened to us. But we began to see that the rest of the world did not share our view. In their eyes, we were no longer like everyone else. Somehow we had changed. An invisible barrier had been erected and we were on the other side. We were no longer *normal*.

Why is it that we in America are so afraid of disease?

People were always afraid of us. I could sense this. It was as though they felt that we had been touched with a curse and that too close contact might contaminate them or give them a glimpse of an unpleasant reality they wanted to avoid having to face.

We have such an ideal of physical perfection in our twentieth-century American life: eternal youth, health, shiny teeth, firm breasts, luxuriant hair, everything deodorized and polished. It is as if repeating over and over that we are perfect will make us so; as if, by presenting a perfect outside shell, everything will be perfect inside. Any deviation from this shining ideal is to be avoided, and, if it is not possible to avoid, then only glanced at sideways, quickly and guiltily, before fleeing. By thus setting aside and avoiding those who are different, do we not create fear and even loathing? Do we not shut away a perception of God's purpose and deprive ourselves of wholeness and reality?

Early in our experience I realized that the world would accept us—and Bobby—only to the extent that we did not bother them too much. That is, if we pretended. If we looked like them and acted like them, it would be all right. We had to remake ourselves in their image; they did not reach out to understand our world. Our world frightened them, with its echoes of pain, helplessness, and desperation. I mean, what would they do if we actually broke down and wept in front of them? They were afraid of such responsibilities. And I, sensing this fear, realized that to maintain any contact at all, we had to cheer them up. We had to create an atmosphere of calm, of matter-of-factness, so that they would not be afraid to approach us. If we looked cheerful, if we looked in charge, they could risk the contact. And so I found myself constantly reassuring people, soothing them, by explaining that they had no need to be afraid, there was nothing to it, really.

I withdrew behind this façade of confidence. No one would know, I vowed, the despair. In fact, the more despairing I felt, the more I tried to project calm. I think it is impossible ever to shed this habit. When I felt most totally pessimistic, which was most of the time, I argued for optimism. (People still keep saying to me, "But you are so sunny, so energetic!") This elaborately erected façade was necessary, because if I had allowed what I felt to show, it would, like a terrible force unleashed, have destroyed me.

But, behind the façade, how I hated it all! I got sick of being asked, "How are you?"—that all-purpose, meaningless formula that sets up barriers of false interest between us. There is only one answer: "I am fine." Any other answer is unacceptable. Imagine the startled surprise if I had answered, "I am in despair."

How I resented their questions, those questions which ignored the fact that I had feelings, questions that made me feel like some kind of strange specimen. They examined me with their curious, prying remarks like, "That's funny. I thought it was only a royal disease." Or, more callously, they would say importantly, intelligently, to Bob: "Oh, yes; your wife passed it on to your son." Or to me, "You gave it to your son, isn't that right?" Or, "Doesn't that mean you are afraid of every scratch? Isn't he going to die? Aren't you terribly frightened? Don't you feel guilty?" (And when I tried to explain, defensively, that over 40 per cent of the cases had no history whatsoever, most of the time my questioner would look at me as if I were lying and say, huffily, "Why, I never heard that!")

Over the years, we learned to explain, to give little mechanical lectures, as if none of these questions hurt . . . and we taught Bobby to explain.

Then there was pity. People drench you in it, which is not at all what you need. They whisper behind your back, "Oh, poor parents! Oh, poor child!" From well-dressed ladies with smoothly organized lives, over and over I heard the same refrain: "I just don't know how you do it. I know I couldn't." As if I had wanted to cope, as if anyone wants to struggle and suffer for the pleasure of it. I felt like hitting them. Instead, I thanked them for their concern. But I hate pity. It is a weak emotion, an easy, socially acceptable emotion, one that all too often serves simply to keep us aloof from one another and from the demanding, disturbing realities of human anguish. Compassion is what is needed. But compassion demands stronger emotions: love and courage, sacrifice and discipline.

I grew to hate society, that fat, happy, untormented society that did not want to see me. They were well. They were happy. They could make plans, they had a future. Resentment curdled my soul and came boiling out in unreasoning angers—I would shout at drivers in other cars.

Later, of course, as I began to look beneath the surface, I found that no one's life was simple. But then I felt alone and defiant

—that it was me and my family against the world. I withdrew. More and more, I longed to retire and find another level of understanding, a place where I could nurse my wounds and not have to put on a bright face. There seemed to be two ways: to leave the world, to hide. Or, to do battle and conquer and achieve power, which is another way of being left alone to feel and act as you like. I got so sick of hearing, "Poor Sue; she has such a hard life," that I vowed that one day those same people would say, "Lucky Sue; she has the most interesting life of anyone I know."

The ostracism and isolation were almost harder to adapt to than the disease itself. More than ever, we needed the help and comfort of close human contact. We needed friends. In our situation, they were essential. But old friends whom we had loved were far away. New ones became harder and harder to find.

To be sure, all along the way we found many well-meaning acquaintances. Many people offered individual acts of kindness, moments of understanding and help. For these, I was always grateful. But there was something in their personalities, or in mine, that stood in the way of intimacy. I guess most people just didn't want to become involved—too many problems of their own. I had the feeling, too, that people were a little embarrassed by my intensity, that they found something a little uncouth and excessive about it. The whole thing was to remain cool, and at least outwardly in control of one's emotions. Unfortunately, I was neither cool nor in control.

Hemophilia had wiped out any interest or ability I might have had for superficial relationships. It sharpened my need for knowing the essentials and made me impatient with social trivialities. I wanted to know about the loves, the hates, the struggles of others. But in the suburbs you don't easily talk about these things. Where we lived, the women talked about the PTA and their children's activities. How could I participate in conversations about children's activities when my child could never join them? I was not interested in small talk, or chatter over coffee. I could never make plans ahead. I couldn't go out for lunches. I hated bridge. Anyway, I keenly felt the one-sidedness of these relationships. The people I knew had trouble occasionally. We seemed to be having trouble all the time.

We were monotonous with our eternal problems. People respond well when there is a single crisis. They send flowers, they send cards, they break away from work to come to visit . . . as long as it is temporary. But when somebody is always sick, people tend to lose interest. They grow bored asking, "How is Bobby?" and always hearing the same answer, "It isn't good; he's sick." Very soon there are no more cards, no more telephone calls, and worse, no more visits.

In any case, whom could I ask to go to the hospital in the middle of the night? Whom could I ask to shoulder such fatigue, such responsibility? I hesitated to impose this even on my own parents. Through the years, they did occasionally come to spell us, but I could see the fatigue and strain these days caused my mother. To spare them, I had to remain in control.

We had no money, so I could have no help, not even a person I could hire to come in for an afternoon just to sit and read with Bobby while I took a walk. There was no one to take him for an outing, no uncles, no aunts, no cousins.

I cannot remember a single friend who was near us in the early days of Bobby's illness. My college friends were all conducting lives of supreme normality. My catastrophe only confirmed in their minds the fact that I had always been "different." We were living in a modest apartment development populated by people totally unrelated to us in background or interest . . . it was as though we were living on an island.

In that apartment development, there was a little grassy area behind our ground-floor kitchen door. To protect Bobby and to keep him from roaming once he began to walk, Bob took a little piece of land under our window and proceeded to try to erect a little fence around it. One husky, beer-bellied neighbor swaggered over aggressively and snarled, "That's not yours." Bob tried to explain the problem. The neighbor fixed him with a look of contempt, but Bob stiffened and kept digging his fence post hole. The neighbor finally backed off, growling. In this minuscule yard, Bobby played in a sandbox and then in a tiny plastic wading pool. Other children stood outside and watched. Bobby was very friendly and always wanted them to come in and play. Very rarely, their parents allowed them to. Bob sat nearby and pretended to read his book and be invisible.

By the time we were able to move out of that apartment into a little house, I didn't want to know anybody.

Living with hemophilia was to live off balance all the time. I learned that there was only one thing I could absolutely count on and that was that I could never count on anything. Not plans, not vacations, not hopes, not anything. All of us, without realizing it, live mostly in the future. At least half of our lives is consumed in thinking and dreaming of tomorrow. With hemophilia, there is no tomorrow, at least never a tomorrow you can rely on. And certain it is that, should you begin to count on tomorrow, to permit yourself for one moment a timid confidence, the disease, as if it were malevolently conscious, will plot to destroy your plans and your fragile confidence—just to show its power.

This tantalizing promise of normality was the most exhausting part of living with hemophilia. I felt helpless, in the hands of a merciless monster who operated by rules totally mysterious and illogical. Almost everyone can cope with a crisis, so long as it lasts a short time and is not repeated too often. The human soul can survive and adapt to the most difficult condition, so long as this condition is stable and its outline clear; so long as the victim knows what he must fight. But with hemophilia there is no status quo. Unpredictably, everything could change drastically from day to day, even from hour to hour. Bobby might be well and running about happily in the morning, only to be in horrible pain a few hours later. Try as I might, like the father of Sleeping Beauty, to hide all the spindles in the kingdom, somewhere where I least expected it a spindle lay waiting.

We were living in a disordered world, a world without reason. I learned that no case was like another case, that there could be no way at all to predict what Bobby would or would not have to go through by examining the experience of others. The experience of others only deepened the questions. Everything might hang on totally irrational factors: the season, Bobby's mood, chance, luck. Quickly, in such a world, you grow superstitious. You look for signs. You begin to search for any kind of explanation, however odd; you begin to search for miracles. And you learn never to talk about good fortune, because it is Bad Luck. Something is sure to happen.

The ancient Chinese, I have heard, never talked about good fortune. Instead, they wailed loudly, "Woe is me! How terrible!" when something *good* happened. This was to placate the unfriendly gods who might only be lying in wait for a happy human so that they could strike him down and assert their domination over him.

I quickly understood this philosophy. It seemed that we had only to say "Bobby is fine, thank you," to bring on some new blow. So by silent agreement Bob and I would never talk together about how "well" Bobby was doing, or how "successfully" we seemed to be dealing with a given episode. Even in company, when I was absolutely forced to say out loud, "Yes, he is doing well," I would try to say it as quickly and quietly as possible, and then surreptitiously try to knock on wood somewhere . . . the floor, when nothing else was available. This I did by seeming to bend down and pick up my handkerchief. How quickly we are reduced to reliance on such symbols! For it always seemed that at the very moment I permitted a hope to rise in my soul, the disease would strike again, wreaking the maximum emotional havoc. Try as I might to prepare, a new attack would come from an entirely other direction. It could hit anytime, anywhere. I tried to stay in an emotional state of alert at all times. But no one can stay at peak alert twenty-four hours a day. You weaken, you allow yourself to be happy, allow yourself to grow timidly confident. That is when it strikes. Each time you are defenseless.

There is nothing to do but learn to live with fear, in constant dread of the unknown. Such a way of life does strange things to the personality. Fear can grip and dominate you until you are unable to move in any direction. A person living with hemophilia can finally become paralyzed with fright, like a rat in a maze who has met with an electric shock at every innocent-looking exit until finally he simply turns frantically in circles, afraid to try any more doors.

Interrogators know this technique well. It is by using this fear of the unknown, by being arbitrary, by falling on their victims when they are least prepared, that they erode the personality. A prisoner is made to face an ordeal which, without reason, is suddenly eased, only to have another crisis fall on him again when he has been lulled into the belief that he is the master of his pain and fear. This arbitrary, bewildering treatment can break the will more surely than pain itself.

During a crisis, I was possessed by a strange tense calm. I could fight. I *knew* what had to be faced. Such a strange feeling of release would suffuse me! It made me feel guilty sometimes. I would breathe a sigh of relief; it was only a knee. I knew about knees. The bad time was *after* the crisis, that apprehensive waiting for the next blow, wondering what it might be, from what direction it might come.

It is late at night that raw panic comes. And despair. Lying in bed, sleepless, I could feel my heart pounding fiercely in my chest, dominating the stillness of the night. Waves of anxiety rolled over me. My hands were clammy. Where? What? When? When?

Exhausted by my thoughts, finally I would sleep—only to be pursued by nightmares. Always in these dreams Bobby, or one of the girls, is out of reach and dying. I try to reach them, but I cannot. My limbs are heavy and I cannot lift them. I see Bobby lying on the sand at the bottom of a great, deep dry well. I cannot go down. Or, I am caught in an elevator and he is falling off the top of a building. Or I have lost Susy and I search the streets and she is gone. When I woke from these dreams, covered in sweat and weeping, I would lie in the dark, shaking for hours, sometimes until dawn. These nightmares were so real that I would have to force myself to go into the children's bedroom to see if they were still there, and, even when I saw them and heard them breathing, I did not believe.

Statistics tell us dryly that suicides are most frequent in those dark hours before morning. How I longed for a human voice! But it is unthinkable to call anyone in the middle of the night. Certainly

not after 10:00. One's best friend . . . well, perhaps 11:30. But at
2:00? Who could be so good-tempered? Yet that is when, do what
you will, the fear comes over you. What will be next? Will he fall?
Will it be serious? Can I stand it? What happens if I can't? And
the girls? What if something should touch them?

Sometimes, when Bob was away and I was alone, nearly overcome, I would go and stand by the phone, trying to find the
courage to dial a number, running over in my mind the friends I
could count on. And I would decide there were none. I leaned my
head against the wall, banging it silently, and would sob until I
exhausted myself.

Once I even put my head in the gas oven. But I chickened out.

One thing I knew. I would have to find the courage to let go.
I had to learn to control my overwhelming desire to be awake
every minute, to be alert every second, to try and outthink the child
and Fate. For this was the way to madness—as futile as asking the
rain to stop falling. Trying to get up the courage to step out of the
house was excruciatingly hard. At first, I would make myself do
this only at night, when I knew Bobby would be sleeping and the
risks minimal. But finding babysitters was a serious problem. You
had to gauge their character, their fortitude, their calm. Then,
having judged the complicated human equation for yourself, you
had to be extremely careful how you explained it to them. Many
refused to come. The best were the young student nurses at the
nearby hospital and older ladies with the calm equanimity of age.
But, even to the best among them, you didn't explain too much.
It might frighten them away. No; you had to project calm. We
went out, leaving a paper trail of numbers where we could be
reached at every moment. Then, after the door closed behind us,
I had to fight for control, to make myself go through with it. At
times, during an evening, as talk swirled around me, I was taken
with unreasonable chilling attacks of fear. (Perhaps there is an
emergency. Maybe the phone doesn't work. Maybe she is too
scared to call.) I wanted to get up and go home as fast as I could.
But I forced myself to stay, to sit, to talk.

Wherever we were, when the phone rang I was certain that it

was for us. Almost always, it was. I remember one night we were attending a UN dinner. As we were being served I heard, through the thick swinging doors that separated the dining room from the kitchen, the distant sound of a telephone. I stopped, frozen, in mid-sentence. "It's for me!" I gasped. The ambassador who was my dinner partner was startled, but he saw in my face that my fear was real. Gently, he said to me, "No. Don't be afraid. Surely it isn't." But it was. A few moments later, a servant came through the swinging doors and asked for me.

We had to leave precipitately from parties. Each of the few times that we were able to save up for theater tickets, at the last minute we could not go and had to lose them and forget the cost. So we gave up going. We rarely went to the movies because of the fear that in theaters we might not be found in the crowd. When we did go, we would, like doctors, stop at the box office, explain our problem and then carefully show the usher where we were sitting. Even then, I would hear the telephones ringing distantly at the box office and worry that somehow they had forgotten our instructions. In the middle of the film I would get up and go ask. We began to watch a lot of TV. At least then I could relax— Bobby was in the next room.

Sleep meant giving up vigilance, so I did not sleep. I stayed up until exhaustion annihilated me. I read, I worked, I watched late movies, I wandered aimlessly around the silent, sleeping house. The price of eternal vigilance is fatigue, crushing fatigue.

The days became harder and harder to face. I awoke in the morning with a lump in my stomach and it never went away. Sometimes my first reaction on opening my eyes in the morning was to cry.

Confined. Trapped. My bones ached, my arms and legs felt like heavy weights, too heavy to drag around. It was an effort to move. As if I were in training, I had to tell myself: Walk. Bring your arm into the air. Bring it down. Scrub that pot. Make it shinier. I would meticulously wash and minutely scrape the corners of the kitchen floor, scrubbing on my hands and knees until the sweat poured off my face—physical effort took the pain away a little. I threw myself into cooking, because it kept both mind and hands active. Kneading bread was a blessed release. Push down, slap, push down, slap, down and around, again and again, feeling the tension leave my shoulders as the yeast came alive, and the dough grew silky and elastic under my hands. I beat eggs and sugar together until the mixture was fine and light and lemony and made beautiful ribbons as it fell off the spoon. I made cookies. I chopped things fine and still finer. I composed elaborate menus. They were my only distraction and through them I traveled the world . . . to the places I had already seen and loved and now were denied me, and to those I dreamed of and thought I would never see.

I devised mental exercises for myself. I said to myself, if I can find one beautiful thing each day and study it, perhaps I will get through until tomorrow. So I studied nature around me. I would stand transfixed before a magnolia tree. I would find a flower, and without picking it, stand gazing, gazing, to find the universe in its heart. I would remember that single flower all day. Another day it might be a bird that I could observe from my window, or a sunset, or a cloud. I clung to them.

I found a sweet relief in listening to the more solvable problems of others. I call this the Mary Worth syndrome. People, even those I did not know very well, began to unburden themselves to me. They told me tales of unrequited love, of jealousy, of family bickering and slights. How simple all these things seemed to me! How wise I could be! It gave me a seductive illusion of power. When one's own problems are unsolvable, and all best efforts frustrated, it is life-saving to listen to other people's problems. Some of them you can do something about; and helping somebody is fighting back, almost like being in control yourself.

Yet sometimes, while driving down a road or walking along the street, for no reason at all I would suddenly burst into tears.

And yet . . . I dare not admit despair, because I know that if I do, it will engulf me, sending me whirling down into terrifying regions close to insanity. But it is there, nevertheless, lurking. When

I look in the mirror, I see it there sometimes, behind my eyes. It is closest in the bright days of sunshine, when the air is sweet and the flowers in bloom, when the grass smells cut and the world looks so beautiful and gay, and I know it is not for me. The pain is sharpest then, or when I am with friends and their children are tumbling and running so naturally, not realizing that every muscle movement, every bend of a knee is a miracle. Why should they, why should my friends know? But the weight in my own stomach grows heavier and the monster waits because it knows that victory is closer.

I am happier when it rains or when fog obscures the sharp outlines of the everyday world . . . and when we are in action it retreats . . . as long as one can fight, struggle, work.

Evil is near. Sometimes late at night the air grows strangely clammy and cold around me. I feel it brushing me.

All that the Devil asks is acquiescence . . . not struggle, not conflict. Acquiescence. Accept, accept that I have won, whispers the Devil. You can see for yourself that life is unjust, unfair, that suffering is ordinary. Who is stronger? I am, of course. Just despair, my dear, despair. Only tell me that I am strong, that Evil rules. Your own eyes show you the truth of it. Your own heart feels my grip. Only accept that this is so. Give yourself to me. Proclaim my truth.

I remember one night careening over the roads to the hospital. I shook my fist at the darkness, angry tears burning my cheeks, and I cried "No! *No!*" to nobody in particular. But I felt the reality of the conversation.

Sometime after Bobby's cerebral bleeding, as the pressure grew more intense, I realized that to keep my mind intact, to keep from turning around in my cage like a panic-stricken animal, I had to do something hard, something mentally challenging. It had to be something so difficult that it would, by its own force, wrench my mind away from the unresolvable mysteries that tormented me

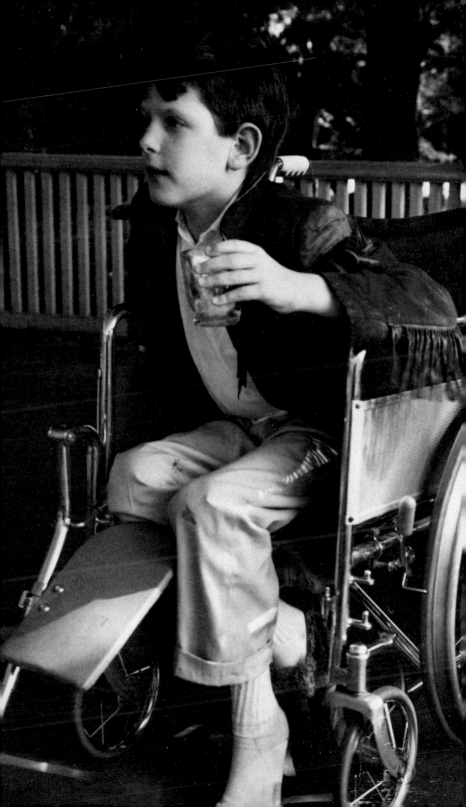

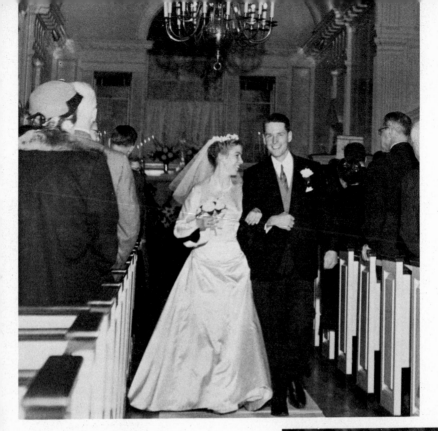

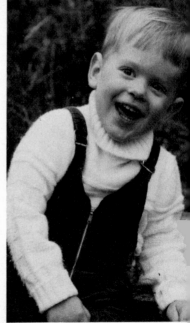

(Overleaf) Spring, 1966. Bobby, age nine, during a period of repeated severe joint bleeding.

(Above) Our wedding day, December 18, 1954, Church of the Good Shepherd in Philadelphia.

(Right) Bobby, age two, before any of his joint bleedings, playing in our backyard in White Plains.

(Opposite, top) Bobby, age eight, Susanna, age six.

(Opposite, bottom) Elizabeth, age two, with Bob.

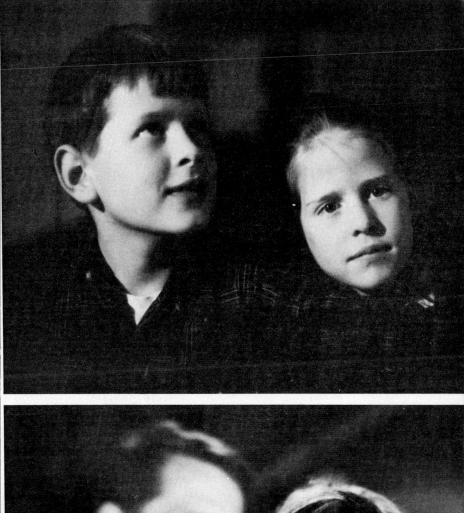
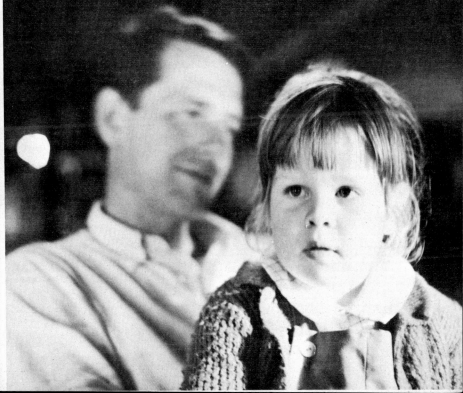

IN MAINE

(Below) The cabin.

(Bottom, left) Bobby and Davey on our beach.

(Bottom, center) Picnicking on the rocky ledges of Conary Cove the summer *Nicholas and Alexandra* was published.

(Opposite, top) Susy wins a ribbon for riding. Bobby, age seven, is wearing his left leg brace. With them are two friends from the Red House, Roger Morse and Davey Gardner.

(Opposite, bottom) Bobby, age eleven, having a transfusion in the doctor's office in Stonington.

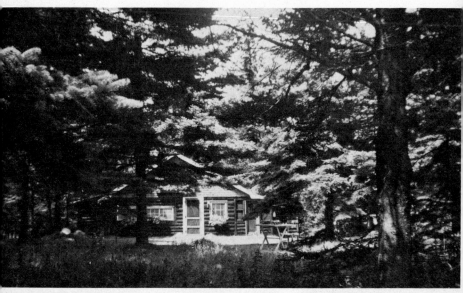

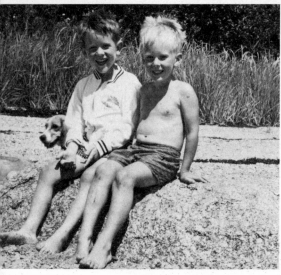

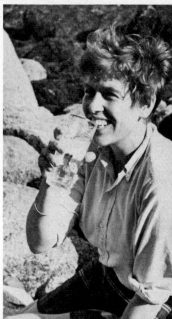

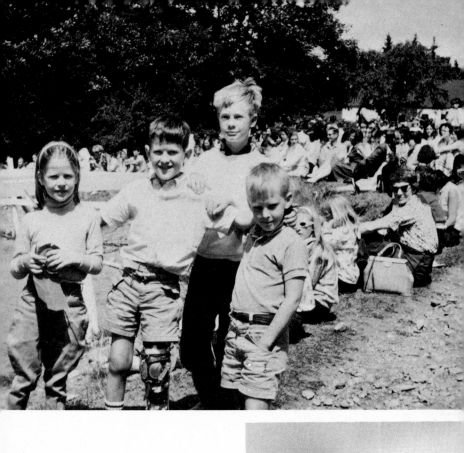

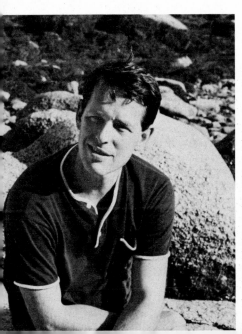

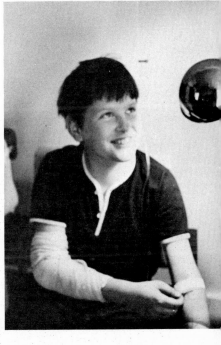

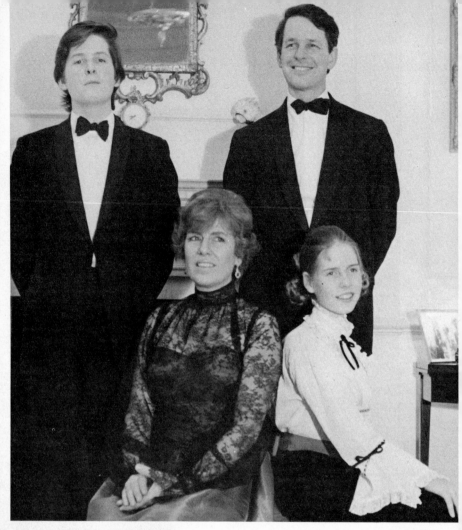

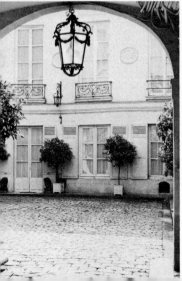

(*Above*) The evening of the London première of *Nicholas and Alexandra*.

(*Left*) The courtyard of our apartment, rue de la Cerisaie, Paris.

(*Opposite, top*) After the New York première. Bobby playing the banjo with Paul Stookey and Peter Yarrow and singing "Weave Me the Sunshine."

(*Opposite, bottom*) At Princeton, to build endurance and strengthen his legs and joints, Bobby lifts weights and swims two to three hours daily.

(*Overleaf*) Bobby today, age eighteen.

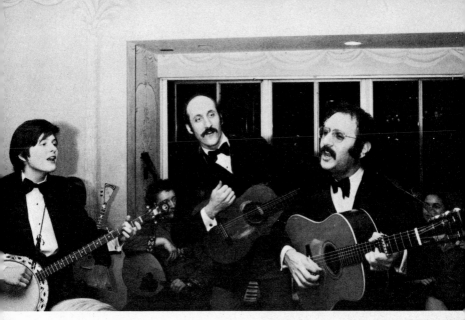

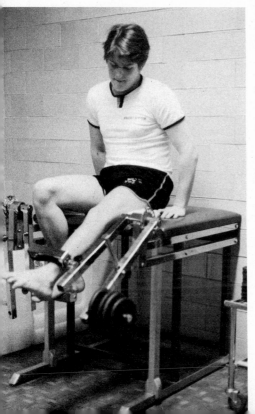

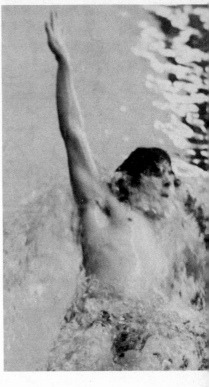

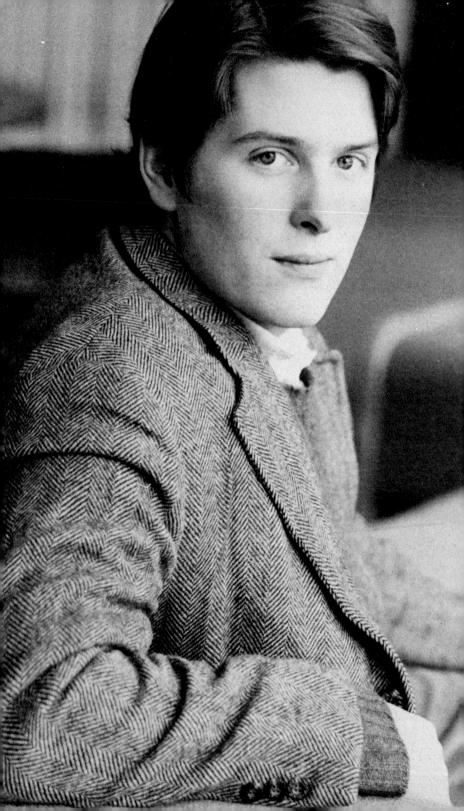

every day. To this day, after it has become the thrust of my life, I do not know what inner voice directed me. But I began to study Russian.

Was it a whispered wish of the Almighty? Was it because my mother, who had lived five years in Russia, had, in my childhood, conjured up for me a picture of color and life, force and passion? I have always loved Russian music and Russian dancing. I cannot remember when I didn't know about great dancers. I studied ballet and wanted to become a dancer. My father did not approve of such a career, and although I studied for ten years it never went further.

Individual Russians had appeared and reappeared in my life. When I was a child, a Russian sea captain from Kiev used to come and visit our house. It was during the war. He was captain of one of the Red Cross ships that docked in Philadelphia. He and my mother sat at the old upright piano in our house and sang Russian songs together. When he came he always brought gifts— but such gifts! Never just one—seven boxes of chocolate, seven dolls. I remember him perfectly to this day, Captain Tsolnikov, with his gray crew-cut hair and his bushy gray mustache.

At the age of five in Paris, my mother took me to the studio of the great Mikhail Mordkin, one of the finest ballet dancers of prerevolutionary days. His studio seemed cavernous and he as tall as a giant. He held a long, slim stick, which he used to fleck the legs of those who were not working hard enough. My mother's stories of his love for the ballerina Balachova stayed with me. For her, their *Swan Lake* was immortal.

Mother had been a friend of the glamorous Balachova. I cut my baby teeth on a small enamel Fabergé Easter egg set with a diamond that my mother wore on a golden chain around her neck. This had been a present from Balachova. They corresponded through the years of my childhood; I dreamed of one day meeting her. The once dazzling ballerina died in poverty and obscurity in a small undistinguished suburb of Paris before I could reach her, yet because of my mother's stories, she remained vividly alive in my imagination.

Why was it that all these people implanted themselves so firmly in my mind when so much else has long ago been forgotten?

Whenever I met Russians, they always looked at me intensely. Often they would hug me and say in their rippling musical accents, "Suzanne, you have a Russian soul." I did not know what they meant. What I did know was that I found something so touching and warm about these Russians, something so full of fantasy, inexplicable and impractical, tender and explosive, that my spirit felt more at ease, more natural with them. They had suffered. You could feel this. Through their experience they had learned the craft of living with grief and unfulfilled hopes and had pierced through to another dimension of life. It seemed that from this plateau they could glimpse even more.

Why I had not started studying Russian sooner, I cannot explain. Perhaps I needed the weight of grief, the challenge of sorrow, to drive me to it. I wanted to pierce through my own despair and gain access to the secrets that the language held. We had no money. I could not dream of private lessons. My children were too small. It was impossible to think of school. Yet one day I learned that the Adult Education Program at the White Plains High School was offering a Russian-language course. The cost: $8 a semester. The sum was modest enough even for us, so I enrolled. When I went to class the first night, I saw a diminutive woman, almost dwarfed by the large desk. Her face would have been quite severe, if not for a broad and teasing smile that crossed her face sometimes, lighting up her dark brown eyes. Her name was Svetlana. I talked to her at the end of the class for a short while. "Suzanne," she said abruptly, "you have a Russian soul." From then on she was my friend.

This study saved my equilibrium and my sanity. Those mysterious characters seemed to be a code that would unlock those qualities of forbearance and faith I had observed. While I worked with them, I could think of nothing else. The language has never disappointed me. It is rich and challenging enough for several lifetimes, a never-ending source of joy, a wonder of human communication. And to me, it has always sounded like music. I have had to abandon my study many times because of the events and pressures of Bobby's illness. I feel frustrated and envious when I see around me students who actually have had the luxury of exams and tests, earphones and professors. My idea of a perfect vacation would be an intensive Russian-language course in Leningrad.

I became a beggar—me, a Swiss, proud and independent, accustomed to relying only on myself and my own energy. Hemophilia turned me into a beggar. We needed things all the time. I would have to ask over and over to leave Susy with neighbors while I went to the hospital. I was begging for companionship for Bobby. I was begging for blood.

Our Protestant-American ethic teaches that if you work hard enough and try hard enough, you will overcome. If you don't overcome, it is because you don't work hard enough or try hard enough. But what happens when you work and try and still cannot change things? What if there is no way to change things? Then what?

Blacks know about this. Russians know about this. I was learning.

For I worked and Bob worked as hard as we could, and we still could not get enough money to care for our child. The most frightening thing, the most embittering thing, is to have a sick child and no matter how hard you try, not to be able to provide for him.

Money was a terrible problem, but the need for blood was worse. This was a need I alone could never overcome, against which energy and pride were useless. Even if I had opened my veins and poured out all my blood, it would not have been enough. In order to survive, I had to depend on the charity of others . . . the life of my son depended on it.

Humility is a hard lesson. As Christ said, the hardest.

I went around begging for blood from everyone I knew. I heard all the excuses. It seems that in the United States every second person has hepatitis or malaria hidden in some dim corner of his or her medical history. Or has a cold. Or is anemic. Or has veins that are too small. The men, usually even more afraid than women, are "too busy." After turning me down, people would often say, "Of course, if you really *need* blood, I'll give it, of course." (We needed it. We always needed it.) What was left unspoken was, "if he were dying . . ." But blood for his day-to-day living, they made clear, that would have to be taken care of by others . . . strangers preferably. So servile and dissembling did I become that I got very good at smoothing over this awkward moment by saying, as if I were profusely grateful, "Thank you. Don't worry a bit about it. If we really need it, we'll call you." Then they were relieved.

One day I realized that I could not ask anymore. No matter how hard I tried to be charitable, no matter how little I showed what I felt, I was too angry and hurt when people turned me down in person. I felt humiliated. I despised their cowardice. In any case, when people are afraid, they also feel guilty and would prefer not to see you anymore. So if I wanted to preserve any friendships at all, I should avoid asking, so as not to embarrass them.

To those who did give, I felt so beholden! I couldn't do anything but smile at them forever, no matter how I felt. If they wanted to stop over and talk for hours, convenient or inconvenient, I had to accept it. Whatever they wanted, I had to grant it. Because I never could do anything in return. The burden of eternal gratitude is intolerable. We needed them too much, too often. They never needed anything from us. It is terrible to be dependent! You cannot love other people when you are dependent upon them for something so vital. But what to do? The need was still there—if not to friends and acquaintances, where could I go?

I tried the church. More out of a kind of superstition than any deep religious conviction, faithfully, every Sunday, I had been attending services in a little Episcopal church not far from us in Elmsford. But this calm, well-meaning suburban church with its chatty coffee hour seemed pale to me. There was nothing there that spoke of passions or trials; only politely ordered doses of morality. While the minister delivered his sermon I would concentrate on the windows, on the ceiling, trying to find some inner peace. It was nice, sitting calm like that for an hour. Each Sunday, as I greeted him at the door, the minister would ask, "And how is Bobby?" He seemed interested. Well, I thought, maybe they might help. One day, after I had been attending the church for many months, I finally permitted myself to approach the minister timidly at the coffee hour and ask, "Do you think it might be possible to put up a small notice on the church bulletin board to ask if those who regularly give blood might give it to the credit of Bobby?" His answer was quick. "Oh no, Mrs. Massie; we couldn't possibly do that! Why, if I permitted you to put up a notice like that there's no telling how many appeals people might want to put up!" I fled that church and never returned.

A few years later, when we moved to Irvington, it happened that the minister of the Episcopal church, David Matlack, was the older brother of a friend I had known in high school. I had heard many good things about him. I sent Bobby to Sunday school, but I never went to church myself.

One night, I ran into him at a party and he said to me, "Why don't you come and talk to me about Bobby? We'd like to help if we can." But I didn't go.

Some months later, I happened to run into him again at a crowded party. He came over to me and said quietly, "Forgive me for asking you to come to me. I should have come to you."

The next day, the doorbell rang. It was a woman from the church guild. The church was organizing a blood drive for Bobby. Did we mind? Did we have any suggestions?

With his gentle words, David Matlack had showed me what I had become. Resentful and proud, I had created my own walls. And I was ashamed, for I saw that it was not humility that I had been learning; it was only bitterness.

Locked in my solitary bitterness, I was no longer noticing that if there were all those people who did not give, there were also many others who, for no reason at all, without even being asked, did, quietly and without fanfare. Sometimes we did not even learn of blood donations until the names were sent to us later. Much of the time we did not know these people personally. They would just hear about us from friends, or friends of friends, or even the newspapers . . . then they went and gave their blood.

And when it comes to blood donations, policemen are soft touches. They never turn you down. I never hear the word "pigs" without resenting it, without wondering whether those who call policemen names have ever volunteered to give a pint of blood. What I have seen is a horde of motorcycle policemen, all strangers, roar up to the White Plains County Center where a blood drive was being held for two Westchester hemophiliacs, one of them Bobby. Neatly, they 'parked their ferocious-looking vehicles in ranks in front of the building. Inside the cavernous hall I saw them, rows of burly men, stretched out like so many pieces of beef, with their blue sleeves rolled up and their helmets on the chair beside them. When they were through, they all got up and roared off again. I don't know why they did it, but I remember.

And there was a Russian friend of mine who gave blood at Christmas "because that is all I have to give."

Bobby might not be alive today but for this unseen, unsolicited sense of brotherhood.

Thanks to Dave Matlack, I saw that it was my own vulnerability that I had not wanted to accept, my own pride that made gratitude such a heavy burden. Once I accepted this, the burden was lightened. Need does not come to everyone at exactly the same time. Good cannot be repaid on a one-to-one basis. It is not a static thing, but a circle, continuously in motion. Almost surely I could never directly repay the help that others were giving us. But, by waiting patiently, the moment would come when I, in my turn, could pass my gratitude along to someone else, someone perhaps whom only I could help. That person might never wish to thank me, nor be able to return my favor in kind.

The process was not like getting and giving Christmas presents, but more like throwing a pebble into the water. It is impossible to see the limit of the ripples that grow in an ever-widening circle until they disappear into infinity. The important thing is to throw the pebble.

And as for friends, was I not being greedy? Why did I ask for so many? What is friendship, anyway?

There are times when you need a friend every day; there are other times when it might be nice to have one but you can make it alone if you have to. The true friend knows the difference. However you try to dissemble it, he always can discern the authentic cry for help. And he is there. No matter what the hour, convenient or inconvenient. He knows that you need him at that very moment

—not tomorrow, not next week. By next week you may be happy, or you may be dead. This quality is the essence of friendship. The French have a good word for it—*disponible*, which means to be ready to be useful, to be *available*. A true friend is always *disponible*. With him, no formal codes apply. There are no hours when you cannot call, no times when you cannot drop in. Happy or sad, he will receive you.

The finest compliment one human being can pay another is to feel that he can lay open his weakness and grief and do this without fear of rejection, safe in the knowledge that his stupidities and intrusions will be forgiven, that both the sublime and the foolish will be listened to. To be a friend takes time, and time is what nobody has. Therefore, real friends are rare. A person can count himself lucky if he has one. I now realize that I was unbelievably lucky: even during my most difficult years, I had two.

I met Janet Dowling at the house of a mutual friend, a college classmate of mine, when Bobby was three years old. Janet is tall and blond with amber-brown eyes and a gentle manner. She went to Connecticut College and she has lived all her life in the suburbs of New York City. There was no reason at all to think that she would understand any better than my college friends did, nothing to distinguish her from the people I had learned to think of as "them." Yet I had met that day an expert in the art of friendship.

Janet is the most giving person I know. She tends to the community around her in countless unspectacular ways. She delivers hot meals to housebound old people. She serves on juries. When someone is sick, she is the one who has time to stop and visit, bring flowers, and send a cheery word. She renders innumerable small acts of friendship to an army of friends and acquaintances quietly, unobtrusively. God knows, most of us must be a terrible disappointment to her, but she never shows it.

To do all this and still manage a large house and a busy household, three children (two of them small), two dogs, a cat, plus a stream of dinner guests, Janet gets up at 5 A.M. every morning.

Yet we have been friends for fourteen years and I cannot remember a single moment when Janet was not there when we needed her. She offered her blood without being asked, and regularly, through the years, keeps right on giving it. Especially when Bobby was small, we needed people to pick up plasma for us. It was hard to ask. A few people offered. Janet was the first. There was a time when we were abandoned by all acquaintances and friends and no one ever invited us to dinner. Janet did. Over the years, Dick Dowling has lavished friendship and generosity on us, but as long as I live, I will never forget that when Bobby was four years old, Janet and Dick invited us to dinner at the Larchmont Yacht Club. We had not set foot inside a restaurant for over a year. We could not possibly have afforded such a luxury. I dressed for this dinner with the excitement of a girl going to her first dance. How glamorous, how exciting it was! No restaurant dinner since then has been as important to me as that one, which was offered when all dreams looked shattered, all ambitions dashed; when the cage was narrow.

With her friends, Janet rides up and down the waves of life. No matter what happens, she is always the same: understanding, patient, sharing triumphs with unreserved joy, and grief with compassion. Whatever happens, she offers herself, to serve. She listens without judging—observing personalities, adapting to their needs, demanding nothing. By now, her company is as natural to me as breathing . . . and as necessary.

They must have been thinking of Elizabeth Campbell Parks when they coined the phrase "black is beautiful." I have been with her, feeling like the Infanta's dwarf, when some awed male would approach her in breathless homage and say, as if surprised by his own temerity before such a goddess, "Excuse me, but I *have* to tell you that you are beautiful." Liz would look a little shy, but would smile her vulnerable, happy smile.

Liz's father was the great cartoonist E. Simms Campbell, the creator of the famous harem girls of *Esquire* magazine. As a child, she lived in Hastings, New York, on a large estate, a pampered daughter of a member of black society. Then her father, in disgust at the discrimination in the United States, moved to Switzerland, where Liz grew up, blossomed, and began to live the exotic life of the expatriate international beauty. Somehow, through it all, she remained down-to-earth, simple, loving; not in the least narcissistic despite the attention lavished on her. The possibilities of a glittering career as a model were spread before her. She turned them all down. "That life is too superficial," she said. With Liz, it is the heart that counts. Appropriately enough, she was born on St. Valentine's Day.

When I met Liz, Bobby was six and she had just married Gordon Parks, the famous photographer-director whom I had known during my *Life* reporting days.

I was down and nearly finished, scraping for pennies, wearing an old coat without buttons, feeling dowdy and forgotten. Liz would come to see me. The door would fly open with a burst of fresh air and I would hear, "Wellll, how are you, you old . . . !" Then she would envelop me in a big bear hug which smelled deliciously of her expensive perfume. ("I throw that on to get the funk off," she'd say. That remark became a household expression, like so many of Liz's imaginative phrases.) Then she would head for the kitchen, throw open the icebox, and nibble whatever she found there. She brought me luxuries I could never afford but which I adored: champagne, pâté, a beautiful piece of Brie cheese, and with them, hopes and dreams for better days.

If I was downcast about our endless scrimping, our empty, unfurnished, windowshade-less house, she'd say, "What the hell, Sue, your house isn't empty, because it's furnished in your own mind!" One day when Bob was away on a story and I was lonely, Liz came over for supper, wrapped in a glamorous, fuzzy, floor-length fur coat, swinging a bottle of expensive Bordeaux. We talked and drank so much that neither of us noticed that the snow had been falling steadily. When we finally looked up, her Jaguar was buried in a snowdrift in our driveway. We were snowed in together for three days. Liz made snowmen with the children, we opened cans, we forgot that there were troubles in the world.

The children adored her. She made them giggle until they nearly burst with pleasure. She played games with them and I would hear Liz and Bobby laughing uproariously over nothing. Bobby wrote in his diary after one of her visits: "I really like Liz Parks. She really helps me." She came to Maine, and we have movies of her celebrating Bobby's ninth birthday. There is Bobby, in his red bathrobe, hobbling around on his leg and doing the frug with Liz, who was encouraging him by saying, "A little more ass action there, Bobby; the camera is turning!"

Without Liz, we would never have known and enjoyed the spark and life of black society. (Alas, I think it is even more exclusive and harder to be accepted there than the other way around.) Her friends didn't know it, but they helped us a lot. We needed them. They didn't need us. Liz regularly offered her swimming pool and every year invited us to her Fourth of July barbecue. There was music and delicious food. We threw melons in the pool to cool them off and the children, like tadpoles, would try to swim after them. And then, in the warm, dark July evening, listening to the fireworks in the distance, we would talk and drink until all the children had fallen asleep, full of multiflavored ice cream cones and baskets of potato chips.

With Liz, gaiety and grace came into our house. She was like an explosion of bright colors. With her gift of laughter, her expansive joy in life, she helped us back to the human race.

There was one place where I found peace.

In the early spring of 1967, after Bob had turned in the manuscript of *Nicholas and Alexandra*, we decided it was essential for us to go to Russia. We managed to scrape up the money by borrowing on our life insurance. It was the first time that we would both be separated from Bobby since the day he was born nearly eleven years before. My mother and father came to look after our household. Dr. Engel and Dr. Newman agreed to remain on call twenty-four hours a day. We left a stack of carefully written instructions. We hoped.

The night before we flew to Leningrad I cried, afraid that the disappointment of seeing the reality of my dream would be too great.

But from the first moment that I looked down from my plane window onto the vast, dark forests below me, I felt a strange stirring of recognition. From the first moment on the ground, when I saw the customs inspector with his gold teeth and the old porter in his shabby boots, I felt absolutely at home. I had an unexplained but powerful sense that I had been traveling toward this land for a very long time.

The first days, Bob and I walked delightedly along the banks of the river Neva, and wandered the streets for hours. We looked in awe at the great city of St. Petersburg, where the drama that had consumed us for three years had actually happened. About the city is the seductive pull of the impossible, a sense of dreams and glory. It is a city where, as one poet wrote, "even in anguish one can live." I fell in love with that city, with that expansive, free sky.

We knew no one, yet I had a sure sense that I was waiting—for what, I did not know, but for something. One day, when we were visiting a palace, by chance we met a poet, and with him went through the looking glass that separates foreigners from Russians and Russian life. It was a kind of miracle.

Beginning with that first trip, and continuing with seven more that followed, I met hundreds of Russians: young and old, working-men, museum people and teachers, poets, artists, dancers, biologists, engineers. I loved them. I knew them. Amazingly, they knew me.

Russians understand the rhythm of despair. They know how to cope with it. Their country has suffered so much that despair is a way of life. So decimated have they been by the double catastrophes of Stalin and war that almost no family is intact: fathers, brothers, mothers, sisters, all have been swallowed up. "Reasons?" said one Russian to me. "Why ask for reasons? It is only Western people who ask for reasons." Perhaps because of the immense suffering through which their country has passed, there is none of the sense of possessiveness that marks human relationships in the West. How can there be, when they know so well that people are only loaned to those who love them; they cannot be held, but can disappear in a moment without reason, without justice, without hope. Russians know how to live with the knowledge that death is near.

The contact I felt was deep and immediate. Hemophilia had been preparing me for ten years for these meetings. They knew the terror of the knock on the door, the telephone in the night, the anguished knowledge that in one awful moment a life might be shattered. The causes were different, but the psychological result was the same. We shared the reflexes of people who live with fear.

I knew what it was to feel suffocated, to be unable to travel, unable to determine my career, to live in isolation from the rest of the world. When I looked at the sorrow written on their faces, prematurely aged; at the drinking, the apathy, the discouragement, I knew why it was, and I felt the greatest tenderness and compassion for them. For me, it was like finding a huge family that belonged to me, but that I had never known existed.

Among them, at last, there was no need to pretend an optimism I did not feel. They understood. No words were needed.

Russians read skillfully the signs of grief. They know the yearning need to release, some way, any way, the daily crushing weight. Do you want to feel the melancholy of loneliness, savor the sadness of life? They will drink with you thoughtfully, sorrowfully, respecting the need for weeping when there are no answers, and no way to change the reality of existence. Do you, on the other hand, suddenly feel an unexplained surge of hope, a communion with the stars, with nature, until the meaning of life and suffering are blindingly joyous? They will walk with you through the night along the river, forgetting that there is a tomorrow with appointed work and duties, joining in the triumphant discovery, singing, laughing, forgetting time.

Is the loneliness so great that you feel yourself floating away ever farther from reality? They will crowd near you, to bring you back, stroke your hand, gently embrace you, crooning soothing words in their musical language, and there is no need to be ashamed to confess the terror of human helplessness. They know that there are some sorrows that never will be healed and sometimes no grounds for thinking that there will be a happy ending. And they also know how vital is simple, warm, human contact to give the strength to go on.

This was what I wanted. This was what I needed. Not pity. Russians have extraordinary strength and stoicism in the face of disaster. I met people who had spent twelve years in prison camps, years in solitary confinement, and who had returned to pick up again, to live again. I wondered at them, at such moral stamina. It was as if they had been able to develop a sort of suspended animation of the soul. It was their calm fatalism that had made them capable of surviving impossible trials . . . and a different, less finite sense of time. "People in the West are always in a hurry," said one of my friends, "but it is the devil who works quickly. It is the devil's work that is quick, brilliant, and flashing. God works quietly and slowly. Look at nature."

In Russia, I saw religion alive; beleaguered, tormented, but alive. In the churches of the Soviet Union I was nearly crushed by crowds in services. I saw strong men standing and singing in church, unashamed of the tears rolling down their cheeks. In a state where great cathedrals have been turned into obscene "anti-religious" museums, where God has been officially declared dead, this was a sublime example of His enduring strength in the hearts of men.

The Russian capacity for compassionate understanding of suffering is perhaps the greatest gift that this great people has to give to us in the United States, lost as we are in our visions of perfection, of being forever healthy, young, beautiful, and strong. The burden of having to disguise the realities of human pain is a terrible one; it destroys many among us.

With my friends in Russia, I talked whole nights away and the talk was of the soul and of destiny. It is impossible to describe the joy and the sense of relief that I felt. These encounters gave me strength. They changed my life and gave it a direction and purpose it had not had before.

With the help and example of my Russian friends, I began to learn patience. Instead of turning frantically in circles seeking answers to my dilemma, I learned to wait and trust in an unknown, ultimate plan. A poet wrote me: "Perhaps we are all only witnesses in a single enormous trial whose outcome is unclear, but certain. We can only occasionally perceive its outline as when behind a driving rain, we can sometimes glimpse the silhouettes of angels."

I glimpsed the silhouettes in Russia. Mysterious, powerful country of my heart, which calmed and comforted me! But this precious source of strength and help was to be taken from me. As I was leaving for my ninth trip in June of 1972, the Soviet government arbitrarily refused my visa. I was to be exiled from the country and the friends whom I had grown in those five years to love so dearly, who had given me so much that was vital to my life, and to Bobby's life. Again, there was no reason, no purpose, nothing but mindless cruelty. So I must wait, as my friends taught me to do.

My energies failed. My soul was in chaos. The Devil whispered sweet poison of annihilation and surrender. Only God remained, my only appeal, my last refuge. I had to trust Him blindly, for I knew that my strength did not suffice and that there was no human comfort to take away my pain.

In the dark night, lying lonely and terrified in my bed, I prayed—rather, I beseeched—God to help me. I did not pray for alleviation or cure; I prayed for strength . . . only strength to go on.

Sometimes, then, I would feel a great calm, a sense of destiny and purpose. I felt that I was only an instrument and that all that had happened, and was to happen, was happening through us and not to us.

In the morning, I doubted. Was it not arrogance on my part to presume for myself a *purpose?* How dare I believe that we had been singled out for such a grace? My eyes had been sensitized to suffering . . . and I saw that the terrible fact was that it was so *ordinary*, so dull and commonplace. It was nonsuffering that was extraordinary. And if suffering is ordinary, how can any individual presume to find meaning in it?

Educated by those nights of Bobby's suffering, I had found the ecstasy of pain. It makes the sun brighter, the stars more brilliant. Pain heightens every sense. More powerfully than any drug, it intensifies colors, sounds, sight, feelings. Pain is like a glass wall. It is impossible to climb it, but you must, and, somehow, you do. Then there is an explosion of brilliance and the world is more apparent in its complexity and beauty.

But what to do with all this new sensitivity when the crisis is over? What to do with the great surge of strength that is not needed now? Each trial strengthens the soul, fills the body with power and the need to act. Yet suddenly, there is also an acute awareness of the sadness in the world, of the grief written on the faces and staring from the eyes of passers-by on the street. It is difficult to kill an insect; even the sight of dead flowers is painful. Sorrow seems everywhere.

You must learn to harness this new sensitivity because if you do not, one further step and it will shatter you like glass subjected to extreme vibration.

I found that I could no longer look without weeping at photographs in the newspapers of mothers in India and Ethiopia and Vietnam, wretched in their poverty, with their starving children clinging to their hollow breasts and their dark eyes full of uncomprehending pain and fear. Those eyes scream at you: "We are all helpless. Life is only blind, random, meaningless suffering."

How could we who had enough to eat, who were always under a roof and slept in a bed, how did we dare to call our feelings painful? What of those millions who suffer and die without any of these comforts? They would consider themselves happy and at ease with everything we had to fight our battle. Compared to their agonies, my little struggle was so ordinary, so small, so insignificant, a tear in the ocean. How dared I think that there was any meaning in it, when such meaning was denied to others who were extinguished seemingly without a trace . . . when suffering was so banal.

And yet the need to find meaning remains.

Why, God, why?

Albert Camus said that he became an atheist because he could not believe in a God who permitted the suffering and death of a single child. The Book of Common Prayer says, "God does not willingly afflict the children of men." But if not willingly, then why?

At an IBM exhibition at the 1964 World's Fair, I watched fascinated for a long time a machine that was randomly hurling a great quantity of small balls into the air. This exhibit was designed to illustrate the mathematical law: the greater the chaos, the greater the order inherent in it. Sure enough, it only *appeared* that there was no order, for no matter what the number of balls and where or how high they were thrown, some fell into an orderly pattern with mathematical regularity. The chaos was only superficial . . . at the heart of it was order.

I could not consider Bobby's hemophilia a punishment. When I looked at my bright-eyed child, full of energy and drive, it was unthinkable that God would meaninglessly visit His wrath upon him. And when I walked along the banks of the river Seine and looked at the luminous sky of Paris, the flower sellers' bouquets, the curve of the trees with their silvery rustling leaves, like stars fallen from the sky, I knew that these, too, were the truth. And I could not believe that this fight, the hope for life, was fraud and a deception.

It was I and I alone in my large family who had been touched with hemophilia. Strangely, from the first I was certain that it was only to be me. The years have proven me correct. My two sisters now have four boys. My first cousins have nine. None of them have been touched with hemophilia. Why had I been so sure?

Could it be to teach us by suffering? The Russians saw in suffering a way to enlightenment. To them, it was not a curse, but a mystery with great potential for good. "Be glad, Suzanne," Svetlana would say to me. "Be glad that you feel deeply. Not everyone can feel deeply." "And remember," she would say, "you are a queen, because you are suffering." In the Soviet Union, a friend told me with respect, "Hemophilia is your family struggle. Through it, you have been able to glimpse the suffering of our Lord."

In time I came to believe. In time I became grateful that we had been given the chance to see and to feel so much. And I told Bobby this: that he had been given suffering earlier than many, but that inevitably, suffering and failure come to all in life. I told him that he was fortunate to have had the chance to meet it when he was young, because those who meet it early are luckier than those to whom it comes later, when it often breaks them. His knowledge and his trial could be for him a strong arm for the future. It could bring forth in him understanding and tenderness for others, teach him discipline and patience.

And if there were no reason? Then why that unexplained calm in the night . . . a calm stronger than fear?

I tried to reject it, I agonized over it, but despite all doubt, the sense of destiny remained. I decided to *believe* that what had happened to us was a challenge and that we must meet it. Bobby must *live*—not as if he had nothing, but with it, using it; even if there seemed to be no purpose, even if that purpose was to remain hidden from us, unknown to us, perhaps to remain unknown to us forever.

As for myself, I finally learned to pray: "I am Yours. If it is Your will that I should survive, then keep me as Your instrument." And this has sustained me and dictated my actions and my life.

Chapter 13

R M

There are two levels on which the battle against hemophilia or any chronic disease is fought. The higher level has to do with the human spirit. The other has to do with money. Treatment of hemophilia and other chronic diseases costs a very great deal of money. People who are concerned with hemophilia, either because of a child in their own family or because they are working for the Hemophilia Foundation, spend an enormous amount of time scrambling for money. If they don't get it—such is the health-care system of our rich and powerful nation—hemophiliac boys will not be adequately treated.

The Hemophilia Foundation exists primarily to raise money and supply blood for hemophiliacs. Founded in 1948 by Robert Lee Henry, the father of a hemophiliac, it was, until quite recently, a small, haphazardly run organization whose chapter offices were staffed mostly by volunteers—not infrequently, the mothers and grandmothers of hemophiliacs. They were sincere, dedicated, persevering people. They worked hard running cake sales, raffles, bingo games, luncheons, theater parties, and door-to-door solicitations. They raised money, but only in driblets, a few hundred dollars here, a thousand there. Compared to the need, it was hopelessly, pathetically, frighteningly inadequate.

Later, the foundation tried to reach a wider public by using spot television commercials. Everything about the disease and the foundation had to be encapsulated into sixty seconds. ("Hi. I'm a hemophiliac. You know, the people who can't stop bleeding . . .!")

Sadly, these messages were frequently inaccurate, even harmfully so. Some of them deliberately played on the oldest and wrongest hemophilia cliché: that hemophiliacs can bleed to death from a scratch. "Watch," said the boy on television as he simulated pricking his finger and making it bleed. "Don't worry," he said. "It's nothing serious, but a year ago this could have put me in the hospital . . ." Of course, it couldn't have put him in the hospital if anyone had the sense to wrap a Band-Aid tightly around it. But there it was, this ignorant stereotype that all hemophiliacs spend their lives fighting to erase from the public mind—there on television, with the endorsement of the Hemophilia Foundation.

Bobby was upset and indignant about this commercial and he telephoned the foundation to protest. The official he spoke to was surprised and hurt. "But," he said, "the air time and the ad agency work were donated. They were free."

The problem is that, in America today, most charities are an intensely professional big business, which run on the basis not of need but of names. It is not just whom you ask, but who does the asking. Polished professional fund-raisers in dark, conservative suits appear before corporate public relations vice-presidents or even corporate boards of directors asking not for hundreds or thousands, but millions. Better yet, they persuade the wives of giants of industry to go and solicit their husbands' business colleagues. In this milieu, bingo parties, door-to-door solicitations, and lurid TV commercials are in bad taste. Nobody wants coins or even dollar bills. Checks, big multizeroed checks, are the objective. Any campaign in which two-thirds of a fund-raiser's goal is not met by a few dozen top contributors is an automatic failure.

For most of our experience, the Hemophilia Foundation had no contact with this affluent world. The hemophilia population was small and scattered; the little foundation chapters, made up almost exclusively of parents, were almost totally absorbed by the problems of getting blood. The few hemophilia families who did possess power and wealth took pains to hide the illness and wanted no part of the foundation. (There is a persistent rumor that a famous film actress has a hemophiliac son whom the world has never been allowed to see.) People like this sent their private doctors secretly to hemophilia specialists to learn all they could; they bought blood

and plasma privately and administered them in private circumstances. None ever accepted any obligation to help others, less
blessed with money, to cope with the disease.

For all successful medical charities, a Great Name acting as
Patron is a necessity. In Britain, the royal family parcels out these
duties: If you are lucky you get the Queen; less lucky and you get
Princess Alexandra or the Duchess of Kent.* In America, movie
stars and sports heroes play these figurehead roles, allowing their
names to be used on letterheads and making annual TV appeals.
("Hi. I'm Big Moviestar. Did you ever stop and think what it
would be like to be sick? All the time? . . .") For the public, the
important thing is that somebody famous is endorsing the disease,
touching it with the glamour of his name, and making our donations a kind of personal favor to him. The archetypal Hollywood
figurehead is Jerry Lewis, who, of course, is not a figurehead at all,
but a dedicated man whose twenty-four years of work on behalf
of muscular dystrophy have brought $100 million to the care of
people suffering from that malevolent disease.

In this celebrity sweepstakes, the Hemophilia Foundation has
done the best it could. One of the first to allow his name to be used
was Basil Rathbone, an accomplished actor but for me an unhappy
choice, as in my subconscious I always thought of him as Sir Guy
of Gisborne, the villainous role he played in my favorite boyhood

---

* The royal patron of the British Hemophilia Society is the Duchess of Kent.
But even with the support of the Duchess and the British National Health
Service, the society still works hard to raise money. My favorite fund-raising
story was reported in a letter to the society:

Dear Sirs:
   I have much pleasure in enclosing a cheque for £20. This was raised
by a small group of karate experts, members of the Meridian Karate
Club, who with their bare hands and feet smashed an upright piano into
small pieces.

                                        Sincerely,
                                        R. D. Franks
                                        (Apsley, Nottingham)

film, *The Adventures of Robin Hood*. In my mind's eye, "A Message from Basil Rathbone: Dear Friend: Recently I have become aware . . ." became A Message from Sir Guy of Gisborne. Probably this had nothing to do with it, but Rathbone played mainly villains and an appeal from a villain is less likely, on the face of it, to persuade than an appeal from a hero. In any case, the message from Rathbone/Gisborne brought in little. Ten years later, Vince Edwards, at the height of his television popularity, became the hemophilia figurehead. "Dear Friends: My television role as Dr. Ben Casey has made me keenly aware . . ." Edwards accepted the role because some jockeys he knew at the racetrack had friends with hemophiliac sons and he wanted to help. But still money only trickled in.

Then, in the early summer of 1964, lightning seemed to strike. Richard Burton held a press conference in New York to announce that he and his new wife of two months, Elizabeth Taylor, were setting up the Richard Burton Hemophilia Fund. The Hemophilia Foundation was beside itself with glee. For two years, while they had made *Cleopatra*, abandoned their respective mates, and stormed ahead with their passions, the world had read about their doings, day and night. Not all the publicity had been favorable, of course. There were even some cynics who felt that the Burtons' sudden surge of philanthropy stemmed less from a generous impulse in the mercurial Welsh character than from the urgings of a clever press agent in need of a better image for his clients. Nevertheless, smudged or pure, the Burtons were Very Great Names, and the Hemophilia Foundation hurried to make the announcement.

The press conference was held in a medical auditorium in Mount Sinai Hospital. Most of the seats were filled with hemophilia parents, children, doctors, nurses, hospital orderlies—the word had spread. Sue and I, arriving early, had to find seats near the back. There was a long wait, then a flurry of activity, and suddenly, surrounded by the familiar and highly pleased faces of hemophilia doctors and foundation officials, there stood the short, husky figure of Richard Burton. For a few seconds, we all craned our necks awaiting the arrival of his wife, but then a disappointing bit of intelligence rippled through the room: "She's not here. She's not coming." It didn't matter because only a few minutes later we all were reeling from the impact of something that Burton had just said.

In his rich, resonant, glowing, incomparable voice he told us that he himself had hemophilia.

"I've been a bleeder all my life," he said. "My case has been mild, but even in mild form it has been extremely dangerous to some members of my family. I had six brothers and four sisters. Two of my brothers were powerful Welsh coal miners. When I was about eight, they had their tonsils removed and, suddenly, it seemed they were about to die from bleeding. After that, I knew we bled easily, but I still never heard the word 'hemophilia.' Until recently, I had no idea that it could be so severe a problem."

What, the reporters wanted to know, were some of the problems he himself had had with the disease?

"Well, when I was seven I had a tooth out. Later, I broke an arm playing football. A year and a half ago, as I was coming out of Paddington Station, I was attacked by six Teddy boys who kicked me around with their steel-tipped shoes. Now (Burton was at that time playing *Hamlet* on Broadway) I sometimes get cut in the dueling scenes with Laertes. When he nicks me, I bleed more than when I nick him." Burton suddenly switched on his Shakespearean voice and declaimed, "And if you prick me do I not bleed?" He cackled. "Even today I have to be careful in the morning when I shave. God bless America for the electric razor."

Nobody laughed. We were bewildered. First, we had seen in the flesh Richard Burton. The hemophiliac. Or, as the mind struggled to grasp the implications: the hemophiliac Shakespearean actor. The hemophiliac husband of Elizabeth Taylor. Then, thrust along by the compelling power of that majestic voice, we had been given other vivid images: a Welsh child suffering from hemophilia having a tooth pulled, his mouth filling with blood! A hemophiliac boy playing football and having his arm broken! A hemophiliac traveler attacked in a train station and kicked into a mass of bruises by Teddy boys! A hemophiliac actor leaping about a stage trying to avoid being cut by a sword!

Reality dawned. Behind us a chair scuffed and I heard a disgusted adolescent voice: "He's a phony!"

I turned and saw the son of one of the officers of the local hemophilia chapter. His crutches were leaned against his chair. "He doesn't have hemophilia," the boy said, looking at Burton. "He doesn't know anything about it."

On stage, the doctors looked uncomfortable. Dr. Richard Rosenfield, a hematologist, stepped forward and explained that there were degrees of severity in hemophilia and that Mr. Burton perhaps had a very mild case or some other mild coagulation disorder. Burton, unembarrassed by this discussion of his case, continued. "Elizabeth couldn't be here today, but she has agreed to become chairman of the Richard Burton Hemophilia Fund." Copies of a statement by Mrs. Burton were handed around. She said:

> I am proud of the creation of this Fund in Richard's name. We have both known how serious hemophilia can be and are challenged by the opportunities for service to the many thousands of hemophilia sufferers. We are planning programs which will bring the story of the Hemophilia Foundation to the public. We want to help with special events and affairs, TV and radio, and records— in any way we can be most useful. We'd like to feel that one day we will have helped to conquer this illness.

Burton elaborated on his wife's statement. "We'll do poetry readings for hemophilia," he said. "If Elizabeth feels comfortable and if they are halfway successful, we'll do recordings and TV shows. We'll mobilize our famous friends. We'll get dollars, pounds, Swiss francs."

On that hopeful promise, the press conference ended.

Unfortunately, that initial press conference was also the high-water mark for the Richard Burton Hemophilia Fund. When *Who's Afraid of Virginia Woolf?* opened in New York, half the proceeds of the première, about $7,000, were given to the Hemophilia Foundation. But there were no poetry readings, no TV shows, no records, no famous friends, and, other than the sum mentioned above, no dollars, pounds sterling, or Swiss francs.

The point is not that some actors, like all of us, forget their good intentions, but that the system is wrong. Why should movie stars be asked to bear the burden of our national irresponsibility on health? What is truly foolish is for Americans to continue to rely so heavily on the good intentions of show business folk to raise the money we need to pay for the treatment of diseases that, day after day, relentlessly ravage our lives. Whether a movie star remembers or not.

As for the individual families, most of us were in even worse condition financially than the struggling Hemophilia Foundation. The medical bills and other expenses that go with hemophilia are almost impossible for most people to imagine.

Take our expenses, for example. Bobby was getting an average of one hundred transfusions a year. To give the transfusion—that is, to put a needle in his vein—doctors charged anything from $4 per transfusion (Dr. Jerry Wessel on Deer Isle), to $27 (Dr. Jack Rheingold in Washington, D.C.). Dr. Engel charged $10 for transfusions in the office and $15 for a transfusion at home. Other doctors, acting as consultants in orthopedics or hematology, charged $15 a visit. The cost of fresh-frozen plasma and cryoprecipitate was $13.50 per bag. As an infant, Bobby had one bag of fresh-frozen plasma per transfusion. When he was ten, he received six bags of cryoprecipitate per transfusion.

There were other direct medical costs. Visits to the Hemophilia Clinic cost $8. One autumn Sue drove Bobby into New York twice a week for half-hour physical-therapy sessions in the office of a private muscle specialist. This cost $10 a session, $20 a week. Later he switched to Blythedale Hospital in Westchester, where the cost was $4 a session, three times a week. X-rays, needed frequently to monitor what was happening inside the joints, cost $20 to $60. When Bobby couldn't walk, we rented a wheelchair at $15 a month; then, when we realized that this condition was semi-permanent, we bought a child's wheelchair for $300. When he outgrew it, we bought a bigger wheelchair for $500. (Twice, within the first two years, the new wheelchair broke and collapsed with Bobby in it. He was unhurt but this meant two $50 repair bills, plus $15-a-month rental fees for substitute wheelchairs.) Crutches for use in places a wheelchair couldn't go cost $30. Bobby's first left leg brace cost $125; the next cost $198; in all there were five for the left leg, two for the right leg, and three for his elbows. The pulleys and weights he needed for traction cost $75; later, he needed a home exercise stand which cost $350. His special orthopedic shoes, to support the ankle and diminish torque on the knee, cost $125 a pair; he had a new pair every year.

There were other costs, not directly medical, but directly attributable to Bobby's hemophilia. He could not walk to the school bus or climb on and off it, so, for a year, until he came under a state transportation program, we paid for a private school taxi twice a day. The school-home intercom cost $104 to install, and the service was $44 a month; we kept it for three years. He needed extra clothes because the friction of the metal braces underneath wore the cloth out quickly. There was even the big, expensive color television set I bought as soon as I was able because Bobby spent so many days at home and so many hours staring out at the world only through the medium of television.

How did we pay for all of this? Obviously, I could not pay it all myself and we do not have in America a system of government health insurance. Instead, we have private insurance plans, some nonprofit like Blue Cross, and some designed for profit, like the group major medical plans offered by Prudential, Equitable, Mutual of Omaha, Travelers, and dozens of other huge insurance companies. The trouble is that these insurance companies—whose essential purpose is profit, not health care—do their best to exclude exactly the people who need help most, the chronically ill. They pick and choose among the population, seeking people they consider "best risks." Obviously, hemophiliacs and the other seven million chronically ill Americans are the poorest risks of all. The fact that they are going to need help, and lots of it, is certain.

In this situation, the insurance companies have compromised. They are willing to accept the chronically ill (a "pre-existing condition," they call it) as part of a group policy issued to a corporation or other organization that also has plenty of healthy employees. But they will not issue policies to any chronically ill person on an individual basis. It would be impossible for Bobby to walk in off the street, a free individual citizen, and sign up for any kind of medical or health insurance. And it has been impossible for me, as his father, to find any individual coverage for him. The only way I have been able to get it has been to work as an employee for a company that has a group plan.

That it is impossible for an American hemophiliac to find individual major medical insurance I know, because on two separate occasions, fourteen years apart, I have tried to get coverage for Bobby. Both times, I was rejected with exactly the same arguments. My first attempt was in 1959, when I saw an ad for a Mutual of Omaha major medical plan of the kind that this and other insurance companies still spread across the pages of American newspapers and magazines. I wrote for the brochure. When it arrived, it looked hopeful: "Health insurance years ahead of its time . . . Lifetime sickness benefits . . . Can never be canceled. . . ."

A few days later, a salesman sat in our living room.

"Now, Mr. Massie, just a few questions," he said, writing my name and address on his questionnaire. "You're in good health, your wife's in good health, the kids are O.K., of course. Now . . ."

"My son has hemophilia, but otherwise he's fine," I said.

"He has *what?*"

"Hemophilia."

"Oh, my! Well, of course, if there are any pre-existing conditions, we have to eliminate that member of the family."

"Without Bobby, I don't want the insurance."

The salesman reached for his hat. "Look, Mr. Massie . . ."— he was backing out the door—"believe me, we'd love to solve all the problems in this country, but we're in business, you understand. . . ." The air in our driveway turned blue with gas fumes as he gunned his motor and roared away.

Fourteen years later, nothing has changed. When we came back from Europe where all hemophilia expenses are cared for by French government health insurance, I contacted a salesman from the Equitable Life Assurance Society. I called him because, while we were in Europe, the Equitable had set up a group major medical plan for the members of the Authors' Guild. The first thing I learned was that the Authors' Guild program had been discontinued. The results they had had with authors were disastrous, the agent told me feelingly. "You wouldn't believe the number of times authors get sick or are out of work. We lost a bundle," he said.

Nevertheless, I asked, do you have an individual plan even if the premiums are higher?

"Oh, yes," he said, and we agreed to meet.

When he came to our house, he and I had almost the same dialogue as I had had fourteen years before. Confronted with the fact of Bobby's disease, the salesman said that there was only one chance in a hundred that he would be covered. Besides, he added, by applying for health insurance, the fact that he has hemophilia will get into his records, making it impossible for him to buy life insurance later on. Why not forget the health insurance and buy life insurance for him before the company finds out?

I thanked him, explaining that we wanted coverage for Bobby's health, not his life.

"Under our present system, there's just no chance," he said, wishing me well.

Actually, to say that individual medical insurance for hemophiliacs has never been available is not entirely accurate. There once was a plan offered by the Continental Casualty Company of Chicago. The premium was $15 per year, and here were the terms: After twenty-one days in the hospital, during which time the policy would pay nothing, the company would pay $5 per day for hospital room and board expenses, plus a single lump sum of $50 for all other hospital expenses. It was caricature—but we took it for a year. Almost nothing was better than nothing.

The result of all this is that through most of our lives Sue and I have worked as employees so that Bobby's medical bills would be partially covered. We have had Blue Cross to cover our hospital bills and a New York insurance plan called GHI (Group Health Insurance) to cover our doctors' bills. Their coverage was grossly inadequate because most of Bobby's medical care was handled outside actual admission to a hospital, thus relieving Blue Cross of any obligation, and because GHI's reimbursements were always far below the level of the doctors' fees. Nevertheless, they provided an essential base.

On top of this, we had the group major medical plans of our employers. *Newsweek*'s plan was with Prudential. The employee paid the first $300, after which Prudential paid 75 per cent of all costs up to a maximum of $5,000. My next magazine, *U.S.A.** *1*, had a better plan with U.S. Life Insurance Company. After a ninety-day waiting period, and a $100 deductible, they paid 80 per cent up to a maximum of $10,000.

When Sue went back to work at Time Inc., she was covered under a Travelers group plan that had a deductible of only $50, but paid only 75 per cent of our medical bills up to a maximum of $10,000.

For most employees, these plans provided substantial protection. But not for all employees. The hitch was the $5,000 or $10,000 maximum. One couple, who were friends of ours, had a son with epilepsy. Both worked at Time Inc., the husband as a *Life* photographer, the wife as a senior researcher. Within a few years, they exhausted the husband's $10,000 maximum. Travelers would not reissue a new policy to him. And they never permitted the wife to hold a policy at all. Had we stayed in our jobs, we soon would have had the same difficulties.

The point is that our insurance structure in the United States actually runs counter to our traditional American values. Supposedly, ours is the country of individual initiative; each citizen is exhorted to get out on his own, develop his own capacities, work for himself, become a Horatio Alger character. Yet members of hemophilia families and other chronically ill citizens cannot exercise the supposedly deep-dyed American privilege of working for themselves. No private insurance company will cover the individual hemophiliac who wants to work for himself. He is forced to go to work for somebody else, simply to get into a major medical insurance plan.

There is an even crueler irony. Because of his disease, the chronically ill citizen cannot get insurance for himself and therefore he must work for a company and be covered by a group plan. But sometimes, in a vicious circle, the company is afraid to hire him because of his disease. Or there are even cases where the company has been willing to employ the person in question, but the insurance company has objected and, by threatening to raise the company's rates, forced a rejection of the application for work.

I feel strongly about this because, throughout Bobby's life and my own working career, I have been strongly affected by it. So are millions of other Americans. But even those lucky enough to have escaped unscathed, if they really stop and think about our American system of paying for health care, will realize that something is very wrong.

During Bobby's childhood, most of the physical and psychological burdens were in the home and they fell on Sue. But there were three absolutely essential requirements that only the outside world could supply: doctors, blood, and money. The first two depended on the third, and the third—money—depended on me. It was up to me as the family wage earner to find a way to pay the bills.

I had grown up with a kind of strangely schizophrenic view of money. My family didn't have any; my grandfather had been a minister and my father a schoolmaster. In general, we thought that people who did have money, or were busy making it, were slightly vulgar. By osmosis, it was impressed upon me that a gentleman did not talk about money; a gentleman didn't even think about money.

At the same time, a second idea was also being drilled into me. That was "Be Independent, Stand on Your Own Two Feet, Don't Be Beholden to Anybody." The trouble was that when I went out into the world, I discovered that the two basic tenets with which I had been equipped were mutually antagonistic. If I disdained money, how was I going to be independent? In time, of course, I learned that in order to display a properly contemptuous lack of interest in money, one had to have some—perhaps even quite a lot —tucked away somewhere. And I learned that for me the only solution was to give up some of my cherished independence and go to work.

This is a path trod by many an idealistic young man. It is a useful experience, part of growing up. But for me it was abnormally difficult. I still hadn't resolved the philosophical conflict of money versus independence when hemophilia changed everything. Suddenly I was completely dependent on the thing I had been taught to despise: money. I was totally responsible for the survival and welfare of a family one member of which had a very expensive disease. Out of this tangled confusion of principles and pressures came other emotions: resentment and fear. The truth is that during most of the years I worked as an employee, I both overly resented the power my bosses held over me and worried excessively that I would lose my job.

When I left the navy in 1955, I wanted to teach history or become a lawyer and go into politics. But that meant three more years of study in graduate school or law school. I was twenty-seven, Sue was pregnant—perhaps later.

Journalism seemed an excellent compromise. Seen from my romantic and largely academic perspective, it appeared to be a blend of history (current history) and literature (current literature). It was a respectable profession, or at least a semirespectable semiprofession. In those days, some of the glamour of the great reporters of the Second World War still touched it. And, it was a way to work with ideas and still be paid a salary.

It didn't take long for me to discover that journalism was not much interested in me. I had fifty-five interviews in various newspaper and magazine offices and no one offered me a job. Thus, ironically, I who disliked even talking about money almost went to work in a bank. I was saved at the eleventh hour and became—although the words sound grand for the minion I was—a magazine journalist.

What I didn't know was that I was boarding a sinking ship. Of the four national magazines I worked for, three are no longer around. One by one, the huge general-interest magazines, *Collier's*, *The Saturday Evening Post*, *Look*, and *Life*, capsized and went down like great, leaky leviathans.

I worked for two of these giants, *Collier's* and the *Post*, and Sue worked for *Life*, so we were eyewitnesses to a good deal of this mayhem. When *Collier's* sank, I went to *Newsweek*, the only magazine I've ever worked for that's still afloat in its original form. I was hired there by the Back of the Book editor, Frank Gibney, who edited copy behind a closed door with his radio playing classical music. While in the navy in Japan, I had read his book, *Five Gentlemen of Japan,* and when I applied for a job, I mentioned that I had liked it. Approving my taste, Gibney took me on and assigned me to reviewing books.

I'm afraid that I went into journalism with fuzzy ideas and ambitions. I never had any desire to be a hard news reporter and cover a regular beat, or to advance, desk by desk, to the managing editor's chair. From the beginning, I wanted to sit further back and take a longer view. This was why the news magazines, which wrote the news in the perspective of a week rather than a single day, appealed to me. And, of course, on a news magazine, the longest view was the one exercised by the book department.

There were two of us in the department, Wilder Hobson and myself. Between us we were responsible for producing four or five reviews a week. Wilder did the fiction; I did histories and biographies. When Wilder was away, either on vacation or on a leave of absence to write a novel of his own, I did everything.

Being with Wilder in those early days of my career and Bobby's hemophilia was great luck for me. Wilder, who was in his fifties, was a gentleman, a marvelous wit, a superb raconteur, and a graceful writer. To me he was also a friend. Bobby's hemophilia was diagnosed on my third day of work at *Newsweek.* Reeling under this shock, I was incapable of work. Most people at the new office were too embarrassed or frightened to mention my catastrophe. But Wilder and Kermit Lansner, our editor, asked me to talk to them about it, tried to reassure me, and told me not to worry about the job. For many weeks, Wilder took most of the work from my shoulders.

And Wilder made me laugh. We convened on Wednesdays to sort out the assignments for the week ahead. This was a performance, conducted as a kind of private theater, with Wilder as the star. The seventy books sent us every week by publishers were placed in three piles: a small pile of Likelys, a larger pile of Possibles, and a sad mountain of Out of the Questions. Before his tiny audience of two editors, a researcher, and me, Wilder would pick up books one by one, and hold forth. If he knew the author, he would tell a tale. If not, he would read aloud, often irreverently, from the jacket copy. Reputations were punctured, bombast mocked, pretension debunked. We quaked with laughter. There was very little to laugh about in my life in those days, and the mirth Wilder provoked was a wonderful way to release tension and slough off strain.

After I had been writing reviews for about six months, the editors created a new feature for the books department; it was called "A Talk with the Author." Once or twice a month I would take my notebook and pencils and call on an author whose new book had just been published. I interviewed James Jones, Teddy White, John Gunther, Cornelius Ryan, Vance Packard, Ayn Rand, Amy Vanderbilt, Fanny Hurst, Erskine Caldwell, John P. Marquand, John Creasy, Sloan Wilson, Peter De Vries, and Jules Feiffer. Teddy White was the most fun; I liked Erskine Caldwell the least. From John Gunther I learned three work rules that I have adopted myself: "Use scissors and stapler to structure notes. Never write on both sides of a piece of paper. All happiness depends on a leisurely breakfast."

I did all of my reading and writing at the office. (The presence of one—and then, when Susanna was born, two—toddlers in a small apartment, plus the constant tension of worrying every minute about Bobby's falling and hurting himself, made it impossible for me to work at home.) *Newsweek*'s books, theater, movies, and television critics—five writers, and two researchers— were all crammed into a tiny compartment where we worked under the kindly and sophisticated eye of Kermit Lansner. When he chose to write—a cover story on Picasso, for example—Kermit could write better than any of us. But it was as an editor that he shone. He did very little editing with a pencil. If a story or review was off the track, he called the writer in to discuss it and then, with a word of encouragement, sent him off for another try. After one of these sessions, I always felt that I wanted to do a better job, just to please Kermit. Later, with other editors, I felt the lash.

In this little office sitting all day in a badly worn, incomparably comfortable green leather chair I spent two peaceful office years. When *Newsweek* moved to more modern quarters on Madison Avenue, I did my best to persuade the office manager to bring along my old leather chair—to me a symbol of England, stability, and gentility. He said that it wouldn't match the new, standardized plastic chairs the management was buying for everybody and would make the office look funny. In those days, I did as I was told. The chair vanished and I spent my remaining years at *Newsweek* sitting uncomfortably.

Secure and content as I was in my niche, nevertheless after two years I was ready to leave. I like to read, but, reading interminably, gorging myself on newly published, mostly mediocre books, the taste was going out of it. The real reason, though, was money. Book reviewers were paid less than most other writers on the magazine. The editors looked on our little cultural cubbyhole as a kind of backwater, a refuge for burned-out older writers who couldn't be trusted to meet a hard news deadline, and whose services, therefore, merited smaller salaries. It was true that three of the critics next to me were men in their fifties from whom the years had extracted a toll. A hundred thousand sheets of clean white paper rolled into a typewriter, waiting for that first typed sentence, five thousand deadlines, half a million cigarettes, a thousand bottles, too much pressure, the mind beginning to blur, a long rest, a new job with less strain and diminished stature . . . they had all followed that path. But the damage was done. At fifty, they were worn out. Within a few more years, all three were dead: two by sudden illness, one jumped from a window. And yet, in the heart, I found them a better breed than the driving, compulsive news writers and editors on the floor below.

Just at the moment that my restlessness was becoming acute, a new foreign editor took over at *Newsweek*. He was an Englishman, lanky, blond, talented, wreathed in ambition. He was building a new foreign staff and I was invited down to see him. My goal, I said, was to be sent to *Newsweek*'s London or Paris bureau, explaining frankly that because of Bobby's illness and the need for good medical care, we couldn't go anywhere else. He said that he understood, that he would work it out, but that he wanted me to write for a while in New York to get the feel of the department. Three years later, I was still in New York, still writing for him, still waiting to be sent to London or Paris.

The work week in the news sections of *Newsweek* was bizarre and exhausting. It was not that we did more work than people in the Back of the Book; it was just that we did everything in a more concentrated period of time. Supposedly, we worked a five-day week, Wednesday through Sunday. In fact, during the first three days we did nothing, and the entire week's effort was jammed into the last two days before press time. The reason was logical: Writers assigned stories at the beginning of the week never bothered to write them because there was an excellent chance they would be killed to make room for later-breaking stories.

The week began around 11 A.M. on Wednesday morning when writers (mostly male) and researchers (exclusively female) gathered over coffee in the foreign editor's office to listen while a story list was made up and preliminary assignments handed out. Here was none of the humor and wit of Wilder's performances; this was all deadly serious, the world was in our hands, we were mini-foreign ministers analyzing the fate of nations. Emerging from this meeting, we sent cables to the overseas bureaus asking for their contributions, and then, for two and a half days, we did nothing. We came in late, went home early, and spent the intervening hours wasting time. The older writers went out with each other for three-martini lunches; the younger ones, who couldn't afford to go out, sat in the office eating lunch from brown paper bags.

The last two days of the week were frantic and all-devouring. On Saturday morning we arrived at the office early and began to churn out copy. Two stories before lunch—if there was time for lunch—two more during the afternoon and early evening. The editor would appear, beckoning: "The story's all right, but you've got the wrong lead. . . ." By 10 P.M. perhaps you could slip out for supper. Then back to work as a fitter. That meant sitting down with a layout man and laying out the story, word by word, line by line, column by column, into the magazine. If it was too long (it was always too long) you trimmed or whacked or lopped. It was always painful; the carefully balanced story you had handed in at noon was reduced, by midnight, to an awkward, distorted lump. But it had to be done. And over the years it was a hard but excellent school. I learned to write short stories and longer stories, to cut lightly and deeply, to use different styles, tones, and points of view, and to do all this no matter what was happening around me at the office or what was going on in my head about my worries at home.

At 2 A.M., sometimes 3 A.M., we crawled across the street to a hotel for a few hours' sleep. Red-eyed, we came back on Sunday morning, rewriting to keep up with the news, refitting to make room for fresh stories. Finally, in the early afternoon, we drifted away, a procession of stumbling zombies. For me, it was Grand Central and home.

The work at *Newsweek* broke down all the normal rhythms of life. The slack period of the early week, followed by two days of intensive effort, left me exhausted; I understood why men were burned out after a few years. The weekends didn't help; instead of the pressure of work, I felt the heavier pressures of hemophilia. For it was at home that the vitally important battles of our life were going on.

Sometimes, I quailed before these crises at home. In the middle of the night when Bobby would call from his room, "My knee hurts. I'm bleeding," I would be hit by nausea. In the worst crises, when he screamed in agony, I could scarcely stand it. Every cry wrenched me and horrified me. I began to sweat, to pace up and down, clenching my fists. Susy, hearing those awful cries, would come running out of her room, her little face terrified. Comforting her, I tried also to calm myself. Then I would begin to work, to defrost the plasma, to help with the transfusion, to bring extra pillows—anything not to feel so impotent.

But sometimes, after the doctor had left, the pain went on for hours. Sue was sitting beside Bobby's bed, holding his hand, smoothing his brow, letting him know through the red mist of pain that the human being he was closest to was there. What could I do? Nothing. Only work. Write, to earn money to pay for whatever help, medical and otherwise, I could find. Work, for me, meant rolling a piece of clean white paper into a typewriter and waiting for something to come out of my head. Suppose, one day, nothing came. On my ability to find words to put on those clean white sheets, usable words, words an editor would not reject, words that eventually would be put into the magazine—on this depended my ability to help Bobby. If I couldn't write, I would lose my job. I had seen it happen: writers who couldn't produce were fired and no one cared why or what was happening to them at home. And grueling and underpaid though my job was, I knew that to others from the outside it looked desirable. My desk at the office was near enough to the foreign editor's door to see the endless parade of hopeful young men going in to apply for a job like mine.

So, in order to keep my job, in order to earn money, I had to write. And in order to write, I had to sleep. Filled with nausea, guilt, and desperation, I went back to bed and threw a little switch in my head. While Sue sat up with Bobby, I slept.

Along with worrying about Bobby, I worried about Sue. The best antidote for her would have been to go back to work. We couldn't even consider it; there was no one else we would trust with Bobby. A night by ourselves in New York—dinner, the theater, parking, and babysitter—cost $50; it was out of the question. Even a temporary respite, a chance to do something else, relax and temporarily forget, would have helped her. But we couldn't afford it. Only twice in ten years did she really get away by herself. Once, she went to her college class reunion, leaving me the Daily Schedule. It read:

6:30 A.M.	Bottle, Susy.	
7:30	Bobby wakes. Bottle, then change and dress him.	
⎧ 8:30–9:00	Breakfast, Bobby.	
*⎨ 10:00–10:30	Bath, Susy.	Do wash somewhere
⎩ 11:30	Bottle, Pablum, Susy.	in here.
12:30	Lunch. Bobby.	
1:15	Toilet and nap, Bobby.	
⎧ 3:30	Bottle, Susy.	
⎨ 5:30	Bath, Bobby, then bottle and supper.	
*⎩ 6:00–7:00	Bottle and Pablum, prunes, Susy.	
	Change Susy's clothes and bedding.	

* Crisis Areas

The reunion lasted only a day and a half, but it was too much for me. When Sue arrived home on Sunday night, she opened the door to hear strange sounds. The children were in bed and I, exhausted but pleased with myself, was leaning back, having a third drink, and enjoying *The Magic Flute*. I was quite oblivious to the fact that I was listening to a 33 rpm record at 45 rpm.

The only other time was when she went to Paris in 1960. We had met in Europe and it had been our hope to go back there. But there had been Bobby's hemophilia, sinking magazines, and *Newsweek*, which had promised to send me there but never did. Sue missed France greatly, and that spring I borrowed $500 from a bank and bought her a plane ticket. When I gave it to her she burst into tears.

For me, Maine was the deliverance. I loved the trees, the starry nights, the water. Sue feared small boats, but for me a few hours in my little wooden sailboat, the sails bending to the wind, the hull knifing and plunging, the waves crashing against the bow, the bubbles hissing as they slid along the leeward side and foamed off astern—this brought peace to my soul.

But when weekends or vacations were over, I had to go back to the office. I remember the sinking feeling I had when the phone would ring in the office and it would be Sue, her voice tense. "Bobby is bleeding. I think he may need a transfusion."

"Are you sure?" I hoped she would say, "Well, maybe not." She never did because she never called unless she was certain.

"Shall I come home?"

"No. I'm taking him to Dr. Engel."

". . . I'll take an early train."

Then I would put my head on my desk, rub my face with my hands, go get a drink of water, walk around the office corridors, come back, sit down, and try to write about some distant event.

Looking back, I don't understand how we survived financially. *Newsweek* then was in the hands of a pair of Scots, father and son, who shared the same name, and the belief that the way to make a profit was to keep costs low. Writers' salaries were an item of cost.

Looking for ways to save money, I retired from the *Newsweek* Retirement and Pension Plan, which had been taking $22 out of my monthly check. I resigned from the New York Newspaper Guild and saved another $6 a month. There had never been a strike in the history of news magazines and our dues were used mainly to finance strikes at the daily newspapers. The one time I had asked for Guild help they had botched it so badly that I was lucky to keep my job.

To ask for a raise was an act of daring, compelled by desperation. There was always the danger that the thing might backfire. Suppose you had just gone beyond some invisible line ("Just how much do we really need Massie, anyway?")? It took a lot of fortifying talk at home ("We just can't live on this . . .") and a lot of comparative research ("If Jones makes this much, and I produce more stories than he does, then I deserve more than I'm getting . . .").

One day when I was thirty, writing four or five foreign stories a week, and had seen a string of raise appeals postponed or rejected, a nice young fellow with no writing experience whatsoever was brought into the office, introduced as a newly hired writer, and given the other desk in my cubicle. We talked and he told me how pleased he was with his salary. He should have been; it was much higher than mine. Furious, I wrote out my resignation, left it on the foreign editor's desk, and went home. That night a soothing telegram arrived, bringing with it a money order for $10 and the suggestion that I buy a bottle, calm down, and return to the office in the morning for a chat. I returned and found that my walkout had had an effect; my raise was granted. But I was warned, "That was a theatrical trick. I had to stick my neck way out for you. Don't put me in that position again." I promised that I wouldn't, knowing that if I ever left again, it would be for good. Then I called Sue to tell her the good news.

Supplementing the money trickling in from *Newsweek* in those early years, we had two sudden, wholly unexpected windfalls. One was from a lawsuit, the other from a quiz show. The lawsuit grew out of a plagiarism of an article I had begun working on at *Collier's* and which, when *Collier's* sank, I sold with *Collier's* permission to *The Reporter*. My article was on Ogden Reid, Jr., the president of the *New York Herald Tribune*. It was inadvertently plagiarized by *Esquire* and a magazine writer named Theodore Irwin. But the real perpetrator was a young public relations man named William Safire, who had taken a copy of the first draft of my article and turned it over to Irwin as material he could use. I sued, and Safire's firm offered me $1,000 to settle out of court. Urgently needing money, I accepted.

Much later, the subject happened to come up when I was sitting around with John Denson, the crusty old newspaperman who then edited *Newsweek,* and later, when the Reids sold it, was to edit the *Herald Tribune.* "You settled for chicken feed," he growled. "You could have gotten ten times as much."

In fact, although I didn't tell Denson, the reason I had settled was that, when the trouble erupted, I went in and told the younger of the two Scots, who advised me—strongly—to settle quickly for whatever I could get. "We don't want *Newsweek* people mixed up in this kind of thing," he said. Unready to risk my job, I obeyed.

About the same time, willing to do anything legal to make extra money, I shuffled into the line of open-faced young men who waited outside the door of the producers of the television quiz show *The $64,000 Question,* hoping to get some use from their store of generally irrelevant information. Like all successful commercial products, this one quickly began to spin off duplicates. One was called *Hi-Lo,* and I was selected for it. I have forgotten the rules, but I remember being shut up in one of the famous glass isolation boxes and asked to name all the people who die in *Hamlet* and to describe the manner of their deaths. I did it and in five minutes I won $1,000, two months' pay at *Newsweek.* When the check came, Sue and I looked at it with wonder, having never seen or held in our hands a sum that large. Unfortunately, *Hi-Lo* was a summer replacement and the show ended that night.

The only solution was for me to work on weekends. I had two days off, Monday and Tuesday. Monday morning I slept, exhausted by the strain of the weekly closing at *Newsweek.* But in the afternoon, I sat down at my own typewriter and tried to augment our income by writing free-lance articles. At first, I worked in our bedroom with the door closed while Sue shushed the two young children outside. Then one winter as a Christmas present, she used her ballet earnings to have a room built for me in our unfinished, unheated attic. It was freezing in the winter and stifling in the summer, but in spring and autumn it was fine. I have always liked the smell of attics anyway—the woody scent of old beams mingling with the musty fragrance of old trunks, old letters, and books becoming for me a tantalizing link with people who lived in the past. The neighborhood children were intrigued. Once, floating up the attic stairs, I heard a strange child's voice asking Bobby, "Is your daddy still up in the attic?" It was one more thing that made us odd.

The trouble with my free-lance career was that I chose subjects that I thought were interesting (two famous World War II American battleships about to be scrapped; the postretirement career of Britain's eccentric Field Marshal Montgomery) and then went ahead and wrote articles without even talking to an editor. When I submitted them, editors responded that they thought the writing was good but the subject "not right for us."

I tried children's stories. One spring afternoon when Bobby was four, he and I went into a patch of woods near our house, sat down in a grove of saplings and, together, we made up a story about "The Lion Who Tried to Fly." In it, I was trying to say something about him and to him. Children's book editors weren't impressed: "Too contrived . . . animals who try to fly are a dime a dozen."

Eventually, one of my stories worked out. The newspapers were filled with stories about all the Harvardmen swarming into Washington to work for President Kennedy. I realized that a surprising number of important New Frontiersmen were also Rhodes scholars and began counting heads. When I had enough, I proposed an article to *The New York Times Magazine*. They bought it: $90.

Finally, I found steady weekend work. Having developed a certain craft for writing book reviews, I proposed myself as a reviewer, first to the Sunday *New York Times Book Review* and then to *Saturday Review*. Both took me on. Thereafter, I spent the first day of my weekend reading the book, the second writing the review. For each review I was paid $40 or $50.

Meanwhile, my chances of going to *Newsweek*'s London or Paris bureau seemed to be getting nowhere. Every time I brought it up, the bureaus were fully staffed, the budgets were set, the men overseas were doing well. Then a vacancy would occur, I would once again present my candidacy, and the job would go to someone else. I was offered Nairobi, then Bonn, but the medical situation in both places was unsatisfactory for Bobby.

In the autumn of 1961, *Newsweek* offered me a chance to become a bureau chief right in New York, at the United Nations. The catch was that it was not a fulltime job. I could go to the UN on Wednesday and Thursday, but by Friday, when the office tempo was picking up, I was expected to be back at my desk, writing. My story load remained the same.

Nevertheless, it was worth it. I arrived on the day Dag Hammarskjöld was killed in a Congo plane crash. The succeeding months were filled with drama in the Security Council, the General Assembly, the corridors, and the vast, constantly changing theater of the Delegates Lounge. The American ambassador was Adlai Stevenson; it was a pleasure to stand even on the fringes and watch this urbane and warmly human American statesman.

Nineteen sixty-one was also a year of change at the top of *Newsweek*. The magazine was bought by Philip and Katharine Graham, who owned the *Washington Post*. An efficient young editor, Oz Elliott, took charge. Kermit Lansner became one of his two deputies.

Almost immediately, everything about the magazine—the writing, the layout, the covers—began to improve. Nevertheless, by early 1962 I wanted to leave. I had been on the magazine for five years, in foreign news for three. I was tired of the miserable pay and the grinding work week, tired of waiting in vain to be sent to the London or Paris bureau, and tired of sitting at a desk writing about people I never saw. A news magazine writer, functioning as a human machine, processing raw copy filed by correspondents into finished magazine columns, never really sees anybody except his office colleagues, his fellow commuters, and his long-suffering family.

Just at this time, I heard about a new magazine called *U.S.A.**1* being started by a young *Time* writer named Rodney Campbell. It was to be a monthly news magazine with quality color photography and approximately twelve full-length, by-line articles in every issue.

It seemed exactly what I was looking for. Along with everything else, the total anonymity of *Newsweek* writers in those days had become increasingly frustrating. All my book reviews, both raves and blasts, had been unsigned. Most of my foreign stories, even long cover stories that had taken days of hard work, were anonymous. I was proud of some of these stories and it was humiliating to have to go around among my relatives and friends and say "I wrote that." (Most news magazine writers felt as I did and, about two years after I left, both *Newsweek* and *Time* began to sprinkle names of their writers much more generously through the magazines.)

Along with a regular by-line, there were other attractions to *U.S.A.*1*. One was a 30 to 40 per cent increase in salary. Another was a chance to get out of the office, to travel around on stories, talking to many different kinds of people—politicians, doctors, admirals, depending on the story I was working on. It was relaxing and refreshing to plunge into their worlds, even for a few weeks.

Perhaps there was something else in my eagerness to take this new job: a subconscious desire to escape, even for a while, from the heavy responsibilities and anxieties of my own world. Later, in doing research for a magazine story about hemophilia, I discovered that sometimes fathers of hemophiliacs simply ran away. Some did so by divorce or abandonment of their wives and sons; others by retreating into work or other activities outside the home. The effect on the boys, throwing them into an even closer relationship with worried mothers, was almost always devastating.

I never thought of leaving for good, but I remember the enormous feelings of relief, almost lightheartedness, with which I left for the airport to go off on a story. At night in some motel after a good expense-account dinner, telephoning home to describe my day and learn how Sue was managing, I felt guilty. Often I would leave out some particularly interesting experience or glamorous detail because I thought the contrast with her life at home would be too painful for her to hear.

In those years, I usually managed to rationalize my exuberance and consequent guilt at leaving by telling myself, "I have to leave because of my work. Otherwise the family will sink." Sue was wiser. She said simply, "It's good for you to get away." Slowly—much more slowly for me than for her—we have come to realize that when one of us needs to leave for a while—a few days, a few weeks—it is not a rejection of the other. We always come back. It is simply the necessity to breathe different air and think different thoughts.

U.S.A.*1, while it lasted, was a joy. Operating from three or four rooms in the Beaux Arts Hotel near the UN building, surrounded by piles of newspapers and cups of three-day-old coffee, nine writers struggled to produce twelve major stories a month. It was a chance to follow my own interests, write at length, and develop my own style. I wrote six full-length articles in four months, on East Africa, on Mississippi, on Franco Spain, on the Common Market, on twenty-nine-year-old Teddy Kennedy's first race for the Senate, and on the 1962 America's Cup race.

My best effort was a profile of the State of Mississippi. I talked to people on all sides: the leader of the White Citizens Council, the majority leader of the legislature, bankers, judges, newspapermen, Medgar Evers of the NAACP; and when the article was published, I got nice letters from all of them. But these letters arrived to find *U.S.A.*1* collapsing. The capital needs for starting a new magazine had been underestimated, the stock market had plunged, and the original investors were unwilling or unable to put up new funds. The money ran out and, five months after I had joined, I was out of a job.

This time, I had two choices. *Newsweek*, which for all those years had hesitated to send me to London as a member of the bureau, now offered me the job of London bureau chief. I was tempted, but I also had what seemed to us an even better prospect: the chance to continue doing full-length by-line stories, this time for *The Saturday Evening Post*.

I signed on as a contract writer to write eight articles a year. I was not on the staff, so for the first time in my career I had no major medical insurance coverage, but I decided—and Sue encouraged me—to risk it. I was paid by the article and I began in a rush; my first year at the *Post* I wrote nine stories. I went back to Mississippi and covered the riot at Ole Miss when James Meredith entered the university. I did a second profile of Teddy Kennedy as he entered the Senate. I did a major story on hemophilia, and a report on the debate over aircraft carriers between the navy's admirals and Secretary McNamara's slide-rule Whiz Kids.

One of my most interesting assignments had to do with Lady-bird Johnson. In 1964, when the Johnsons had been in the White House for about six months, Mrs. Johnson agreed to allow the *Post* to print one of her speeches the same week she was to give it. This meant writing the speech well in advance. To facilitate matters, the magazine offered to send along a writer who could help gather material and draft ideas. The decision came suddenly. One morning the White House telephoned the *Post* and asked that a *Post* writer be on board the President's press plane that night to fly to Texas. I was the writer chosen. That night I was sitting by myself in the back of the press plane, watching with interest the veterans of the White House press corps as they guzzled and ruminated.

The next morning a small helicopter landed in a vacant lot near my hotel in Austin, I got in, and we clattered away over the dry, scrub hills of central Texas. On landing I was met by Liz Carpenter, a key member of the Johnson entourage, who functioned as Mrs. Johnson's chief of staff, press secretary, shield, and filter. Mrs. Johnson was busy and Liz suggested that, while I waited, I go for a swim in the President's pool. "In the men's side of the pool house you'll find a lot of extra swimming trunks. Take any one that fits." Undressing, I stared at the suits. Who had worn them? Dean Rusk? Robert McNamara? Chancellor Erhard? A few minutes later, floating on my back, I saw a surprised face peering at me over a hedge. The owner yelled at me to get out quickly. It was a Secret Service man, who wanted to know who I was and how had I gotten into President Johnson's swimming pool. I explained.

Not long after, Mrs. Johnson came out of the house, wearing a bright crimson sweater and slacks, gave me a friendly smile, and asked if I minded going for a drive while we talked. I was surprised by how small, delicate, and attractive she was. With her dark hair and luminous eyes, she looked like a young woman. I know people who photograph handsomely, but who are surprisingly colorless in the flesh. Mrs. Johnson is the opposite.

We got into one of the Johnsons' famous white Lincoln Continentals, I in back with Mrs. Johnson, and Liz Carpenter in front with the Secret Service man who was driving. We began to drive slowly around the ranch. From time to time, Mrs. Johnson would ask the driver to stop so that she could admire a favorite view or watch a doe grazing in a meadow. Before we had gone far, Liz Carpenter pressed a button in the part of the car where the glove compartment usually is. A door opened; there was a small bar with ice, paper cups, and bourbon. Liz began pouring and handing.

Rolling over the dirt roads, a cup of bourbon balanced precariously in my lap, we began to talk about the speech. Mrs. Johnson was concerned about the misuse of a great national resource: the talents of American women. She wanted to urge women to take a more active part in public and community affairs, at whatever level was possible. She felt that, far from detracting from her family role, an active woman became that much more interesting and attractive to her husband and family.

I asked whether there were some women she knew personally who might serve as dramatic examples of the kind of involvement we were talking about.

"Yes, there are," she said. "Let me tell you about one woman. I went to college with her at the University of Texas. Her second child was born with cerebral palsy. After several years of fighting this fact and carrying her child to many, many doctors, she accepted it. She discovered that there were different degrees of this illness and that some victims could be helped. So she went to work. She brought together the Crippled Children's Society, the Junior League, a church, and the city fathers. We now have a clinic in Austin. Hundreds of youngsters come from hundreds of miles around to be helped. Behind every achievement or success is one dauntless person who keeps gathering together the strength that makes the web of success. It wasn't easy for this mother to overcome her shyness and reluctance and ask other people to involve themselves in her problem. But she did it. She turned her personal misfortune into an advantage for hundreds of other affected parents and for a whole community."

I was surprised and touched. Mrs. Johnson could have answered my question by naming any number of successful women she knew, but the one who came to mind first was the mother of a handicapped child.

She continued: "I know another girl, living in Philadelphia, whose child was born with cataracts on her eyes. This child's eyes are so bad that she has to sit within a few inches of the TV screen to be able to see. Normally, a child like this might be institutionalized. But this mother did not want her child set apart. She organized a group of women who spend their summers typing school textbooks in extra-large type so that this child and others with a similar problem can sit in class with normal children and follow the lessons in their special books."

We drove for two hours. It started to rain and Mrs. Johnson asked the driver to stop in front of an old wooden house somewhere on the ranch. The house was empty, but it had a wide porch with three or four rocking chairs. We sat and rocked and looked out across the hills, now misty in the rain. I could see how refreshed and excited Mrs. Johnson was just by being there; talking about the hills and the deer and the wild flowers, her eyes glowed and her voice was warm with affection.

The special radio in the car crackled with a message from the ranch: President Johnson was in the helicopter on his way back from Austin. "Oh, my," said Mrs. Johnson. "He'll want his supper as soon as he gets back. I have to get home right away to take care of that."

In Austin and then at the White House, the speech took shape. Flying back to Washington, my suitcase and typewriter acquired official tags saying "Trip of the President," which I managed to keep for years until they faded beyond legibility. There were a number of changes, but on June 24, 1964, the First Lady stood up in Detroit before 3,500 women of the American Home Economics Association and gave the speech.

During this brief working acquaintanceship, I never mentioned our own problem with Bobby to Mrs. Johnson. But three years later, when *Nicholas and Alexandra* was published, I sent Mrs. Johnson a copy with a note saying how touched I, as the father of a hemophiliac, had been by her feelings about medically afflicted children and their parents. She read the book, and in March 1968, she invited Sue and me to dinner at the White House.

Later, as we grew to know Mrs. Johnson, we came to admire her greatly. Her special quality is to be enormously friendly and democratic and, at the same time and in the best sense, regal. She sits very straight in her chair. She listens with complete attention to whoever is talking, but if she notices that someone present is not included, she gracefully makes an introduction and gently shifts the subject to one in which everybody can participate.

Given a choice, she once told me, "between lying in a hammock under an apple tree with a book of poetry, watching the blossoms float down, and standing on a platform before thousands of people, I don't have to tell you what I would have chosen twenty-five years ago." But her life demanded more. To me, she seems a permanent First Lady.

One problem faced by all *Post* writers during that period was that editors' heads were rolling so fast that there was a new man to deal with almost every time you came into the office. You were given a story assignment by one editor, you discussed it with him, got his ideas, went out, wrote the story, and brought it back to turn in, only to find that he was gone and another man was sitting in his office. The new man might not like the story at all and that was just too bad for you. Writers were paid only when their stories were "accepted."

During my first two years at the *Post* I wrote nineteen stories and fourteen of them were published, a reasonable percentage. During the next two years, I wrote only eight stories and only four of these were published. And instead of doing stories that I thought were important and interesting, I found myself dispatched to write about a Chicago musician who thought he was a billionaire, a New Jersey inventor who had built a flying submarine, an animal keeper in the Pennsylvania mountains who kept the last of the Lobo wolves.

Sometimes I worked for weeks on an article only to have it rejected. Our fragile security began to dwindle away. The last and greatest of these disappointments came when I turned in a long article that had absorbed three months of my time. Prince Yussopov, Rasputin's murderer, still alive at seventy-eight, had come to New York to sue CBS for a television play about the assassination. The trial was in a New York courtroom. For me, this meeting of opposite worlds was rich in drama and fascination. The *Post* thought so, too, on assigning me the article. But when I turned it in, they had changed their minds. The article was rejected.

Despairing, I came home and said to Sue, "I just can't go on like this. What am I going to do?" She looked at me, her blue eyes glowing with anger and determination, and said, "Bob, it's time for you to write a book."

Somewhere among the other hopes and dreams that had been buried when hemophilia came into our family lay my hopes for a career.

After college I had worked for two years at Time Inc. In those days, the Luce publications each year imperially scoured the country for promising college girls. Five acolytes were chosen and offered a chance to be "trainees." In 1952 I was one of the last group of that now extinct species. We were put to work in a wide variety of jobs throughout the magazine empire. We roamed through clip desks and photo labs, editorial departments and production desks, worked in the research morgue, wrote answers to letters to the editor, learned about printing and production, and generally hung around learning what we could. The pay was minuscule, but the useful editorial experience I picked up during those months has proved to be pure gold ever since. The pinnacle we were aiming for was the exalted position of "researcher" (never "writer," although we were expected to learn to turn out masses of written material; in those days, as if it were an immutable law of nature, writers were always men, researchers always women. The few women who became editors were so rare and so odd that they were treated as if they were another gender entirely). At the end of nine months I became a researcher for *Time* magazine. There was something a little monastic and ingrown about the *Time* atmosphere and I longed to go where the action was, so I managed to get myself transferred to *Life*, first as a photo editor and then, at last, as a cub reporter. I got there just in time for the last great free-wheeling days of the old *Life*. Glamorous photographers like David Douglas Duncan, Eliot Elisofon, and Gordon Parks swung in from assignments all over the world. Draped with expensive cameras, wearing suitably mussed trench coats, they roamed through the halls, flirting with the girls and trailing clouds of sophistication and *savoir faire* behind them. But just as my assignments started to pick up, I got married. Then Bobby was born. End of career.

For five years I gloomily scanned the *Life* Table of Contents page and watched as my old pals climbed the masthead and got by-lines, while I was tucked away in an obscure suburb with a husband who worked late at night and on weekends and was often out of town. No help. No money. Two small babies. Two or three loads of diapers in the washing machine every day. Dishes (no dishwasher because we couldn't afford one). Laundry. Ironing. Cries. Screams—and all those transfusion trips. Not much time for intellectual musings in that schedule. Where was that faraway girl who had had so many dreams?

Under the circumstances, even to *dream* of continuing my own career seemed utter madness. If free-lance writing is difficult for a man, it is even more difficult for a woman . . . and a woman with children? The essence of a free-lance career is to be available any time, for anything. Under the circumstances, the very idea was ludicrous. Nevertheless, there was something in me that doggedly wanted my own self. An ambitious me.

My road back to a career started with ballet. I had always loved it; I had danced since the age of six. I began teaching ballet to little children in the local public school auditorium. For two years I drilled a series of little pupils in the first five positions. I played a lot of good music for them, told them stories of the great ballets, and tried to instill in them a respect for the discipline and devotion of professional dancers. Until I could find a babysitter, Bobby sat outside the classroom and waited for me. From this effort, I earned about $200 every ten weeks, minus babysitting fees. I used the money to build a writing room in the attic for Bob.

Still, how could I get back into journalism? I loved to cook, so I tried cooking. I sent recipes in to magazine contests. I thought up cookbook ideas. Nothing. Suddenly, when Bobby was six, a break came. Bob had just joined *The Saturday Evening Post* as a contract writer. The first story he was assigned was an article on the frantic social whirl of the diplomats of the United Nations. He had just begun working on it when he was pulled away and sent, instead, to cover the story of James Meredith's entrance into the University of Mississippi. I told Bob I would take over the UN story. I worried a lot about leaving Bobby with sitters, but I knew it would be mostly night work. I persevered; I knew a chance when I saw it.

Every night for three months I put on my one sensible black dress and a pair of white gloves, fetched the babysitter, and drove off to New York for a marathon of parties. I learned to dance the Ghanaian "High Life," I skulked around the cavernous halls of the Soviet Embassy under the mammoth portrait of Lenin, drinking vodka and jockeying for the caviar while I listened to Eastern European diplomats griping about the boorishness of the Russians. I met my college hero, Adlai Stevenson, and found him as charming and witty as his publicity. I found that the Saudi Arabians and the Argentines gave the most lavish parties (champagne, hams, pâtés, turkeys, and caviar), and the Americans the worst (salted peanuts and Scotch whiskey). Best of all, I made friends who are now scattered in diplomatic missions all over the world.

I wrote about it all and then turned my story over to Bob, who reworked it and handed it in to the *Post*, explaining what I had done and asking for a double by-line. The *Post* refused. "She is not one of our contract writers," they said. Bob fought so hard that they finally gave in. The story ran with the by-line "By Suzanne and Robert Massie."

It was a victory, but there the road ended. I kept studying all the magazines trying to find *somebody, somewhere,* who would take a story. In the process I got more and more disgusted at the simpering quality of the women's magazines. Their reader was me, the lady with her hands in the dishpan. They were my only contact with the outside world, and what were they feeding me? Gooey stories, gooey pie recipes. At night, when Bob came home and told me of the *Ladies' Home Journal*'s sagging circulation, I would snort, "Well, I know why." I nagged him with ideas about what should be done until he finally said, "Look, don't tell me. Write it." I sat down and banged out eighteen pages of reasons why women were not interested in women's magazines and what should be done about it. Bob sent it off to the editors of the *Journal*.

Weeks later, one summer day I was picking raspberries in Maine when I was fetched back for a telephone call from the editor of the *Ladies' Home Journal*. "We want more," he said. "Can you come to lunch?" "I am in Maine," said I. "We'll fly you down," said he. Overwhelmed by this unusual attention, I flew down from the fresh seacoast of Maine into the hot, muggy streets of New York for a bizarre evening with the two top editors of the *Journal*. Drinks. Dinner. Nothing was said. At about 2:00 A.M. they finally got down to business. "We like your ideas. Will you write us some more?" "How much?" I asked. "$2,000," they said. (For my ideas! A fortune!) Nevertheless, I kept my head enough to ask, "If I do it, how much will I have to do with implementing my ideas?" Nothing, they said. No, thank you, said I, and flew back to Maine.

Then something happened to change my mind. Several months before, we had seen a beautiful Victorian ark of a house in Irvington-on-Hudson. It was crumbling and badly needed repair, but it had *land*, magificent trees (including a huge chestnut; Paris!), lilacs, and a wide porch where you could sit looking out over the Hudson River, watching the boats go by. There were wide rooms with high ceilings and an old rope-operated elevator installed at the turn of the century, perfect for a boy in a wheelchair. I had fallen in love with it. But the house was not for sale.

Suddenly, a few days after my evening in New York, our real estate agent called us in Maine and announced that the house was on the market. Excitedly, Bob clanged the bell to summon me back from the point. I arrived panting, thinking something had happened to Bobby. On the spot, without any idea how we would raise the money, we phoned back to say, "We'll take it."

I called the *Journal* back and capitulated. I wrote forty-three pages in three days, pouring out my ideas and suggesting a new editorial approach to women's magazines. In those pages I put forward the revolutionary concept that women were interested in . . . *men* . . . not just in cream pies (a series, please, on the most sexy and dynamic men in all fields, with pictures), that women were interested in reading about each other and particularly in the accomplishments of successful women in the so-called "men's fields." (Let's have a story on the career of a woman brain surgeon.

Will a woman ever make partner at Sullivan and Cromwell? Etc., etc.) And lots more. All these ideas are dreadfully old hat now, in the days of the *Cosmo* centerfold and *Ms.* and consciousness-raising sessions, but in 1963 they were quite daring. They bought it. In June of 1964, the *Journal* breathlessly announced on its cover: "WOMAN—THE FOURTH DIMENSION—A Special Issue" (note the "Special": it was not meant to be thought of as a regular practice); then the subtitle: "A Daring New Concept to Expand Your Life" (that is, being more than a wife and mother). How quaint it looks now! But I had made my point and my bargain, I had my $2,000, and we had the house. Its thick walls and its land were a haven and a fortress in an unfriendly world. And the sunsets! We lived in it empty because we had no money to buy furniture. People were very curious about the two crazy writers with a hemophiliac child who had moved in. They came to call or even to peer into the windows of our empty, curtainless, furnitureless rooms. But with the sunsets and the river, who needed furniture?

And then too, the *Journal* asked me to expand on one of the 110 story suggestions in my memo and to do an article on the personalities and problems of the women career diplomats at the United Nations.

I went back to the UN. That year, Madame Pandit, the younger sister of Prime Minister Nehru, had just been elected the first woman president of the General Assembly. I interviewed her in her hotel room, a tiny, gray-haired lady in a sari, playing happily with her grandchildren, and she confessed to me, "When I made this first appearance on the platform and looked down at all those men, it made me a little drunk with joy!"

Interestingly, I found that the most important career diplomatic positions held by women were held by women from underdeveloped countries. "Because," said Miss Eugenie Laurens, the Counselor of the Indonesian Mission, "we couldn't be choosy. The number of trained intellectuals is limited. We cannot permit ourselves the luxury of choosing a man over a woman." In "developed" countries, the score was dismal—the United States and the Soviet Union the worst. From all over the world, from South American, Arabian, Indian, English, Canadian, and French ladies, the message was the same: "We have to work harder and have twice as many qualifications to stand our ground."

But at least they had careers. For me, it was back to the dishpan and the Grand Union. Every chance I had, I would sit down and dash off another story suggestion. I kept firing them all around town one after another, like paper planes, tailoring my style to each different magazine. I sat for hours outside editors' offices, terrified, hopeful, steeling myself for the turndowns ("Well, it's very interesting but I'm afraid it's not for us"). What I wanted to do was to write about ballet. I *needed* to. I knew it would be therapeutic. These were among the most painful days of Bobby's illness, I was living each day on the edge of despair, and I knew that ballet would help me to survive. Whenever in my life I feel absolutely miserable, if I can only go to a good ballet, I am nourished, transformed. There is something so tenderly beautiful about those dancers who, chrysalis-like, emerge for a brief moment to glow like many-colored butterflies. In difficult moments I would close my eyes and I could photographically recall those moments in ballet which had most touched me. But we couldn't afford tickets. So if I wanted to go, somehow I had to persuade *someone* to let me write a story.

Ballet was not as popular then as it is now. No national magazine would agree to any kind of story on the subject. "Too esoteric," said editors. "But," I pleaded, "the girls are beautiful, the men are handsome. I can make it interesting, you'll see. Give me a chance." "No," they decided.

While I was looking for assignments, occasionally I had lunch with an old *Time* or *Life* colleague and listened wistfully as they told me about their trips and stories. How I envied them the warm security of their comfortable salaries. Many of them had moved to Time-Life Books, which was churning out one series after another. But the answer to me was always the same: Sorry, no part-time work. No free-lance stories. One day Bobby's godmother, Valerie Vondermuhll, who had been on the lookout for something for me, called and asked if I could come in and help out temporarily to close a photographic essay on hurricanes for a Weather volume for Time-Life Books. Somebody had gotten sick. Hurricanes? It was *money* and I snapped it up. It happened to be the early fall hurricane season, so I spent a turbulently interesting few weeks talking each day on the telephone with the men of the hurricane watch in Florida and tracing hurricane patterns on the weather maps in the weather station high up in Rockefeller Center. The real dividend was that I was able to bring intricate weather maps home to Bobby, who was in bed. He was absolutely delighted with them.

Just as this short assignment was ending, I happened to hear that a photographic essay on genetic disease in the Health book was bogged down; no one could imagine how to tackle the subject in pictures. "You see, Sue," the researcher explained to me earnestly, "it's really impossible, because all of these people are *pathetic* cases." She didn't know I had a son with hemophilia. I charged in and offered myself for the job. It was an editorial challenge; it *was* difficult to find ways to show the subject in pictures. In thirteen pages we proposed to cover five of the best-known genetic diseases: muscular dystrophy, cystic fibrosis, epilepsy, diabetes, hemophilia. My biggest problem was to get the photographers *not* to see the subjects as "pathetic" through their lenses. At first Fritz Goro, one of *Life*'s best science photographers, was terribly upset and depressed at the sight of boys twisted with muscular dystrophy. I soothed him, reassured him, and was able to convince him to look for the spirit and the will of those boys instead of letting his camera see only their bodies; this is a question of the photographer's eye, not his lens. He succeeded brilliantly. In four weeks we managed to catch up the delay and finish the essay on time. It is the journalistic story that I am proudest of professionally.

As it happened, just as I had taken on the genetic disease essay, my biggest break finally came. A *Post* editor who had liked my story on the UN ladies finally decided to take a chance and let me do a full-length profile of George Balanchine and the New York City Ballet. It was to be the first ballet story ever assigned in the *Post*'s history. I was ecstatic. Balanchine, Georgian-Russian choreographer genius of ballet, had been a hero of mine ever since I had eagerly hung over the third balcony at the City Center in my college days.

It was ironic, but when that longed-for moment came for me finally to meet this hero, I was pregnant. It was said that the very sight of a pregnant woman offended Balanchine's aesthetic ideal of the female shape. Never mind. Things never happen at the right moment. Lumpy, I haunted the rehearsal rooms watching Balanchine at work with his lithe dancers, unsuccessfully trying to cover myself up with a huge coat but painfully conscious of my bulky self reflected from a hundred mirrors.

As every ballet lover, I knew that not many years before Balanchine had suffered a great personal tragedy. His young wife, Tanaquil LeClercq, one of the most brilliant ballerinas of the company, had been stricken with polio and was left crippled and unable to dance again. In sorrow, Balanchine left ballet for one year to devote himself to her and her care. I had been strictly warned by ballet officials that this was one period in his life that was never to be discussed in an interview. So when we sat down to talk over dinner one night, I was careful to bring up every subject but that one. Yet as we talked, he asked me about my own family and I mentioned that we had a child with hemophilia. Suddenly he brought up the subject of his wife's illness and the acute problems they had faced. It turned out that we knew the same doctors. We compared exercises and orthopedic problems. What he said about his fight, and his attempts to apply the discipline of ballet to the terrible challenge of illness, was so touching and personal that I never wrote about it, but his experience and advice stayed with me. It helped me to preserve my determination during the years of disciplined exercise it took to restore Bobby's bent leg.

The Balanchine story meant a great deal to me. I was painfully anxious that it be good. During the last weeks of my pregnancy I worked feverishly to finish the first draft before I would have to leave for the hospital. When I came home, I stayed up every night for ten days to finish the final draft, getting up from the typewriter every four hours to nurse the baby.

Proudly, I turned it in. Great, said the editor. Then, silence. One day, weeks later, Bob was at the *Post* and saw someone working over my copy. To fill a hole made by a story they had killed, the editors decided to cut my story to half its assigned length. I was horrified, and drove furiously into New York, where I stormed unannounced into the editor's office and fought to save what I could. But the damage was done. The new version was garbled and sensationalized. I was mortified. I tried to apologize to the ballet people for what had happened. They were polite. Thereafter I hated the *Post*. And when it sank a few years later, I knew precisely why.

Knowing what had happened, a publisher asked to read the original version of my story and, on the strength of it, asked me to do a book on Balanchine. But, by that time, there was no longer a question of a free-lance career for me. We desperately needed a steady income. Bob was writing *Nicholas and Alexandra* and had given up his contract at the *Post*. It was a great gamble—a family gamble. The book was more important to us than anything else; it could mean our freedom. But one of us had to have a regular job that provided major medical insurance or we could not survive. So, after nursing Elizabeth for two months, I went back to being a researcher at Time-Life Books. With a tiny baby, it was impossible for me to work every day. I knew it, but kept silent until I was solidly signed on the job (temporary workers were not eligible for insurance). Then I managed to persuade the head researcher to permit me to come in only three days a week. I did a full week's work by working on the train, on weekends, and never taking a lunch hour.

The job was a good one, and extremely useful for our main project, the book. I became the senior researcher for a Time-Life book on early Russian history called *The Rise of Russia*.

I spent happy days working with a professor at Columbia University and reading in the Columbia Library. Along with my own job, I was able to do a great deal of research for Bob. Then, my trainee days were invaluable. I knew how to find everything in that huge Luce organization. I had friends among the hard-working, unsung, specialized people: researchers in the morgue, men in the photo lab, artists in the layout department. They all helped me. I could lay hands quickly on obscure facts in reference books. I knew how to use the photographic library, I could use the copying machines. Like a mole, I quietly tunneled my way, bringing back what was most useful for Bob.

Those were hard days. I almost never slept. I woke at 6:00 A.M. and went to bed at 2:00 or 3:00 A.M. Many nights, when Bobby was in pain, I didn't sleep at all. I worked at Time-Life during the day and then, bearing my load of history books, would come home to find Bob writing in the library. I would make dinner, do the dishes, and then start reading and editing pages Bob had written during the day. I had no help, other than a babysitter, so I spent my weekends cleaning the house and doing the wash and ironing. I planned meals and marketed a week ahead, baked Christmas cookies and birthday cakes when the seasons demanded. When Bob's advance from his publisher was used up, my small salary was all the money we had, and I remember the sinking feeling of seeing the bills and wondering how we could pay them. Bobby was bleeding in his joints; during the last month of the writing of *Nicholas and Alexandra* he needed twenty-five transfusions. Bob was exhausted; he began having severe headaches from the strain. He was so absorbed that days passed with him shut up in the library, constantly playing Russian music as he wrote. The children barely saw him. One day Elizabeth looked at the closed door from behind which she heard music and uttered her first word. "Daddy," she said knowingly, and toddled away. I worried about having to be away from her so much. But I needn't have. She was wonderfully cared for by our babysitter, a motherly lady named Mrs. Connors, who had raised six children of her own. Mrs. Connors hugged her, fed her chocolates, and sang her Irish songs. Elizabeth has turned out to be the calmest and most easily affectionate of our children.

And despite the problems, it was an exciting time. All our professional experience, our education, our imagination, the best we had to give, was coming together on this one project . . . and we knew it.

Meanwhile, at the office, the early Russian history book was coming to an end. Time-Life Books, always searching for new subjects, had been planning a food series for over a year. Knowing about my cooking experience, they asked me to write a master concept for the series. I was whisked away from Russia to an isolated cubicle and began to write about food. I wrote a long memo proposing an overall concept for the multibook series. Then I outlined two books in detail, the cooking of provincial France and Russian cooking, as examples of how the concept could be expanded. I finished, I was congratulated—and sent back to my old job. A few weeks later, I passed an editor's office and noticed a stack of several hundred copies of my memo. I went in to ask if there might be a job for me. The chief editor looked at me coldly and said, "Oh, you did a very good job on those memos, but did you ever really think that we would make a woman the head of a series?" However, he continued, perhaps Bob would like to write the book on Russian cooking? I could help him perhaps—"in my spare time"—while I worked as a researcher on another project. Bob refused. I quit.

A grand gesture, considering that at the time we were penniless. But fate stepped in to help. A few weeks before, I had gone to *Gourmet* magazine to try to sell them an article. I had given my food memo as reference. To my astonishment, they rejected the article idea but proposed that I become their managing editor. I accepted. I was there only five months. On August 21, 1967, *Nicholas and Alexandra* was published, and overnight our life was dramatically changed.

Chapter 16   S M

People always ask. The discreet approach the subject sideways, as if treading on eggshells. "But," they ask, "do you have other children?" The direct just say, "Weren't you *afraid* to have other children?" (The answer to that is a dry "yes.") The tactless say, "Do all your other children have it too?" The self-important accuse, "Don't you feel you have a responsibility to society?" Directly or indirectly, what they all want to know is how I felt about having other children—me, a carrier of hemophilia.

The genetic factors are clear. Once hemophilia has declared itself in a family, with each succeeding pregnancy four possibilities exist: a normal girl, a normal boy, a girl who will carry the hemophilic gene but be normal herself, and a hemophiliac boy. Some families have several children and only one hemophiliac boy. Other families have two, three, or four hemophiliac boys. The risk with each pregnancy is 25 per cent—one in four. No accurate method exists to predict if a child will be afflicted. No reliable carrier test exists. The tests there are raise more questions than they answer.

But dry facts do not decide the issue, nor do statistics affect the human heart. Once a genetic defect has appeared, the decision whether or not to have other children is made in the silence of the soul. It is a most intensely personal choice—one that neither medicine, nor the state, nor the church should be able to dictate to any individual.

When I learned that Bobby had hemophilia, I grieved, but I never felt guilt. I am told that many women do. I did not. Perhaps it was because it was such a bolt out of the blue. How can anyone feel guilty about being hit by lightning? My husband helped. Never once did he make me feel that I had failed him. Guilt was simply not one of the problems I had to face. Bobby's hemophilia never affected my conception of my worth as a woman.

At first, after Bobby was born, I was too overwhelmed and frightened even to *think* about whether or not I wanted other children. Susy came before I could make any conscious decision; she brought with her new life and courage. But to make the *intellectual* decision, to actually *plan* to have another child, took many years.

Early in our search for facts about Bobby's disease, I had heard a story that affected me very much—so much, in fact, that even before Susy was conceived I think I had already unconsciously made up my mind. Perhaps this is why it did not occur to me to look for an abortion. It was the story of a very determined and positive man. He was organized and strong and, as men can be, absolutely determined that he *would* conquer by sheer will the disease of hemophilia which had struck his son.

In those days—and it was not so long ago, only thirty years— very little was known about hemophilia, and less was done to help. This man fought in the courts and insisted that his wife be aborted of any other children. He won and she was. He did everything to help his only son; when there was a body of medical thinking that believed warm climates might be beneficial, he moved his wife and son to Florida. And his son grew. He surmounted crises, he managed school and, as he was very intelligent, went on to college. The organization, the determination, had won. Or so it seemed. I do not know what the wife thought of her legal abortion, how the son felt growing up alone, or how lonely the man was in his defiance. The walls of defense had been erected. And yet, one day a tumor grew, and because the boy was a hemophiliac, an operation was impossible. At twenty-one he died. And there were no other children.

I thought long and hard about this. Will was not enough. It was impossible to order the future. Hemophilia had already taught me the lesson that man is not in control of his own destiny. The more he believes he can order it absolutely, the more it slips from his grasp and veers out of control. There are moments when man's control looks absolute—those are precisely the moments when it is least secure. I looked at Bobby and knew that his happiness would not be increased by living alone, with parents hovering over him, cut off from the companionship of brothers and sisters as well as from other children. If anything, he needed brothers and sisters *more* than did a normal child. For Bob and me, the odds were quite good: three out of four. All we needed was the courage to face that fourth possibility.

And there was hope. I saw how quickly life was changing around me, how knowledge was expanding each day. How futile to presume to predict the world as it would be when my children were grown! It seemed at least possible to dream that with better methods of control, hemophilia could one day become a disease as controllable as diabetes—and few people consider this a disease for which sterilization and abortion are necessary.

And if I had a girl? Well, even if she were a carrier, she might not marry, or she might not have children, or, who knows, by then she might be able to decide the sex of her child.

Thinking all this over, I chose life. That was only sixteen years ago, and medically we are already much further ahead, with the picture more hopeful than I could have imagined. Then it was an instinctive reaction, which I suppose came from contemplating the stars and the flowers.

Still, courage did not come quickly. It took years before I felt strong enough emotionally and physically to face the prospect of another boy with hemophilia. By then we all wanted another child. We decided to go ahead.

People *do* try to make you feel guilty. When I told people I was having a baby, I braced myself for their questioning looks. Some even said what they were thinking out loud—"Do you think it is . . . *wise?*" Nina Bisordi, who went on to have three healthy children after having had two sons with hemophilia, told me that she was afraid to go to hemophilia meetings during her pregnancies because she was so criticized. Bill says doctors came up to him and said, "What's the matter with you? Are you crazy? Didn't you learn anything in medical school?"

I was pregnant when I went to work on the genetic-disease story at Time-Life Books. During all the months in which I was most emotionally sensitive, I was plunged more immediately than ever before into a soul-searing examination of the problems that our personal decision posed to medicine and to society.

Never before had I clearly understood the magnitude of the problem of genetic disease. In the course of my research I leafed through thick medical books that listed thousands upon thousands of possible genetic defects. Their number and the infinite variety were terrifying. Reading those books, normality seemed a miracle— the exception, not the rule.

I went from interview to interview, I talked with doctors and parents about their problems and struggles—some so agonizing that our problems with Bobby faded in comparison. How alone they were! Locked into their own particular tragedies, isolated in little islands, competing against each other for public attention and for money—somehow we had lost sight of how many problems we all shared: the ignorance of the outside world, the staggering financial burden, the painful forced isolation from the world of the "normal." If only we could find ways to fight the common problem— genetic disease—together! Counting only the diseases that our story covered, over five million people were affected. Together, what power those numbers could give us! We could elect representatives, we could insist on money for research and treatment. Instead we were fragmented and weak. Like a modern Tower of Babel, we did not communicate with each other.

Each day I saw fresh tragedy: children with twisted bodies waiting for certain death, children who struggled for breath; agonies of patience and suffering that met only failure and defeat. And yet, at the same time, often in the same buildings, I visited research laboratories where men and women, undiscouraged, were dedicating their lives to investigating the mysteries of genetic defects. I went to the Muscular Dystrophy Institute; it is a modern, fully equipped center for research and care built largely from funds raised by the devoted efforts of a single man, Jerry Lewis. There I talked with a warmly compassionate doctor, himself a victim of cancer of the throat. He had learned to talk again by using a voice box and pushing air up from his stomach to make sounds. There was hope and vitality in that hoarse voice in which he spoke to me about the future. "Genetic disease," he said, "is the great medical problem of the twentieth century. In the nineteenth century it was bacterial disease, and we conquered that. We must now conquer genetic disease. A breakthrough in one will be a breakthrough in all. When we understand the flaw in the genetic chain that causes muscular dystrophy, we will understand the basic chain of command and we will also be able to understand, perhaps, what causes hemophilia." At the institute he took me to meet two Hungarian doctors, a quiet and scholarly couple, who were intently working with a gigantic microscope—it seemed almost as big as the room—through whose extraordinarily powerful lenses they were studying the structure of molecules. What a strange and magnificent world was unfolding in those stainless-steel rooms only a few floors up from the bustle of New York traffic. The future was there, in slides of human proteins that looked like rainbows and northern lights; the universe they were probing was as distant and mysterious as that of outer space.

Seeing the pain, the sorrow, the battles so often lost, the distances yet to be traveled in research, the idea is inescapable. Why not abort? Why not sterilize? Again and again during those months I heard doctors discussing this highly sensitive question. How tempting, how tantalizing is the idea of controlling life! It is the ultimate power, the victory of man's scientific knowledge over the forces of nature. Why not clean up the world, eliminate the cost to society, create a race of supermen? How chilling these conversations were! There was something that reminded me of the dark light of Nazi science. (They did not know it, but I was painfully aware that they were talking about *me*.) The idea appeals greatly to the orderly minds of some men of science. It was an English doctor who wrote in 1971, "I do not think we should encourage or enable genetic cripples to multiply their kind and spread genetic abnormality through the population."*

---

* The best response to this sort of thinking came from Dr. Alfredo Pavlovsky of Buenos Aires. Speaking at a hemophilia symposium in New York he said: "We cannot recommend the sterilization of all carriers since there are not yet any sure tests to individualize them and we run the risk that while we are busy trying to eliminate this disease, the hemophiliacs, who already have their own societies, may come to the conclusion that some of us ought to be eliminated because we are too fat, too big, too ugly and by transmitting to our offspring our own defects, we shall spoil the beauty of the race."

Thank God, the majority of doctors admit that such ideas trouble them greatly. The problem is, Where do you begin? No geneticist knows for sure how many genetic disorders are inescapably built into human beings. The English geneticist J. B. S. Haldane demonstrated that the sterilization of the unfit would have very little influence on the proportion of harmful genes scattered through the population; by the same token, the multiplication of "outstanding" genes, fewer in number, would have even less effect. Even if all genetic misfits were sterilized today, the rate of mutation assures that at least a third of the next generation would be affected by new cases of genetic disorder. In a significant number of genetic disorders that have recently appeared, there is no previous family history. Some researchers believe that this mysterious unexplained mutation is influenced by entirely new and rapidly changing environmental factors such as drugs and radiation.

Perhaps, even very soon, premarital genetic counseling will be routine. No doubt this will be useful and helpful. But I couldn't help thinking, as I heard those discussions among doctors, how glad I was that I had not been counseled *before*. For one thing, it is such an uneven relationship—the doctor, wearing a white coat and radiating scientific superiority, advising an untechnical, uninformed, frightened lay person. There is little training for such counseling in medical schools today—doctors are left to their own prejudices. Much of what passes under the guise of medical counseling really consists only of saying no; of advising the safe way, the way of least resistance. Not long ago, I attended a medical symposium and heard a famous geneticist talk learnedly about the need for "objective" counseling in cases of genetic disease. Fine. Then he concluded his remarks with this highly subjective sentence: "I cannot imagine a family who would not *wish to avoid* the emotional and financial stress imposed upon them when a hemophiliac is born."

I wonder. Suppose someone had talked to me this way? Suppose I had been told before I was married that I was a carrier of hemophilia and therefore should not have any children? Suppose I had been advised to adopt children? Personally, I am profoundly grateful that I was not told . . . that I did not have to make the decision of whether to have or not to have Bobby. Looking back at myself, a newly married young woman, unfamiliar with the feelings of a mother, I think, had I been asked, I would have said no. No one wants to suffer. Everyone is afraid of challenge and sacrifice. This is normal and human. If someone had asked me, "Do you want to walk through fire?" the answer would have been no, of course not. I am afraid of being burned. Yet once in the fire, I fought to get through it, and it is at least possible to think that the experience left me stronger. It is not struggle but the unknown that we fear most. If genetic counseling is to be meaningful, then not only must those counseled be informed of the purely scientific facts, they must also be encouraged to believe in themselves, in their own capacities to live and grow. They must be counseled not only to *fear*, but to be brave enough to live with a question.

Without questions, would we ever search for answers? A child with a genetic illness is a perpetual question, pushing us to seek answers to this dilemma of nature and God.

It was with all these vivid impressions that I waited for my third child.

I thought I was strong and hardened, but as the time drew closer I grew frantic. I had no one to care for Bobby and Susy. What if I had to leave at night and abandon them? Dr. Callahan suggested, "Wouldn't you feel better if you knew when the baby was coming?" My sister had three days off for the Washington's Birthday weekend. It was decided that she would come to watch the children and the baby would be induced a week early. The birth would take place on a Friday and I would go home on Monday. During my labor, visions of children in pain mingled with the threatening faces of doctors. As in a nightmare, while I was in painful contractions, a doctor came in and brusquely asked for a piece of the placenta to check it for hemophilia research. It was horrifying. I was afraid!

Elizabeth was born on that Friday, February 19. She was a lovely, plump baby with reddish-blond hair and round, rosy squirrel cheeks. It was a short but wonderful weekend we spent together at the hospital. I sat rocking her and looked out at the East River.

The river was wide and blue, dotted with boats large and small, boats calmly trusting themselves to the unseen currents that were carrying them out to a wide sea. Alone and at peace with the world, I gazed on the face of my new child. The future was in her eyes— and they were beautiful and clear.

Chapter 17

For Bobby, what could I do? I would have given anything to make him well, but I had nothing to give. It is the oldest maxim of torturers that the surest way to break you is to torture someone you love before your eyes. The loved one's pain becomes yours; it is even magnified because you are responsible for it. If you really want the pain to stop, you can say something, find someone, do something, to make it stop.

I was helpless. I couldn't find anything. When he needed my blood, I could lie down and they could take it from my arm and put it into his. I could look for specialists, track down the latest medicines, the most effective techniques. I could pay the bills. I could try—how often I failed!—to be comforting to him and to Sue. Nothing really helped.

The only thing I could do was to write about it. Of all the magazine articles I proposed, the one I most wanted to do was a story about hemophilia. Somehow, I needed to tell other people about it. To explain was a way to relieve the strain, to strike back. I don't know whether all people are affected this way; I expect in some degree they are. But as a writer, I know that to have a shattering experience like this is to feel an overwhelming compulsion to write about it.

From my earliest days as a journalist, I proposed this story to editors. In 1958, I wrote to the *Reader's Digest* (the letter was 1,200 words, half the length of a *Digest* article), proposing that Sue and I describe together our day-to-day life as young parents struggling against the disease. The *Digest* demurred.

During my five years at *Newsweek*, I hovered over the medicine section, urging them to do a story on hemophilia. The answer

—difficult to rebut—was, "We are a news magazine. We need a news peg. Let us know when there is a real medical breakthrough." There weren't any real breakthroughs, so *Newsweek* never did a story.

Finally, in 1963, I did write a hemophilia story for the *Post*. I visited doctors in Washington, D.C., Chapel Hill, Philadelphia, Boston, and New York, and my article was a survey of the medical, social, and psychological aspects of the disease. Along with the main hemophilia article, I submitted to the *Post* a subsidiary story, hoping they would print it as a separate boxed-off story, side-by-side with the main article. It was called "The Most Famous Hemophiliac" and was a brief four-page sketch of the life of the Tsarevich Alexis. As always with magazines, there was a space crunch and the Tsarevich box was quickly eliminated.

Nevertheless, my own interest in this small historical figure was growing. For years, I had heard the story of Rasputin and the Tsarevich. But it was only in outline—brief, remote, indistinct, blurred. Historians passed over it quickly, usually in no more than a sentence or two. Somehow to me, both as the father of a hemophiliac and as a product of the rigorous historical discipline I was trained in at Oxford, this treatment seemed inadequate. Surely, in those early days when no medical treatment for hemophilia was available, there must have been moments of terrible anguish for the parents of the boy. And surely, if someone was able to help him, that man or woman, no matter who, would wield enormous power. In any case, I wanted to find out.

I began using my lunch hour to visit the New York Public Library. In the years that followed, I came to love the Public Library. With its massive columns and broad steps flanked by recumbent lions, I think it is the handsomest public building in Manhattan. I love its old high-ceilinged corridors and reading rooms, its marble floors, the heavy wooden tables and chairs, polished to a glow by contact with thousands of bottoms, elbows, and arms. I liked studying the people who sat across the long reading tables—students, elderly women, men in retirement—turning pages, sifting piles of books before them, making notes, their faces absorbed in following some thread of knowledge.

It was exciting for me to step up to receive my pile of books.

Some of them were old and leather-bound, their pages crumbling. I carried them off like treasures to my seat. Often I sat there through lunch hour and beyond, shamelessly cheating my employers. I began coming in on my day off, sitting through the bright morning sunlight flooding in through the tall windows, the drowsiness of noon, the fading late-afternoon shadows that crept up the wall and merged into twilight. Then I would look up, and outside the sky of the city would be a rich, dark, early-evening blue. Reluctantly, I would pack up my papers, get my coat, and walk to Grand Central to take a train home—always reluctantly. There was more life for me in those pages than in the streets I walked through.

There were dozens of books to read. It seemed that everyone who left Russia because of the Revolution had made his or her first dollar, pound, or franc by writing a book. Grand Dukes, Grand Duchesses, government ministers, generals, diplomats, tutors, ladies-in-waiting, all contributed to a flood of memoirs published in the 1920's. But since then, no one had been much interested. Often, the desk would hand me a copy of a book that had stood on the shelves for forty years and that no one had read before. I learned to carry a knife in my briefcase so that I could slit new pages neatly.

It was not difficult to find significant material on Alexis' hemophilia. In the wartime letters between the Empress and the Tsar, there were constant, specific references to their son's condition. In Nicholas' letters to his mother, the Dowager Empress Marie, there were further descriptions of the boy's illness. In the memoirs of the Tsarevich's Swiss tutor and the reminiscences of the Empress' close confidante Anna Vyrubova, there were moving accounts of the parents' struggle. All of this gave a very different picture from the one I had always had.

It was Sue who suggested that the material might become a book. One day after breakfast, we went into the library and talked all morning. At first, I was dubious. "How can I?" I kept asking. "Why can't you?" she kept insisting. I went over with her again the fresh material I had found in the letters. "You see," Sue said, "nobody knows this. It has been completely ignored. You could change people's thinking about this whole subject."

Then, as she talked about Russian history, Russian literature, the Russian church, the Russian people she had met, I began to see that there was a book that could be done and that only we, as parents of a hemophiliac, could do it. I don't think either of us ever lost that first vision. From the first, we felt a strong sense of fate carrying us along.

When I had written a prospectus, I asked Teddy White for his advice on publishers. He recommended Atheneum, which had published his enormously successful *The Making of the President 1960*. Atheneum was willing, and we settled on a contract that called for delivery of the manuscript at the end of eleven months. An advance of $2,500 was to be sliced into quarterly payments.

Because the more I read about Russia the more I wanted to read, the book went slowly. By the end of the contract period, I had written only the first part, less than a quarter of the book. Then, beginning in March 1966, I began to slave. All day, shut up in my library, sitting in an old Lincoln rocker which Sue had bought in a junk store but which curved nicely to fit the small of my back, with my old college typewriter on my lap, I rattled away. At night when Sue was home from work, we went into the library, started an antique tape recorder which could record for hours, and with its spools spinning before us, discussed what I had written. The next morning, when she was back in New York, I replayed the tape, made notes, and began rewriting, incorporating these new ideas into the manuscript. Sue was a splendid editor. She was never negative, although she had a clear idea as to what was wheat and what was chaff. Frequently, when I was deeply bogged, she lifted me out and set me running again. Her own ideas were fresh and provocative. Of all the professional editors I have worked with, she is the best.

But editing was only one of Sue's contributions to the book. She suggested and did the research for the sections on the "silver age" and on early Russian history. She gave her feeling for Russia, her knowledge and love of ballet, of Russian myths, fairy tales, the church, and the workings of the Russian mind. When émigrés shake their heads and say they can't believe that an American writer could have so much understanding of Russia, the credit is mostly Sue's.

Every day, during her lunch hour, Sue worked on the book. She combed files and libraries for research materials, biographies, speeches, old news clippings. She tracked down hard-to-find, invaluable books. She looked for pictures, searching through all the picture collections and photo libraries in New York, as well as a number of émigré trunks. She did a fifty-page style list of Russian words so that the transliterated spelling from Russian into English would be uniform and correct. The dust jacket, using the white, blue, and red Imperial Russian flag and the double-headed eagle Romanov crest, was her idea and she worked with a Time-Life artist, Ladislav Svatos, a recent Czech émigré, to create an exact design.

For Sue as much as for me, it was a total commitment of three years of work. Hers was more than the contribution of a devoted wife; a devoted wife would not necessarily have had her professional capacities. And it was far more than the help of a professional editor; a professional editor would not have poured in love, imagination, belief, and hope. . . . In sum, quite simply, we created it together.

Now our roles were reversed. Sue was at the office; I was home. But the comparison is misleading. I did little for the children; I scarcely saw them. Nevertheless, for Elizabeth these years were pleasant. She was insulated from her nervous parents by the warm and friendly figure of Mrs. Connors. It was harder for Susy and Bobby. Bobby, sometimes in school, sometimes upstairs alone in his room, had only his books, his games, the television set. Susy, who was then in the third grade, went almost unnoticed.

"I never saw either of you," she remembers. "When I came home, I couldn't talk to anybody. You were always in a bad mood, Daddy. You used to shout at me through the closed library door, 'Leave me alone! Don't interrupt me! I'm working.'

"Mother came home late and I was already undressed. My life then was school and Mrs. Connors. She made our dinners and was there all the time.

"For me, the book was the sound of the typewriter and Russian music coming out of the library. And you and Mom talking into the tape recorder late at night. And all those pictures spread out on the floor.

"I remember that we didn't have any money. All of your friends who had daughters gave me hand-me-down clothes. I remember wondering, Why do they have to work so hard? Why don't we have more money? Why does it have to be our family?"

Even then, of course, I knew that the family was under terrible strain, but having embarked on this long and risky voyage, there was no turning back. If we made it, then, as Sue said, everything would be better. If we didn't, then I would go back and get a job and we would try to live like other people. Either way, if we could only survive the months ahead, things would get better.

In the middle of this ordeal, in order to cheer up the children I issued this promissory note:

> When this book is finished, I promise:
> 1) I will take my children out to dinner.
> 2) I will take my children to see *The Sound of Music*.
> 3) I will buy my children a color TV set. All this I do faithfully promise to do because my children are good children.
>
> Robert K. Massie

By mid-September 1966 I was supposed to be finished, but I wasn't. My publishers were chilly. Also, they were nervous. A book on the Romanovs had appeared in England. Plunged into gloom, with this other book hanging over me like a sword, I kept going while Sue tracked down the book's origins and exposed it as a fraud, written by a forger. Six weeks later, on November 1, I finished. (I wasn't really finished; I intended to rewrite Part I, but the publisher had a completed manuscript, which made him happy.)

Through Christmas and into January I rewrote. On January 17, Sue delivered the finished 900-page manuscript to Atheneum. There was still more for me to do: with so controversial a subject, I thought it essential to include extensive notes on sources. Working on the notes, I found myself beginning to crumble. I had headaches that kept me in swirling, weightless darkness for twenty-four hours. I couldn't concentrate. Writing to Atheneum, I said, "I have been working on the Notes, but it has been extraordinarily difficult. Not editorially, but mentally and physically. I just sit in my chair staring at pieces of paper and my mind wanders everywhere, insolently refusing to focus on the problems at hand. . . ."

Financially, we were sinking. I had no income at all between November and March. Sue's salary covered less than half of our living expenses. On my plea, the publisher gave me another $500, which Sue rushed to the bank. It was like throwing a glass of water on the Sahara. Our bills were unpaid and our credit was poor. "We sincerely regret that we have been unable to pass favorably on your recent application . . ." wrote the credit managers on their mimeographed stationery.

Then, suddenly, in March, our lives began to change. The Literary Guild selected the book as its September offering. A month later, the *Reader's Digest* decided to make it a condensed book. We were suddenly catapulted from penury into having at least two years of guaranteed income.

This good news was tinged with sadness. On the day that I heard that the Literary Guild had accepted my book, my uncle and godfather, Hardin Massie, who suffered from emphysema, slipped into a coma.

An old-school gentleman, a marine officer in both World Wars, Hardin knew about courage under fire and for this reason he had taken a special interest in Bobby. I found that I could write to him freely. "All I care about," I said in one letter, "is seeing that my son, who is a very gallant as well as a charming little boy, has opportunities to which his exceptional intelligence entitles him. He overcomes difficulties which would easily have crushed me. This week, he came and calmly said that some of the boys on the playground had been yelling 'Leather Legs' at him because of his braces, and just as I was turning red with a kind of helpless rage, he said that, by the way, he had just been elected vice-president of his class. Incidentally, because he has been working so hard on his therapy, he has been taking off his braces for a few hours at a time while playing outside. This week, for the first time in his life, Bobby climbed a tree. I can't express to you what this meant to me."

From the beginning, Hardin was fascinated by the book I was writing and he kept sending encouragement and little checks "for the pot" as he put it. "Knowing you are concentrating on your book," he would say in his letters, "I have eased off writing, as I didn't want to burden you with answering. . . ."

When the news came from the Literary Guild, the first person I called was Kit Massie, Hardin's wife. She was in his hospital room. "Tell me all the details," she said. "I'm going to try to tell him." Kit doesn't know whether Hardin ever understood. I hope so. It hurts finally to have reached a point where I could justify his confidence and think that he never knew.

Through the spring, I worked on the galley proofs, the maps, the genealogical tables, and the acknowledgments. In July, we went to Maine. Sue commuted three days a week to New York. I stayed behind, watching the children, restless and brooding. There was a lot of fog that summer which hindered sailing. I passed the time sawing logs and splitting them into stove wood (we cooked as well as kept warm with the wood from the forest around us). At the end of July, Bobby and I flew down to New York to appear on a TV program for Hemophilia Day at Yankee Stadium. An appeal for blood was flashed repeatedly on the scoreboard and I spoke for three minutes between the two games of a doubleheader. But only six people actually made their way to the Bloodmobile van parked outside the stadium and donated blood.

On the afternoon of Bobby's eleventh birthday, Thursday, August 17, in the middle of the annual birthday party with all the Red House children, my publisher telephoned me in Maine to say that the book would be reviewed on the front page of the Sunday *New York Times Book Review*. The review was favorable; we were both happy.

The days that followed were filled with excitement, surprise, and bewilderment. Like swimmers in a powerful, fast-flowing stream, we were swept along, unsure of our bearings, unable to reach the shore, wholly preoccupied with the essential problem of simply staying afloat. There were hundreds of reviews in newspapers and magazines all over the country, and later, all over the world. By myself or with Sue I was interviewed on innumerable television and radio programs in New York, Boston, Chicago, Washington, Philadelphia, Toronto, and Nashville. (After watching me on the *Today* show, my mother wrote: "You were most impressive, really excellent, but why did Hugh Downs keep leaning over in front of you and getting the back of his head in the picture when it was a closeup of you? I was quite annoyed with him.")

There were three thousand letters. They came from friends, classmates, cousins (real and imagined), hemophiliacs, mothers, fathers, and grandparents of hemophiliacs, doctors, lawyers, judges, businessmen, ministers, priests, nuns, housewives, grade-school children, high-school students, college students, graduate students, professors, university presidents, librarians, authors, publishers, editors, admirals (British and American), mayors, congressmen, senators, Members of Parliament, ambassadors, a former American Secretary of State, titled and royal persons from across Europe, and the First Lady of the United States. Of all of these letters and messages, I remember two most clearly. The first was a telegram that arrived the week of publication from three Russians in Leningrad saying, "The book has been published. We are with you in your happiness. Be sure." The other was a letter sent from Kabul by the American ambassador to Afghanistan. He wrote: "A few months ago I was bitten by a dog and while I hung my injured arm over the wash basin to let the blood drip slowly and waited for the doctor, I started to read the book. As the doctor was fairly slow in coming (it was late at night), I got quite a bit of it read . . ."

In September the whole family went to Nashville to enact a delightful version of Home-Town Boy Makes Good. There were autograph parties in the bookstores I used to loiter in as a teenager. There were parties that became a kaleidoscopic blur of old classmates, old teammates, old teachers, and old girl friends. The nicest time was when Bobby and I went canoeing with Jack May on the Harpeth River. It was a warm, lazy, Indian summer afternoon, with no noise except the dip and splash of paddles as we glided in the brown water under the overhanging branches. The river still seemed wild, looping through the harvested farmlands, spotted here and there with unpainted cabins and rusting barbed-wire fences. Here, in this rolling country, I had hiked as a Boy Scout, swum in the river, looked for arrowheads and Indian mounds. Now, only a few miles away, the new towers of the city shimmered and modern expressways girdled a growing metropolis; but here, on the river, it was the same as it had been thirty, and perhaps two hundred, years before.

All that fall the telephone rang incessantly. Often it sounded at the same moment as the doorbell; neighbors were coming by with books—sometimes a pile of five or six—to be signed as Christmas presents. Complete strangers telephoned to ask me to lunch or to invite Sue and me to dinner. People wanted me to help them get their manuscripts published. University libraries wrote to ask that I donate my papers and correspondence. Editors wrote proposing magazine articles. Publishers wrote proposing books. Suddenly, I found myself in demand as a lecturer at colleges, prep schools, high schools, church groups, hemophilia chapters, women's clubs, the Friends of local libraries. . . . It was heady, dizzying, disorienting—like a steady diet of too much champagne. After a while, I began to long for the days in my library, looking up from the typewriter and out at the trees.

The Russian émigrés liked the book. The surviving Romanovs endorsed it; so did Stolypin's son, Yussopov's daughter, and a host of others who had seen and survived the upheaval.

Despite this praise, I was disturbed as Sue and I began to be invited to dinners and dances with the émigré community. Few of these descendants of princes, still calling themselves prince and princess, seemed to grasp the reason for which the book was written. With rare exceptions, they showed not the slightest interest in hemophilia. When Sue mentioned this once to one of these ladies, she countered indignantly, "But hemophilia is not even a *Russian* disease." Ironically, this was precisely the argument given sixty years before by St. Petersburg ladies in talking about Alexandra and Alexis. We were back again, full circle, with nothing learned, nothing understood.

If the Russian émigré aristocracy showed little interest in hemophilia, that was not true of members of the interlocking European royal family, all descended in some degree from the "Granny" of European royalty, and the first royal hemophilic carrier, Queen Victoria. Two great-grandsons of the Queen, Earl Mountbatten of Burma and the Duke of Windsor, both showed interest and sympathy.

I met the Duke of Windsor in a New York restaurant during an evening arranged by Serge Obolensky. We shook hands and he straightforwardly gave me his opinion: "Mr. Massie, I enjoyed reading your book, but I don't think you were quite fair to my father (he was talking about King George V's role in the British government's decision on whether to rescue and offer asylum to the Russian Imperial family). You know, it wasn't my father who refused to send a ship for them. He was extremely fond of his cousin Nicky. It was the politicians, particularly that awful Lloyd George, who refused to have the Tsar come to England. Later, after the Bolsheviks murdered that whole family, my father was so shocked that he refused to see the first Russian ambassador when Great Britain recognized the Soviet Union. He stayed up-stairs at Buckingham Palace and sent me down to accept the man's credentials. Afterwards, he wanted to know what the ambassador looked like. 'Probably had a beard with a bomb underneath,' he said to me."

The Duke was very short and thin, almost a miniature. His white hair still had a touch of blond, there were the sad, pouched eyes, the blue tie with white polka dots tied in the famous Windsor knot. The Duchess was there, tiny and radiating energy from her intense blue eyes. It was obvious that she made him happy. She told him where to sit and, worrying out loud about his heart, tried to order his dinner. But the Duke didn't like her choice—very lean meat and a small piece of cheese—and ordered quenelles in rich sauce and, later, his favorite dessert, rum raisin ice cream.

We talked about the Russian family and the Duchess asked him, "David, didn't you give an allowance to your Russian cousins during the time that you were king?" He said that he had. They both asked about hemophilia. The Duchess said, "Well, they'll surely find a cure soon. I'm sure of it." The Duke, however, kept asking questions. I was going on and on about plasma fractions, and spleen transplants, and home transfusions, and then at one point I stopped and said, "I'm giving you too much of a medical lecture." He leaned forward and touched my arm and said, "Oh, no; please go on. What a wonderful thing it is to know so much and care so much." So I continued as the two celebrated black pug dogs leaped in and out of their laps. I almost forgot that this simple, elderly but still elegant, handsome, and exceptionally charming man had been the king of England.

Inevitably, along with letters from the real Romanovs, came letters from the false ones—fat, bulky envelopes, containing twenty scrawled pages beginning, "I am the third child of Nicholas II, Tsar of Russia . . ." One lady signed herself "Mrs. J. Edgar Hoover, Her Imperial Majesty Catherine III Romanov-Hoover, Diplomatic Agent Five Star A.G., Chief of Mission for President Lyndon Baines Johnson." Most of the letters were pathetic, but sometimes these people and their devoted supporters become disconcertingly rude. Let anyone express a degree of skepticism and they become furiously angry; they attack and insult. Once, in France, I made the mistake of agreeing to appear in a televised debate on the merits of the Anna Anderson case. (Mrs. Anderson is the lady who has claimed for more than fifty years that she is the Grand Duchess Anastasia.) The French love this kind of historical mystery, and the program had millions of viewers. Four supporters were opposed to four skeptics, myself among the latter. The problem was that the supporters were all fanatics, what the French call *cultistes*, absolutely convinced that the lady was Anastasia. Any expression of doubt ("Why is it that the lady does not speak Russian?") drove the *cultistes* into a fury. While one elderly survivor of the Russian court was expressing her doubts, the *cultistes* went into contortions of off-camera sneers, snorts, headshaking, and handwaving.

In the end, of course, nothing was proved, although no doubt the large audience was entertained and titillated. Whether the evening—or, in fact, any of these interminable shenanigans involving self-convinced grand duchesses and tsareviches—was worth the further desecration of the memory of long-dead Russian children is another question. Personally, I think we should let Olga, Tatiana, Marie, Anastasia, and Alexis rest in peace.

As the days went by in that extraordinary autumn, with so many new faces—some famous, some strange, some merely curious about us—crowding into our lives, we met Sam Spiegel, the formidable producer who had made two successful movie epics, *Bridge on the River Kwai* and *Lawrence of Arabia.* He was interested in making a film out of *Nicholas and Alexandra.*

Mr. Spiegel invited Sue and me to lunch at the St. Regis Hotel. He is a short man with a prominent nose, unusually large, almost liquid, brown eyes, and a husky voice with a middle-European accent. He exuded a sweet cologne blended with the smell of expensive Havana cigars. The lunch went well and we were invited to Mr. Spiegel's Park Avenue apartment, hailed as dear friends, given drinks, shown the hallways lined with splendid impressionist paintings, the projection room in which screen and projector slide into place at the touch of a button, the bedroom with an acre-sized bed, and the bathroom hung with Daumier gravures. When we went down the elevator into the lobby, my agent, who was with us, beamed. "Sam is definitely interested."

We waited.

My birthday came in January, and Sue and I were in the kitchen doing the dishes when the phone rang. It was a telegram wishing me a happy birthday, signed, "Affectionately, Sam." A few days later, Sam Spiegel made an offer and we accepted.

In the end, the film did not live up to our hopes. It had a splendid English cast but a shallow script. For all the money spent on sets and costumes, the film lacked depth of emotion and it had almost no feeling for Russia. But everything is relative: thus we were happy that it was as good as it was and, at the same time, disappointed that it wasn't better.

Above all, one important thing happened: the story of a hemophiliac was up there on the screen, the subject of a major film. Millions of people saw it and, hopefully, took away from the theater more understanding of the disease and perhaps a bit more sympathy for its victims. In a remarkable way, the vicious disease that had attacked Bobby and ravaged our lives had also provided us with the weapons to fight back.

One thing that seems to happen to fathers of hemophiliacs is an overwhelming desire to conquer the disease personally. Perhaps it is something deeply male: when the home and young are threatened, the father's role is to go out and destroy the enemy that threatens his family. In any case, this urge is almost a compulsion. I have felt it strongly in myself and seen it in others. Robert Lee Henry, a New York lawyer, whose only son Lee was a hemophiliac, decided in 1947 that "I'd lick this disease all by myself." He founded the National Hemophilia Foundation. Twenty years later, George Stone, a Texan, whose sons Randy and Skipper are both hemophiliacs, decided that the Hemophilia Foundation and the Red Cross were too heavy with bureaucracy to act decisively. He founded the Component Therapy Institute, whose purpose is to encourage the separation of blood into its different components, thus—among many other advantages—making more AHF available for hemophiliacs.

I seem destined in life to be an observer, not a builder. But even this has utility, not only in a general way (I could write stories about the disease and make people more aware), but also in the selfish sense that, as a journalist, I could get in to see doctors, researchers, and all kinds of officials and bureaucrats who probably wouldn't have taken the time to see a mere father. Thus, wearing two hats, I was able to keep myself reasonably well informed as to what was going on in hemophilia research and what the chances were for a significant breakthrough that might radically improve Bobby's life.

For most of his life, the most important possible breakthrough has been the development of an AHF concentrate or fraction. The dream, which persisted through all the years of "miracle cures" and of people saying "Surely they will find something very soon," was of a concentrate so powerful that a small daily injection, perhaps not necessarily even into a vein but simply under the skin, would prevent all bleeding. The hemophiliac, with his daily shot of AHF concentrate, would then be like the diabetic with his daily shot of insulin. This was the dream.

But there were other even more immediate and urgent reasons than the daily preventive shot for developing an AHF concentrate. Hemophiliacs needed a concentrate simply to ensure survival. For the first ten years of Bobby's life, we treated his bleeding episodes in what was then the routine way: with transfusions of fresh-frozen plasma. Sometimes, even with "normal" bleeding episodes, we had trouble getting enough plasma into Bobby to stop the hemorrhage. But for the hemophiliac who had a serious accident, or acute appendicitis and needed major surgery, the prospects were dim. In order to control his massive bleeding, so much plasma had to be poured into the patient's veins that, very often, the circulatory system simply could not take it; the patient's heart would fail from circulatory overload. (In a few desperate life-or-death cases of this kind, Dr. Tocantins resorted to what seems an almost medieval—and, at the same time, a highly logical—solution. As plasma or fresh whole blood flowed into the patient through a vein in one arm, an equal amount of the patient's blood was taken out through a vein in the opposite arm. In this way, while the volume of fluid in the circulatory system remained constant, the level of AHF was raised sufficiently to cause clotting.)

Attempts to concentrate AHF had been going on in a number of countries since the end of World War II. In the United States, Dr. Edwin J. Cohn of Harvard had purified AHF in the laboratory. But the Cohn fraction had only four or five times the power of plasma, it was enormously expensive to produce, and its use had been very limited. At Oxford, Dr. Rosemary Biggs and Professor R. G. MacFarlane had produced laboratory samples of AHF concentrate made from both human and animal blood. The animal AHF had great advantages: it was cheap, plentiful, and enormously powerful. British slaughterhouses could supply oceans of pigs' blood and cows' blood, and, drop for drop, bovine or porcine blood has ten times as much AHF as human blood. But there was an insurmountable obstacle: the human body quickly makes antibodies and rejects foreign proteins. Thus, the first injection of animal AHF usually goes well and its massive impact effectively causes the desired clotting. But antibodies form, and any second injection will be rejected, perhaps violently. Each animal fraction, therefore, can be used only once. In the words of a British hematologist: "In extreme emergencies, the two animal fractions give hemophiliacs two extra lives, but they cannot be used in life-long, day-to-day care."

In 1963, when I was writing my first hemophilia story, the most successful AHF fraction in the world was being made in Sweden by the husband-wife team of Drs. Birger and Margarita Blomback. The Blomback fraction had a purification of ten to twenty times the power of plasma and was used regularly to treat severe hemophilia. But the scale of Sweden's problems was different from America's. Enough AHF fraction for all Swedish hemophiliacs could be produced by three people working in a single laboratory.

At that time, the most productive hemophilia research center in the United States was at the University of North Carolina in Chapel Hill. And the single man most responsible for this preeminence was a transplanted Iowa farm boy named Kenneth M. Brinkhous. Over the years, he has gathered a team of pathologists, biochemists, geneticists, and surgeons who individually and collectively have investigated innumerable avenues of hemophilia research. Today, Dr. Brinkhous is recognized as one of the three or four great hemophilia pioneers in the world. Like acolytes, other hematologists, themselves already renowned, come to spend a year at Chapel Hill working with Brinkhous.

Naturally, he was the first man I wanted to see, and arriving at the Medical Center Building of the University of North Carolina, I found him in front of a blackboard filled with equations, formulae, and graphs.

He is an immensely likable man: thin, bespectacled, earnest, friendly, his Midwestern twang unchanged despite almost three decades in the South. We talked a while and then Dr. Brinkhous asked if I would like to meet some of the hemophiliacs with whom he worked.

"Yes, I'd like to talk to them very much," I said.

"I'm afraid most of them can't talk," he said, smiling. "In fact, most of them don't even have names. Only numbers."

He took me to see these unusual patients. We drove out of town, winding through the wooded red-clay hills until we reached a modern brick building beside a lake. Inside was a fully equipped laboratory, an operating room, and freezer storage room for plasma. Out in back were the cages of the eighteen hemophiliac males and carrier females, all beautiful auburn Irish setters. Overjoyed to have visitors, they barked, wagged their tails, and stood up on their hind legs against their cages, just like any other dogs. But the cages were padded and overhead were loudspeakers playing Muzak, which, the keepers had found, helped to tranquilize the dogs. This day, however, they were in full chorus—not only the eighteen Irish setters, but the thirty-two other dogs on the premises, hearty, healthy, tail-wagging mutts who served as donors, assuring the setters a constant supply of canine plasma.

On the way back, Dr. Brinkhous explained that he had happened on the original setter, a female carrier, in Wisconsin in 1947. He imported her to North Carolina and had overseen the birth of hundreds of her descendants. Through the years, the dogs who suffer from severe hemophilia had been of incalculable value. Working with them, Brinkhous pioneered what should have become the standard technique in transfusion therapy with fresh-frozen plasma. His basic rule was: Be aggressive. Don't hold back. As soon as an animal shows the slightest sign of swelling, or joint stiffness and limping, treat intensively with plasma. Later, in autopsy, they discovered that dogs treated this way showed little evidence of the joint damage normally caused by repeated bleeding.

Along with developing techniques in plasma therapy, Brinkhous was using the dogs in trying to develop an intramuscular injection of AHF—one that would not require getting into a vein. He and his colleagues had worked out a method for identifying which females in a litter were carriers of the defective gene. He had proved that hemophiliac females, hitherto thought to be only theoretically possible, could be bred and could survive. With complicated surgery, involving passing the blood of a hemophiliac dog through the spleen of a healthy dog, they had even found evidence suggesting that the spleen has something to do with the presence—or absence—of AHF in the body.

But the most important work being done in hemophilia research, Dr. Brinkhous felt, concerned "the isolation and purification of the AHF fraction. Here at Chapel Hill," he said, "we have achieved fractions thirty to forty times the potency of fresh-frozen plasma. But we have only done it in small batches for use in catastrophic bleeding situations in our own hospital. What we are looking for is something that can be of general use for hospitals, doctors, and hemophiliacs everywhere."

Leaving Chapel Hill that spring of 1963, I found that Dr. Brinkhous was largely alone in his search. Other researchers were pessimistic on the prospects for any widespread use of AHF concentrates. There was too little of it and what there was cost too much. Dr. Raphael Shulman of the National Institutes of Health, whose project was testing the efficacy of the Cohn fraction in major surgery, told me that "with fraction, we can do any kind of surgery we could do with normal patients." But the cost of covering a tooth extraction was $1,000; enough fraction to cover abdominal surgery was $8,000. This was too expensive, even for NIH.

Dr. Martin Rosenthal, medical director of the National Hemophilia Foundation, was even gloomier. "For the foreseeable future, AHF fractions will have only a very, very limited purpose," he predicted. "For surgery, fractions are essential—if somebody is willing and able to pay the bill. But any widespread, general use of fractions in noncritical situations—the daily prophylactic shot, for example—still is only a dream of the public relations boys."

That was where things stood in 1963. At home, Bobby was six and just beginning the most difficult years of crippling joint bleeding. We went on transfusing him with the only thing available: fat bags of fresh-frozen plasma. To get 250 AHF units into him, we had to pour 250 milliliters of mostly useless fluid plasma into his veins. Then, suddenly, in 1965, from a completely unexpected direction, came the wonderful news that a simple, inexpensive method had been found for separating AHF from plasma. As a result, a new concentrate was available which could be made without special equipment in almost any hospital blood bank. The researcher responsible for this breakthrough was a remarkable woman, Dr. Judith Pool of Stanford University.

Judy Pool was born in Queens, New York. "Even in high school, I loved science," she says. "I picked biochemistry as my major. My parents didn't take the idea of such a career seriously. My mother was convinced that the only success in life for girls came from beauty. I was plain and my mother was doubtful that anyone would ever want to marry me."

At eighteen, when she was a sophomore at the University of Chicago, Judy married a young political science instructor. By the age of twenty-three, she had two sons. Despite her marriage and children, she continued her career in science. She developed a technique using an electrode to measure the electrical potential of a single muscle fiber within a membrane; her technique is now used all over the world. When her husband was offered a professorship at Hobart College, she followed him, although it meant giving up her own work. But when he developed tuberculosis and required long hospitalization, "it seemed a good time for me to go back to Chicago and my attempt to have a career in science."

"Accident determines everything," she believes. "During those years I worked in a school for retarded children, I was a secretary, I taught English and physics, I went to the Hoover Library in California and worked on propaganda material, I worked at Stanford on a cancer research project involving nutrition . . . anything that came along. Then, in 1953, someone at Stanford was looking for a Fellow to do research in blood clotting. I knew nothing about blood clotting, but they wanted a full-time researcher and I wanted a Ph.D.

"In research, accurate measurement is almost everything," she continued. "Sometimes it takes five years to get an exact assay. And you have to work in your own style. In working with fresh-frozen plasma, I was shocked to find how low the levels of AHF were.

I wondered why. I would stay for hours in front of the centrifuge. One day, while plasma was infusing into a patient, I wondered whether it was losing AHF activity during the forty minutes this took. I took a sample of freshly thawed plasma before infusion, and a sample from the same plasma at the end of the infusion. There was much more activity in the final sample than in the first, but in the very last drops the assay seemed to fail me. These drops looked so different; they were full of threads. I was terribly depressed.

"Then, I began wondering: Could these threads have anything to do with it? I centrifuged the last drops, got a concentrated lump of threads, analyzed the threads, and found that they were very rich in AHF. Then, using different combinations of temperature and length of time in thawing, I began trying to get a residue of AHF. I found that when frozen plasma is slowly thawed in a cold atmosphere of five degrees centigrade, and then the liquid plasma is drained from the bag, it leaves behind a soft, white residue rich in AHF." Dr. Pool called this residue cryoprecipitate (precipitated by extreme cold), or cryo for short.

Besides enormous concentration of AHF, cryo had other great advantages. It could be left in the plastic bag, refrozen, and stored for up to a year without losing potency. It was so cheap and easy to prepare that any hospital equipped to separate whole blood into red cells and plasma could make it. In addition, after extraction of the cryo, the remainder of the plasma, now poor in AHF, could be reconstituted with its own original red cells to re-create a unit of whole blood. Or, alternatively, the plasma, having given up its AHF, could be further fractioned to yield albumin, gamma globulin, etc.

Catapulted by her discovery into the front rank of pioneering hemophilia researchers, Dr. Pool has continued her work in the field. Of her discovery of cryoprecipitate, she says, "I had no greater insight than anyone else. I just happened to be there at the right moment." Did she ever think of getting an M.D.? "No. I'm really a physiologist with a medical side. Actually, I'm very squeamish. I'm fine with an anesthetized animal or a tube of blood. But I'm scared to death of real illness or trouble. I would be terrified if I had to put a needle into a frightened, suffering child."

Blood banks and hospitals all over the world immediately began to make Judy Pool's cryo. It became available in New York in 1966 and we began to use it. We kept the bags deep frozen at −20°C. in a freezer in the basement. When Bobby needed a transfusion, we took the cryo from the freezer and thawed it in lukewarm water while waiting for Dr. Engel to arrive. When the cryo inside the bags had melted to a yellowish, thready liquid, we inverted the bag on a transfusion rack over Bobby's head.

We used a lot of cryo. By early 1967, Bobby was having six bags of cryo automatically with every transfusion, and I was picking up eighteen bags, enough for three transfusions, in every trip to the Red Cross. By early March, I was making these trips once a week. As each bag of cryo cost $13.50, each transfusion was costing $81—excluding Dr. Engel's fee—and each week's pickup was worth $243. In March alone, I picked up seventy-two bags of cryo, which cost $972. Fortunately, during this period Sue was working at Time Inc. From March 1966 to March 1967 we used $5,310 worth of fresh-frozen plasma and cryo. The Travelers Insurance Company, which carried the Time Inc. group plan, paid three-quarters of this expense, $3,982. We paid the balance, $1,328.

Despite the cost, cryo was a great advance and doctors were enthusiastic. Dr. Shulman at NIH and Dr. Biggs at Oxford immediately began using it to cover major surgical operations. Both were delighted with it. "It's here, it's safe, it's cheap, it's easy to make, and it works. What more do we want?" asked Dr. Shulman.

What we, the families, wanted, of course, was a more normal life, and in this respect, although cryo was a major advance, it still had serious drawbacks. It had impurities, which still in a few rare cases caused allergic transfusion reactions. It lacked a measurable strength; you had to guess how many AHF units were in each bag. And, most difficult, because it had to be kept deep frozen, it was awkward to handle and transport. One could not stray far from a deep freeze; we could travel only in sudden dashes, with the cryo packed in dry ice, as we did on our trips to Maine.

And so, grateful as we were for cryo, we still continued to

dream of a stable, dried concentrate, the kind that Dr. Brinkhous was working on, one that could be stored in the refrigerator among the milk and vegetables, so to speak.

In the autumn of 1967, after the publication of *Nicholas and Alexandra*, I had enough time to do what I wanted for a while. Bobby's health was not improving. Constant, repeated bleeding was destroying his joints, and he now wore braces on both legs. When he walked, it was stiff-legged, as if he were on little stilts. For this reason I was anxious to peer into the future to see what was happening in the field of hemophilia research.

Already I knew that Dr. Brinkhous was getting closer to producing his AHF concentrate. *The New York Times* had run a long story on hemophilia and AHF concentrates which featured Dr. Brinkhous and predicted "the day when the hemophiliac may be able to carry a vial containing the vital clotting factor his blood lacks. . . . The hemophiliac might even be able to inject the life-saving factor [himself] with a hypodermic needle."

On the strength of this, and other bright spots appearing on the hemophilia horizon, I proposed an article to David Halberstam and Willie Morris of *Harper's* magazine. They gave me the assignment and, once again, I donned my journalist's hat and began to make the rounds.

During the nine months that followed, I became very excited. Suddenly, it seemed, great strides were being made which promised unbelievable changes. The concentrate had arrived. It was enormously powerful. It could stop massive hemorrhages, cover major surgery, and raise the possibility of prophylactic transfusions. For the first time, hemophiliacs were offered a life not dissimilar from diabetics: not totally normal, perhaps, but so much better than before, that for the hemophiliac and his family it would seem a transformation.

But there was another side of this story, a side that at first I found disquieting and then, as I learned more, deeply upsetting. Two men working in laboratories, one in the hills of North Carolina, the other in a room above the morgue of a New York City hospital, had both created something that could make Bobby's life and the lives of other American hemophiliacs almost normal. And yet the result of neither man's work was to become widely available. In one case, the obstacle was money. The concentrate, turned over to a commercial drug company, was priced far beyond the reach of all but a few American hemophilia families. In the other case, the story was more complicated: a medical pioneer was fighting against the executive bureaucracy of his own organization, the American Red Cross, which in turn was unwilling to compete with a commercial drug company by producing a lower-cost Red Cross AHF concentrate. The victims in both cases were hemophiliacs and their families.

I began by going back to Chapel Hill to see Dr. Brinkhous. I found him happy and optimistic. His laboratory work on his AHF concentrate was completed. He had developed and turned over to a commercial drug company, Hyland Laboratories of Los Angeles, for production and marketing, the technique for making an AHF concentrate thirty times as powerful as plasma. It needed only to be kept in the refrigerator. You could travel with it in a cooler the same way you would take a can of beer on a picnic. Medically, there was no reason it could not be given several times a week, on a prophylactic basis. The only problems Dr. Brinkhous foresaw were availability and cost.

"How much would it cost?" I asked.

"Our rule of thumb has been that it will cost about ten cents per AHF unit," Dr. Brinkhous said.

I did a quick calculation in my head. Bobby was getting about 400 to 450 AHF units of cryo in every transfusion; that meant $40 to $45. And he was having about 100 transfusions per year. That meant $4,000 to $4,500. It was no more than we were paying already for cryo. But suppose we needed more AHF units per transfusion? Or more transfusions per year? Or the cost was higher than ten cents per AHF unit? How would we—how would any of the nation's hemophiliacs—pay for it?

"This is a big problem," Dr. Brinkhous admitted. "We've solved the scientific problem of concentrates, but we haven't solved the social problems. I was talking the other day with an HEW official about the special problems of 'fractional populations' —people whose medical problems are so great that society must make special allowances. I believe that society is going to have to figure out a way to pay for this kind of thing. The families simply can't do it by themselves."

This statement by Dr. Brinkhous worried me. How likely was it that the federal government, which had never done anything for most chronically ill Americans, and certainly nothing at all for hemophiliacs, would suddenly start paying for AHF concentrates? And if the federal government did not pay for it, who would? Who could? Wasn't there some way to reduce the price so that we, the hemophiliacs, could pay for it ourselves?

We spent Thanksgiving weekend 1967 in Washington, partly so that Bobby could be with his friend Davey Gardner, and partly so that Sue and I could attend the annual meeting of the National Hemophilia Foundation. At this meeting, we heard a remarkable speech by a hematologist working for the American Red Cross, Dr. Alan Johnson. Through the early years, when we attended occasional local meetings of the New York Hemophilia chapter, we had heard about a shadowy figure named "Dr. Johnson" who was working on an AHF concentrate. From time to time, we would hear that "Dr. Johnson is making progress." Eventually, we heard that Dr. Johnson had developed an excellent concentrate and tested it successfully on hemophiliacs in surgery. But it was only available in small amounts for experimental purposes or extreme emergencies.

That night in Washington, Dr. Johnson was accepting, on behalf of the president of the American Red Cross, an award for his own work in AHF concentrates. He was not really supposed to give a speech; he was supposed to say thank you and sit down. Instead, he spoke for twenty minutes, talking about the prospects and the challenge of his concentrate. His delivery was soft and hesitant—he is an awkward speaker—but while he spoke, the ballroom filled with people was absolutely silent. He said that a vastly improved program of treatment and even preventive care for hemophiliacs was in sight, using AHF concentrates. He spoke of the need for far greater supplies of plasma, and for the utilization of component therapy, the advanced techniques of separating each unit of blood into five or six useful parts—red cells, white cells, platelets, fibrinogen, gamma globulin, and AHF—so that each patient would get only what he needs and one million units of blood could be divided and used to help six million people.

That morning, the audience had heard doctors from many countries in Europe where medical care programs are better organized, more inclusive and generous than in the United States. They had spoken of their free cryo and concentrate for hemophiliacs, their free special wards, special schools, special camps, special braces, special doctors and nurses, special vacations, special vocational training programs. We were all amazed and jealous, for in the United States we had almost nothing of this. But then, after reminding us of these things, Dr. Johnson said: "This is one approach. It is very costly. And I don't believe it is necessary. You see, instead of special schools and hospitals and doctors, I want to use this concentrate and have normal children."

It was because of these words and the human compassion they manifested that, through all that was to follow, I believed in Alan Johnson.

Deeply impressed by what I had heard, I asked Dr. Johnson whether I could come and see him in New York. His lab is tucked away in a corner of the old Pathology Building of Bellevue Hospital. Climbing the stairs, I smelled the unmistakable odors of the morgue and autopsy chambers on the first floor. Opening Johnson's door, I found myself inside a large room jammed with desks, lab benches, centrifuges, refrigerators, microscopes, textbooks, filing cabinets, chairs. From his desk at one end of this close-packed room, Dr. Johnson rose to meet me. He is a shy, soft-spoken man, whose eyes seem nervous, but whose quiet voice has a steely quality. Born in Washington, D.C., he grew up in Virginia and Wisconsin, graduated from Dartmouth in 1940, went to Long Island Medical College. He was an intern at Bellevue and has never left, advancing up the ladder to professor of medicine. In 1961, he became director of the Red Cross Blood Research Laboratory in New York. He works endless hours, often walking to the lab in the middle of the night from his brownstone on West 12th Street. His companion on these nocturnal hikes is his big, shaggy English sheepdog.

He explained to me that over the years he had developed a series of three AHF concentrates which, according to their potency, he had labeled Low Powered, Intermediate Powered, and

High Powered. He had already discontinued his work on the Low Powered because cryo was better. The Intermediate Powered had most of the same characteristics as Dr. Brinkhous' concentrate, which Hyland was preparing to make. Limited production had begun at Squibb Laboratories under contract to the Red Cross, and he had applied for a license to make large quantities. The High Powered concentrate, with one hundred to four hundred times the power of plasma, was his real hope. It had worked beautifully in the lab, but he was still working to improve it before trying to put it in production.

But Dr. Johnson's concentrate had run into some kind of trouble. It was still not licensed. "The intermediate concentrate is through all tests and has been medically approved all up and down the line. We are waiting for a license."

I asked how long it would take. He said six months.

Something that Dr. Johnson said, or the way he said it, bothered me. Why is it taking so long? I asked. He hemmed—hawed—seemed embarrassed. He was quite unlike the man who had flung out a bold challenge to the hemophilia meeting a short time before. What was the matter? I pursued the point; I pushed him.

Finally, he said, "The real problem is that there is no strong leadership in the national level of the American Red Cross. Our concentrate could have been made available a year ago if we had gotten support from the national level."

Doctors are human. It would be normal for Dr. Johnson to be upset that Dr. Brinkhous' concentrate was being released first and that Brinkhous would gather most of the credit for solving this problem. In addition, it was normal that Johnson should be wary of official bureaucracy. Like so many outstanding scientists, he was a loner, at the head of a small band of dedicated, intensely loyal people who worked for him in New York, quite separate from the main Red Cross headquarters in Washington. Still, what he had said was more than a mere indiscretion, provoked by office politics. It was a serious criticism.

I wondered if the real problem was quality. Was there something wrong with Johnson's concentrate which was keeping it from going into production? The Red Cross itself, in its public statements, had always lavishly praised Alan Johnson's AHF concentrate. And, only a few weeks later, on the occasion of the dedication of a new research lab in Bethesda, Maryland, they were to praise it again:

> Outstanding success has been obtained with the purification of AHF. . . . Both preparations are far superior in yield, purity, and stability to any AHF preparation ever produced. An intermediate purity preparation will soon be licensed and a high purity AHF is now being used experimentally in the treatment of severe bleeding conditions. . . . The director of the Red Cross Research Laboratory in New York, Dr. Alan Johnson, is primarily responsible for this breakthrough.

So the Red Cross was satisfied, even pleased, with the Johnson concentrate. What did other independent hematologists think? "Dr. Johnson's concentrate is absolutely tops," said Dr. James Stengle, chief of the National Blood Resources Program of NIH. I checked with Dr. Rosemary Biggs at Oxford. "Alan's material is perfect," she told me. "It is totally reaction-free, instantly soluble, totally effective. What more could a doctor want?"

So it was not hesitation about the quality of the Johnson concentrate that was keeping it out of production. What was the reason?

Dr. Johnson himself had suggested: "Some people in the administration are opposed to expansion of the blood program. They feel that it is already too big and too aggressive." I went to Dr. Shulman at NIH and asked his opinion. "It's true," he said. "The Red Cross administration worries that it is getting in over its head."

Finally, I asked Dr. James Stengle. "Yes, they are uneasy about it. They feel they are getting in over their heads scientifically. A lot of people in the Red Cross administration came up through the bureaucratic ranks and the world of medicine and science is strange and foreign to them. The blood program, related to research and science, is beyond their ken. General Collins (the president of the American National Red Cross) told me, 'We should not let hemophilia become a major concern of ours.' "

If the head of the organization that collects nearly half of the blood in the United States felt this way, then whose concern should hemophilia be? Perhaps there was something to Dr. Johnson's charge after all.

If there is one thing the American people traditionally associate with the American Red Cross, it is blood. The Red Cross advertises itself as the single largest blood collection and distribution agency in the world. Through its fifty-nine regional blood centers, it collects 40 per cent of the blood collected in the United States. Because of the Red Cross's reputation for making blood available free to those who need it, Americans donate blood freely, millions of pints of it a year, to the Red Cross. They also give their money, over $146 million a year, to the Red Cross.

Disturbed by what Dr. Johnson had said, I decided to talk to the national executives of the American Red Cross.

In Washington, in the white-columned Red Cross National Headquarters building across from the White House, I talked first to the vice-president for blood, Mr. Frederick Laise. His language was cheerful and expansive. As he saw it, it was inconceivable that anyone could question the Red Cross's commitment to blood. "We are spending one million dollars a year for blood research," he said. "A substantial part of this goes into the development of AHF. We are a recipient of public funds and we try to act in the public interest. We think that making AHF fraction available at reasonable cost is very much in the public interest. Assuming that Dr. Johnson's approach is the most efficient and the most economical—and we believe it is—we intend to continue our support for him and apply for a license on his high-potency product at the end of this year, 1968."

When I asked why there would be almost a year's delay (it was then February) before applying for a license, Mr. Laise said that this was a purely scientific matter and suggested that I talk to Dr. Tibor Greenwalt, the newly installed national medical director of the Red Cross. Dr. Greenwalt, whose office was down the hall from Mr. Laise's, said that the man holding things up was none other than Dr. Alan Johnson.

"The application for a license on the Intermediate Power concentrate hasn't moved faster because Dr. Johnson hasn't actively pursued the clinical testing program necessary to support the application. It's up to the individual researcher to get it. Dr. Johnson has been too selective about the cases he has chosen for evaluation. Of course, he will tell you that he hasn't been getting enough plasma or enough money. But that is not our fault."

Dr. Greenwalt went on to describe the autonomy of the Red Cross, in which the national headquarters could only request, not require, local centers to send plasma to Johnson for production of AHF. "Johnson will say he hasn't been getting enough plasma, but he's been getting a thousand units a week and we have a hard time persuading local centers to send him stuff because they are hard-pressed; they need the blood products for treatment of patients on hand." Then, having given Dr. Johnson some hard lumps, Dr. Greenwalt mellowed and began to praise him. "I don't mean to say that Dr. Johnson's concentrate isn't excellent. It is really splendid. The real problem is that Dr. Johnson is a very careful, very conscientious worker. You know, a perfectionist."

In medical matters, especially medical research matters, I am in favor of perfectionists. At this point I was prepared to believe that everybody was right; it was a case of people with good intentions stumbling into each other accidentally. And then, just as I had convinced myself of this, I heard a second strange and disagreeable story about the National Headquarters of the Red Cross. It came from George Stone.

Some months before, George told me, when the question had come up of expanding its blood-research activities, the Red Cross had argued that it could not move faster because it lacked the necessary laboratory space to carry out a larger program. Its Washington lab was tucked into a small outbuilding behind the big columned building with the comfortable offices looking out on the White· House lawn. Needing more space, but worried about the cost, they had dithered.

Hearing about this and anxious to get the Red Cross moving, George Stone picked up the telephone. Within a few days, he had found a modern, three-story brick building in Bethesda, Maryland, with 21,000 square feet of floor space and a very reasonable rent. Originally designed for doctors' offices, the building needed only minor modifications to be perfect for the Red Cross. The owners were willing to rent it to the Red Cross but they wanted an option. Guessing that a decision to take an option might easily get lost in the honeycomb of Red Cross bureaucracy, George Stone plunked down $1,600 of his money as an option on a five-year lease. Then he phoned the Red Cross to tell them that the lab space they needed was available.

"They were mad as hell," he said. "Some of the middle-level guys there were running around flipping their lids. But there was nothing they could do. They had to accept it. It was exactly what they had said they needed."

Six months later, on February 18, 1968, the Red Cross formally dedicated its new Research Laboratory in Bethesda. The chairman of the board, Mr. E. Roland Harriman, was there. General James F. Collins, the president, was there. Mr. Laise and Dr. Greenwalt, along with other notables for the ceremony and speeches, were there. But George Stone was not there because he was not invited. And, he told me ruefully two months later, "I never even got my $1,600 back."

This was pettiness. But even before the dedication, the Red Cross administration had done something infinitely more destructive than simply not inviting George Stone to a ceremony: they had ordered Alan Johnson to close his New York AHF research laboratory and move it to Washington. Dr. Greenwalt, whose command this was, had apparently wrestled himself to a decision. As a scientist, he respected and praised Dr. Johnson's program, but as an administrator he wanted to administer. The little empire that Johnson had built for himself in New York seemed entirely too independent. Now that—thanks to George Stone—they had enough space in Washington, why not consolidate all research activities under one roof?

The trouble was that Dr. Johnson and all of his colleagues were New Yorkers. If Johnson, who had been a professor at N.Y.U. Medical School for twenty-five years, refused to move, as seemed likely, it would all but destroy the Red Cross AHF program. And even if Johnson was willing to go, how many of his team would follow? In effect, the team would be destroyed and the work halted. When Alan resisted, the Red Cross offered an alternative. The New York lab would cease to be an integral part of the

Red Cross. It would continue to do research for them on an annual contract basis; every year, the contracts might, or might not, be renewed. Alan would be able to work only on a short-term basis, making no long-range plans, never knowing whether, six months hence, his whole effort might be stopped.

Two men stepped in to prevent this disaster. The first was George Stone. Deeply chagrined by the fact that the new building he had helped to find in Washington was now being used as an excuse to close down the New York lab, he determined that the dedication ceremony in Bethesda would include an exhibition describing the work of the New York laboratory. "We had a team of professionals working night and day for three days before the dedication. We wanted the Red Cross board members and the visitors to the ceremony to remember three things: There is such a thing as the New York lab. It's doing a great job. It ought to stay."

More important, from the Red Cross's point of view, was the reaction of Dr. Stengle of NIH. Alarmed by what was happening, Dr. Stengle told the Red Cross that he had great faith in Dr. Johnson's work. "The attempt to move this laboratory from New York to Washington was an administrative, not a medical, decision," he told them. "Scientists are where you find them. Dr. Johnson is in New York. If you can lure him and his team to Washington, all well and good. But on no account should you let him leave the Red Cross." Dr. Stengle went to the head of the Red Cross, General Collins. "I told him that he may have an administrative problem running a lab in New York, but that was something they would have to solve. You simply don't cut off an arm—get rid of a brilliant scientist—to solve an administrative problem. This would be medically irresponsible."

For a while, Dr. Stengle's admonition had an effect. For six months, the threat to Dr. Johnson's lab was lifted.

But what was going on here? What was wrong with the Red Cross? Why was it so hard to push them into what seemed obvious directions, directions that they themselves, in interviews and in their publicity handouts, constantly announced and confirmed and reconfirmed? Was it entirely bureaucratic timidity or a matter of papers lying for days or weeks in the "In" box of an absent vice-president? Or was it something more serious? In interviews, people told me that, in addition to everything else, "of course, they are afraid of any controversy." What controversy?

Gradually, as I kept asking questions, I began to get glimpses of things moving beneath the surface. It was not just that Dr. Johnson's AHF program was costing too much, or that his part of the work was behind schedule, or that he refused to move to Washington. There was something worse.

I asked Alan Johnson, whose interest was science, but whose life had become filled with bickering, politics, and disappointment. Wearily, he told me: "Bob, some of the drug companies, especially Hyland, are opposed to the Red Cross making AHF. The Hyland product, developed by Brinkhous, is similar to mine, but it is not as soluble and not as stable. If ours goes on the market, it will adversely affect their sales. Right now, Hyland is trying to get a patent on what was originally my procedure for extracting AHF from plasma. Not long ago, Dr. Shanbrom, medical director of Hyland, told a group of Red Cross people, 'Pretty soon, you're going to be paying a royalty to us.' They are determined to protect their investment in Ken Brinkhous' work. They are determined not to lose business because of us. They even objected to the Red Cross asking NIH for a grant for certain fractionation work which they wanted to reserve for themselves. Hyland says they will charge ten cents per AHF unit. A five-hundred AHF unit bottle will cost fifty dollars. We think we can make five-hundred AHF units for twelve dollars. That's why Hyland is very opposed to the Red Cross."

Within a few days, I heard this shocking accusation again from a different source, in even more appalling detail. The director of blood research of the American National Red Cross was Dr. James Pert. In the scientific hierarchy of the organization, he stood between Dr. Greenwalt, the over-all medical director, and Alan Johnson, a researcher on a specific project, AHF. Dr. Pert was now newly installed in the Bethesda Laboratory procured by George Stone's initiative and option money. Before going to see Pert, George briefed me:

"Only two guys in the Red Cross are really trying to get

something done on AHF: Alan and Jim Pert. But Pert is caught in a squeeze play. He is a dedicated man, whose speciality is freezing red cells, but he's caught between Johnson, whose research he admires, and the Red Cross administration, which is hostile to Johnson. Now they've given Jim an administrative assistant who reports behind Jim's back directly to the top. Jim's ability to survive is dubious."

In the flesh, Pert turned out to be a stocky, red-headed man with bright blue eyes and a quiet voice. He took me around the gleaming new laboratory and showed me the centrifuges, the freezer rooms, the powerful microscopes. When I asked him about AHF costs, he gave me wonderful news. "Our costs used to be ten cents per AHF unit. Now they are down to six cents per AHF unit. I would hope it could go down even further. Remember that we're still operating on a research basis, which is expensive. In volume production, the costs should go down to three or four cents a unit."

I asked whether it was true that Hyland had attempted to oppose development of the Red Cross concentrate. Dr. Pert drew a long breath, looked at me hard, and said yes.

"Hyland is one branch of a large drug combine called Travenol, which also owns Baxter Laboratories and a blood-transfusion maker called Fenwal. It is all the same company, Travenol, with headquarters in Morton Grove, Illinois, near Chicago. Fenwal makes the plastic bags and tubing that we use for fresh-frozen plasma and cryo. For each of these bags, they charge four dollars. In Australia, exactly the same bag costs one dollar. We have to pay the cost because Fenwal is the only supplier. And the worst part is that the plastic they use is poor. In some of our shipments we have forty per cent wastage because the bags crack open at low temperatures. As much as forty per cent of our desperately needed plasma is wasted. To try to prevent this, we began developing a Teflon bag which would be stronger, better, and could be made for about fifty cents. But Fenwal opposed our getting funds for plastics research. I'll tell you, Mr. Massie"—and by now Dr. Pert's face was red with anger—"those Travenol boys are a bunch of———"

Forty per cent of some shipments of plasma donated by the

American people, desperately needed by hemophiliacs and others, wasted because inferior bags cracked? And an American company objecting to development of a better bag?

I went back to Dr. Greenwalt, medical director of the Red Cross. My own temper, by now, was rising. Dr. Greenwalt tried to calm me down. "Look at it this way, Mr. Massie. If you were a stockholder of Hyland or Baxter labs, instead of the father of a hemophiliac, you might feel differently. Then you might be very opposed to the Red Cross getting into AHF concentrates."

Stockholder? We were not talking about toothpaste or cars, but about human blood. "Dr. Greenwalt," I said, "I don't believe that the stockholders of any drug company really want to earn higher dividends out of children's suffering. And in the case of every hemophiliac child whose joints continue to deteriorate because the Hyland concentrate is too expensive and the Red Cross concentrate is unavailable, that is exactly what is happening."

Dr. Greenwalt opened his hands in the manner of a man who regretted the system but was powerless to change it. But he confirmed Dr. Johnson's statement. "Yes," he admitted, "if the top administration feels we are getting competitive with private industry, they may have to re-evaluate our programs."

I went on to Dr. Stengle, whose calm and perspective I had come to respect. "Yes," he said, "it's true that Hyland has opposed the Red Cross AHF program, but from Hyland's point of view this is legitimate. They believe in private industry and have invested their own resources heavily in development of these products. Most Hyland plasma is derived from paid donors, whereas the Red Cross pays nothing for its blood. Thus, they are reluctant to compete with the Red Cross, which can undercut them heavily in terms of price."

So, at last, I had put together what seemed to be the ingredients of this unhappy story:

The Red Cross, which could produce AHF concentrates at lower cost than Hyland, was reluctant to go ahead because this would put them in competition with private industry.

Hyland, for its part, was hoping for brisk sales of its new product: $3 million the first year, up to $15 million a year after that, according to the *Wall Street Journal*. If challenged on the morality of making a profit from blood, they would possibly reply

that, were it not for the profit incentive, no research would have
been done and no product would be available at all. The fact is that
Hyland put up only a percentage of the cost of developing Dr.
Brinkhous' concentrate. Part of Dr. Brinkhous' money came from
NIH grants—that is, taxpayers' money. Meanwhile, in order to
protect its investment, the drug company was opposing a lower-
cost concentrate developed by a quasi-governmental organization
supported by voluntary donations, the Red Cross.

And what about the poor old man in the street, Mr. John Q.
Citizen?—the fellow who faithfully pays his taxes so that we can
have medical research, who generously gives his blood and his
money to the Red Cross as a humanitarian act? What happens
to him when he wakes up one day to learn that his son has hemophilia? With the drug companies concerned with making money
and the Red Cross primarily concerned with not irritating the drug
companies, who is going to help him? Who is going to make AHF
available for his hemophiliac son? Nobody.

Dr. Brinkhous' argument was that the government should pay
the bills. Perhaps, in the end, this would be the only way. But how
soon could the American people be persuaded—as every other
industrial Western people had long ago decided—that health care
was a social obligation, that keeping citizens healthy was every bit
as important as teaching them to read and write or paying them
welfare when they were out of work? And when society did decide
to pay the bill for catastrophic illness, should not society pay the
lowest bill possible? If the Red Cross could make AHF for half the
price of a commercial drug company, should society be forced to
pay the higher price? Was this also the American way?

On all sides, I asked whether these impressions were true. There
were squirmings, qualifications, embarrassment, awkwardness,
"Don't quote me's," but basically, from everyone, the answer was
"Yes."

The next development followed quickly. On April 26, 1968,
the *Wall Street Journal* presented a major, front-page story on
hemophilia, pegged to the fact that Hyland Labs was ready to
market the Brinkhous concentrate: "Hope for Bleeders: End to

Hemophilia Peril May Become Possible." "Medical researchers believe that they are coming close to controlling hemophilia," said the story. "Even more effective preparations are on the way, giving doctors hope that hemophiliacs may eventually be able to control their ailment entirely through periodic injections, much as diabetics use insulin."

Rapidly, the story was picked up by other newspapers across the country. Although the *Journal* article was, in general, carefully and responsibly written, other papers ran the story under headlines such as "Hemophilia Cure at Hand" and "Shots to Cure Hemophilia." One of the most optimistic (and, as was subsequently proven, misleading) statements came in a *New York Times* interview with Dr. Edward Shanbrom, medical director of Hyland:

> Dr. Edward Shanbrom, Medical Director of Hyland Division of Baxter Laboratories, said yesterday that the new concentrate would make it possible for the first time to treat about 90 per cent of hemophiliac cases during visits to a doctor's office lasting only a few minutes. Previously, patients had to be hospitalized to be given the vital clotting factor. . . . Although the company recommends that the concentrate be refrigerated, Dr. Shanbrom said a hemophiliac could safely carry a vial for a day or two in case a bleeding crisis should arise when he was away from home. . . .

Anyone reading this story and the others like it naturally assumed that the problem of hemophilia was almost a thing of the past. Hemophiliacs across the country were elated. My telephone rang with the good news, newspaper clippings and happy letters began to flow in. Friends and strangers wrote, "Did you see this?" "Isn't this wonderful?" "Your prayers have been answered." "We are so happy for Bobby and you and Sue."

The same day the *Wall Street Journal* story appeared, I telephoned the nearest Hyland Laboratories sales center. They told me that the first batches of AHF concentrate would be available in six weeks. On June 11, they finally had some in stock, but only in a single size, 900 AHF unit bottles. The price of each bottle was $150. Stunned, I asked if there were any smaller, less expensive sizes. No, not yet; not for an indefinite period. In Chapel Hill, Ken Brinkhous had told me that the "rule of thumb" cost should be ten cents per AHF unit. Now $150 for 900 AHF units meant

that Hyland was charging almost seventeen cents an AHF unit.
And I remembered Johnson and Pert saying that their costs were
six cents per AHF unit or less.

That same day, I wrote to Dr. Brinkhous. I asked whether he,
as the scientist responsible for developing the Hyland concentrate,
could do something about the price. Obviously embarrassed and unhappy, he replied at length:

There was nothing he could do about the price; that was
strictly Hyland's decision. The real question, he said, was who
would pay. Once again, he suggested that the solution lay in
Washington. "We must get recognition of the plight of the hemophiliac and his family by the health planners in Washington . . .
develop a new factual report . . . present it to an HEW committee."

I also wrote to Dr. Martin Rosenthal, the medical director of
the Hemophilia Foundation, urging him to do everything possible
to encourage, urge, and hasten the availability of the Red Cross
concentrate. Then I began to fire off shorter letters like grapeshot.
I wrote to all the officers of the National Red Cross, urging them
to hurry the Johnson concentrate into production. I wrote to most
of the hematologists I knew, asking them to put pressure on the
Red Cross. I wrote to the Hemophilia Foundation, saying that "in
my view, not enough has been done by either the medical or nonmedical leadership of the Foundation."

Almost everyone replied politely to my gadfly letters. They
promised that licensing of the Johnson concentrate was not far off;
that the product would soon be available. The best of these replies
came in a telephone call from Dr. Stengle. "Go to it, Bob," he said.
"You're on the right track and you'll accomplish more singlehandedly. Your position is correct: with the public giving huge
quantities of blood to the Red Cross, they have an obligation to
practice the most advanced techniques.

"Red Cross production of a lower-priced concentrate is the
only way that holds out hope for your son, because the other
route—special federal government payments for commercial concentrates for hemophiliacs—is just not in the cards. Not for a long,
long time."

Conceivably, the tone of my letters and even the fact of my

intrusion into this medical arena may have seemed out of place. Mr. Cunningham, president of the National Hemophilia Foundation, told a friend that he considered me "a publicity-seeking writer." But I had been a journalist long enough to learn that "Don't make waves" is usually the cry of those who prefer lying at anchor. In any case, I was not a "publicity-seeking writer"; I was an "action-seeking father," and the only way I knew to provoke action was to write letters, make phone calls, ask questions.

During those early summer days, two other episodes helped to goad me on. While I was writing my letters, around the Fourth of July, I was also trying desperately to locate some cryo precipitate. As often happens during holidays—Christmas, the Fourth, Labor Day—the Red Cross had almost none. Their donors go out of town, their reserves dwindle, and they save what little remains for real life-or-death emergencies.

Bobby's problem that weekend was a normal hemophiliac joint bleeding. Ordinarily, he would have had a transfusion, but as no cryo was available, he continued to bleed. We treated him with ice and he spent the weekend, with a pale, drawn face, sitting quietly in front of television. As I paced back and forth through the room to and from the telephone, he cheered me up. "Don't worry, Dad. It's not so bad."

I called everyone I knew in journalism, radio, and television, asking them to do something to dramatize the crisis and attract donors. Nobody could do anything. I tried to call Mayor Lindsay, believing that if he would speak up and, better yet, donate blood himself, other citizens might follow. An administrative assistant turned me down. And so Bobby bled through the weekend until, on Monday morning, a trickle of donors came in, I got some cryo, and Bobby, at last, had his transfusion.

This was one reason for my crankiness. The other was a telephone call I had on July 8 from Alan Johnson. The Red Cross, he said, had decided to close down his New York laboratory. "As of last night, the entire AHF program is to be moved to Bethesda. They have cut half of our staff. No, I am not going to go along with it. And, by the way, Jim Pert has just resigned."

The man caught in the middle of all of this was Dr. Brinkhous. In a way, what happened to him that spring and summer was sad and unfair. For years, he had worked to develop a highly purified, stable AHF concentrate. In the laboratory, he had succeeded brilliantly; his concentrate was ready first. Naturally, he was pleased and proud. But like most academic American scientists, he could not himself produce the product he had developed, or distribute and market it. A private drug company would have to do this and they, not he, would set the prices. They intended to make a profit; this was the American way.*

The tragedy for Brinkhous was that they set the price so high that his triumph was tainted with frustration and disappointment almost from the moment it appeared. Hopes had been raised so high that, when the promised salvation was snatched away, many people, including me, could not help partially blaming Brinkhous.

Dr. Brinkhous tried to bring together the two real antagonists, Hyland and the hemophiliacs. As I was the hemophiliac parent protesting loudest and because, as a journalist, I had the largest scope for making trouble (when journalists publish facts that other people don't want published, they are always considered troublemakers), I was the one selected to be convinced.

Ken Brinkhous proposed a meeting with the president of Hyland Laboratories, Mr. Fred Marquart, so that I could point out, face-to-face, my concern about the high price of Hyland AHF

---

* What we Americans have never done—and it is high time we did it—is to decide whether the buying and selling of human blood and blood derivatives for profit *should* be the American way. In his remarkable book *The Gift Relationship: From Human Blood to Social Policy* (New York: Pantheon, 1971), Professor Richard M. Titmuss asks us to consider the implications. Blood, he points out, is living human tissue in liquid form. If blood is permitted to remain a commercial commodity, what about other forms of human tissue or organs of the body? Should human hearts be sold to the highest bidders? What about kidneys? What about eyes or corneas bequeathed to eye banks? Should they be thrown into a commercial marketplace of flesh?

Finally, following his argument to its logical extreme, Titmuss suggests that buying and selling blood may be unconstitutional: "[In] 1865 . . . the Constitution's Thirteenth Amendment took effect and made illegal in the United States the buying or selling of human beings and presumably of living human tissue as well."

concentrate. Mr. Marquart agreed and a meeting was arranged in Washington for July 19. A few days before the nineteenth, Mr. Cunningham, president of the National Hemophilia Foundation, telephoned to say that he felt that representatives of the foundation ought to be present.

At the meeting, I found Mr. Marquart, Dr. Brinkhous, Mr. Cunningham, Mr. Walsh, the executive secretary of the Hemophilia Foundation, and, to my surprise, two men from the Red Cross, Dr. Chrisman and Mr. Freeman. I hoped that they were there to announce the release of Red Cross concentrates, either free, or at a far lower price than Hyland's. I felt sorry for poor Mr. Marquart. With two men from the Hemophilia Foundation, two men from the Red Cross, and me opposing him, and Dr. Brinkhous neutral, he seemed sadly outnumbered.

The meeting began with Mr. Cunningham assuming the chair, so to speak, and giving the floor to Mr. Marquart. Mr. Marquart produced a chart and went down the list of Hyland AHF concentrate sizes and prices: 900 AHF units, $150; 450 AHF units, $85; 300 AHF units, $50. He explained that at present their yields were only about 15 per cent (that is, from 1,000 ml. of plasma they got only 150 AHF units of concentrate), but that if and when they got better yields, they hoped to lower their prices. However, as long as Hyland had to pay donors for plasma, the price would remain substantially where it was.

To my surprise, Mr. Marquart's presentation was received with understanding nods by everyone but me. Alone, I protested that, no matter how good the product was, at the prices charged it would have little impact on hemophilia. Mr. Marquart admitted that perhaps the price was too high; the proof, he said, was that sales were low and inventories were piling up on their warehouse shelves. This was the odd way our dialogue went; he was talking about sales, I was talking about joints. Sometimes, when I was talking about crippled joints, pain, prophylaxis, and better lives, Mr. Marquart smiled sadly at me and said, "Mr. Massie, you're being mean to me." Everyone else sat silent and looked uncomfortable.

Sandwiches appeared and Mr. Cunningham said that now it was time to hear from the Red Cross. Mr. Freeman cleared his throat and tossed a bombshell. Because the Johnson fraction was

not ready for production ("Dr. Johnson keeps changing his method
. . . Dr. Johnson did not properly prepare the license application
. . ."), the Red Cross was going to make an "interim arrangement"
with Hyland. Red Cross plasma would be shipped to Hyland to
make AHF concentrate according to Brinkhous' formula, not
Johnson's. In return for 21 bags of fresh-frozen plasma plus $65,
the Red Cross could have back a bottle containing 600 AHF units.
If a bag of plasma was worth $13.50, the price we had been charged
for it, this meant that the 600 AHF units cost $283.50 worth of
plasma plus $65 cash, a total of $348.50. This was *fifty-eight cents
per AHF unit!*, more than three times as much as buying Hyland
commercially. I couldn't believe it. Nobody else said anything.

Finally, I said, "Mr. Marquart, all these prices are astronomical.
It means that AHF concentrate can only be used for catastrophic
bleeding situations, just as in the past. What about the *Wall Street
Journal* story and all the other publicity promising that the new
Hyland concentrate meant a new day for hemophiliacs?"

"That was the press," somebody said. "As we all know, the
press can be pretty irresponsible."

"Did the press misquote Dr. Shanbrom?" I asked. I fished in
my papers and read from *The New York Times*. Then I went on:
"I know as a result of my travels around the country that thousands
of hemophiliacs are now eagerly awaiting this new Hyland fraction. They have believed these stories and these quotes. What are
you going to tell them?"

And then, at last, we faced the truth. "We are not going to
have an inexpensive, day-in, day-out concentrate for the kind of
care you are looking for unless the federal government steps in and
picks up the bill," said Mr. Marquart. "Not even from the Red
Cross?" I asked Mr. Freeman. "No," he said, "we cannot count on
any AHF concentrate having a routine, day-to-day use. It will be
used only for catastrophic bleeding episodes as determined by Red
Cross medical consultants around the country."

The dream was over.

At this grim but important juncture, Mr. Cunningham stood
up. He announced that he thought that he had absorbed as much
as he could in one day, and that he and Mr. Walsh had to leave to
catch a train for New York. The others left too, and Mr. Marquart

showed me to the door. "I understand your concern, Mr. Massie," he said, "but my sales people are always against any lowering of prices. Remember, I have to think of them too."

Coming back to New York, I felt defeated. The Red Cross, supposedly the alternative to Hyland, was going to produce AHF through Hyland. (Mr. Freeman of the Red Cross later became a Hyland employee!) Hyland would not lower its prices. And the two top leaders of the National Hemophilia Foundation, who should have been arguing and pleading and pounding the table with me on behalf of the nation's hemophiliacs, had simply sat there, acting as mediators.

Fortunately, it did not take long for the medical leadership of the New York Hemophilia chapter to see through the terms of the Hyland–Red Cross agreement. "We have given the most careful attention to the recently announced agreement between the American Red Cross and Hyland Laboratories," they said in a statement. "This announcement was hailed by the national office of the National Hemophilia Foundation, and chapters were urged to issue press releases headlining the availability of the concentrate. . . . But we fail to understand the economics or good medical sense in trading a 600 AHF unit for $65 plus 21 units of fresh-frozen plasma." Instead, they urged, "we believe that the Foundation should take all possible steps to encourage the American National Red Cross to continue its fractionation program with the utmost vigor."

Incredibly, stories fostering the illusion of a "daily shot" for America's hemophiliacs continued to appear. In August, a month after the meeting in Washington, *Time* interviewed both Dr. Brinkhous and Dr. Shanbrom about the new concentrate. "Dr. Shanbrom foresees a day when patients will enjoy still greater convenience," the magazine reported. "Some batches of AHF concentrate have been made 1,000 times more potent than plasma. Eventually, Brinkhous is confident this will become the standard AHF, so safe and stable that hemophilia victims will be able to carry it around and inject it themselves, into muscle, just as diabetics do with insulin."

The qualifiers in these rosy predictions were "foresees a day" and "eventually." Sadly, hemophiliacs, like desperate people of every kind, ignored the qualifiers to grasp at any hope. Most of them believed that very soon a "daily shot" would protect them from further bleeding. They were mistaken. Even today the "daily shot" still is not widely available because it costs too much. The hemophiliacs continue to bleed.

At this mid-point, the fraction story ended abruptly for me. On August 29, 1968, we sailed for France, where we were to live for four years. Having no alternative, we took Hyland concentrate with us, and thereafter until we qualified for French National Health Insurance we supplemented the French AHF we bought in Paris by importing a steady flow of Hyland concentrate. Our friends and friends of our friends arrived in Paris, their suitcases stuffed with tiny bottles. It was enormously expensive; our first six weeks in France we spent $1,500 for Hyland fraction. And now there were no major medical plans to pay the bills. "What we are trying to do," I wrote Ken Brinkhous, "is perhaps wrong: keep Bobby in school every day. But how many hemophiliac families, including the Massies, can maintain this pace?"

Two years later, as the result of a massive revolt by the membership of the Hemophilia Foundation, Mr. Cunningham and Mr. Walsh resigned from office. They left behind them a financial and organizational chaos it took their successors several years to clean up. But we, the Massies, were not part of this. We were living in France, where French AHF concentrate, produced and supplied at cost by the excellent French National Transfusion Center, cost us eight cents per AHF unit. For all French hemophiliacs, of course, under the French Government National Health Insurance Program, AHF concentrates are absolutely free. And yet France, in terms of per capita wealth and income, is a much poorer country than the United States. It is a question of politics, of national priorities and, deep down, of the national heart. America, the most generous nation on earth in a hundred ways, has kept its heart closed tight against those of its own children who are chronically and catastrophically ill.

By 1974, the time of this writing, six years have passed, but very little has changed. Dr. Brinkhous has retired as chairman of the Department of Pathology at Chapel Hill and been elected to the prestigious National Academy of Science. Dr. Johnson eventually left the Red Cross, which severed all connection with his New York AHF laboratory. After some lean years when the lab's status was touch-and-go, he now has a five-year grant from NIH to work on the important problem of removing the hepatitis virus from blood and blood fractions. He has not lost his interest in AHF; he is working to develop a solid electrolytic process that will extract up to 80 per cent of the AHF in plasma. Most commercial fractionaters still obtain only 15 to 20 per cent yields.

The American Red Cross has all but abandoned the effort to make AHF concentrate from the 40 per cent of the nation's blood donations that it collects. Despite its solemn commitment in 1968, despite fresh and glorious new manifestoes by its Board of Governors ("Humanitarian considerations call for . . . whole blood and components . . . available to all who need them . . . regardless of previous donations or ability to replace . . ."), the Red Cross has simply deserted its AHF project—and the American hemophiliac. In 1973, from 3,800,000 donations of blood collected, the Red Cross produced 2,340 vials of AHF concentrate, enough for the needs of ten hemophiliacs.

Of course Americans should continue to give blood; indeed, they should give a lot more. The current donor group—3 per cent of the eligible population—should be vastly expanded, using whatever persuasions, tax inducements, or other incentives are most effective. But the donors themselves should take far more interest in exactly what happens to their blood. Before giving, they should demand assurance that their gift will not be wasted by becoming outdated, as 28 per cent of the blood now donated is wasted. They should insist that the recipient—be it the Red Cross, a hospital, or a commercial blood bank—promise that the blood will be fractionated into its separate component parts, so that one donation may serve five or six fellow humans. And for those who are willing, the Massie family and the families of 25,500 other American hemophiliacs would be grateful to anyone who insists that his or her donation be fractionated in such a way that the AHF or PTC clotting factors are saved so they can be used to save our children's joints. There are no valid medical reasons why this cannot be done. It is simply a question of making the effort.*

For the moment, the American Red Cross has decided not to make the effort. And the Red Cross's abdication of responsibility has left six commercial pharmaceutical companies in control of all AHF concentrate production in the United States. These companies make AHF for profit. No doctor I asked estimated their profit on AHF concentrate at less than 30 per cent; one thought 50 per cent was a more likely figure. No one really knows, because the companies hide all figures—not only money figures, but figures on amounts of plasma collected and fractions made, on domestic and overseas sales. All this, the companies say, is "proprietary information." Blood is a free market commodity. No government body has the responsibility or power to obtain any information or exercise any regulation except in the area of purity. Today, we pay these companies whatever they ask, for they control Bobby's life.

---

* In modern society, organizations, institutions, and bureaucracies are always demanding that private citizens fill out and sign forms. I think that, in general, it might be a healthy thing if private citizens, before performing certain voluntary acts or even public duties, began presenting forms demanding signed assurances from organizations, institutions, and bureaucracies. A blood-donation form might be an excellent place to start. It could read something like this:

> I am voluntarily donating my blood to (Name of hospital, Red Cross chapter, or other blood bank) on (Date of donation) to help other human beings. In so doing, I demand assurance that it be processed by the advanced technique of component therapy so that my donation will help not one, but six other human beings. I request that one of the components extracted from my blood be Anti-Hemophilic Factor. Above all, I demand assurance that my blood will not be wasted.
>
> I understand that the signature below, of the medical doctor in charge of this blood bank, is my guarantee that the conditions of my donation will be met.

_____   _____
Signature of medical doctor   Signature of blood donor

Chapter 19

Every human being wants to be free, independent, self-sufficient. Learning to break away, to do things for yourself, to make decisions on your own, is an essential part of growing up. For a young hemophiliac, this is hard, perhaps even harder than the pain or the damage to his joints. His life is dominated from the outside. He is subject not only to the limitations of the disease but to a dependence on the kindness, generosity, and sheer physical presence of other people. To have to ask for everything, to have to involve others in even the smallest personal decision, to be always grateful, is a kind of torture from which most of us—without even thinking about it—are blessedly free.

The inner turmoil caused by the linkage of this physical and psychological dependence is very clear in this recollection from Bobby's schoolboy years:

"All through my childhood, there were many, many times when I should have had a transfusion and didn't. Why?

"Looking back, I can see the reasons: plasma was rare and even then I knew it was very expensive. The whole process was disagreeable. But the worst part was having to admit that I was bleeding.

"The decision to announce a bleeding was hardest in the middle of the night when, through a semiconscious haze, I could feel a growing pain in one of my joints. I would realize that I was bleeding. But the idea of walking or limping into the next room and rousing my sleepy and sometimes disgruntled parents who themselves did not enjoy arousing a sleepy and sometimes disgruntled doctor was so unpleasant that I sometimes took hours, alone in the darkness, to make my decision. Too often, it was the wrong one. It was so much easier to doze off again, hoping that I would awake to find that it had all gone away. (I occasionally had nightmares about bleeding in the middle of the night, from which I awoke to find, indeed, nothing.)

"But something more important often kept me from revealing a bleeding to my parents. How many spring days I can remember dashing around while my mother or father warned me that I was overdoing it. How many times I replied 'Don't worry. I'm O.K.' When something happened, how could I admit such faulty judgment on my own part? How could I accept I Told You So? Better to delay as long as possible, to try to distance the bleeding from the event which caused it, so that the two appeared (hopefully) unrelated.

"The hardest thing of all, though, was not admitting it to my parents, or to doctors, but admitting it to myself. A bleeding, I thought, was a failure, a defeat. I refused to have this disease dominate my life so completely. If I bled or if I was in pain, then carrying out every detail of my 'normal' life became all the more important because it proved my strength over it. In effect, I was saying, 'Do your worst. I can still hide it from others, and from myself, and it will not hold me back.' Such obstinacy has perhaps helped me in some areas, but it also led to decisions that were medically foolish.

"I can remember waking up one morning when I was in fifth grade with a severely bleeding left knee. It was 5 A.M. I strapped it into its brace to keep it from bending up, waited two hours until time to get up, doggedly went through the charade of breakfast, and, hiding the pain and filled with determination, I left for school on the bus. Two hours later, I collapsed. I came home, had many transfusions, and went to bed for several weeks. But, to me, the ability to hide pain that long seemed a great victory."

Bobby hated the domination of his life by the disease. All of us were longing to free ourselves from the iron grip it held on our lives. It was a chance meeting in January 1968 that suddenly showed

us the way to freedom. In the months after the publication of
Nicholas and Alexandra Sue and I were making a number of talks
around the country. On a cold, brilliantly sunny day, I flew from
New York to Chicago to be at a Sunday afternoon meeting of the
Midwestern chapter of the National Hemophilia Foundation. Afterward, at dinner, I sat next to Dr. S. Frederick Rabiner, at that time
director of clinical hematology at Chicago's Michael Reese Hospital. In the course of conversation, Dr. Rabiner mentioned that he
had begun teaching parents to transfuse some of his hemophiliac
patients at home.

Dr. Rabiner explained that he himself had first happened on
the idea only a year earlier, when a new member of the Chicago
chapter had come to him with an embarrassed confession. This
man, the father of two hemophiliac sons, had moved to Chicago
from Texas, where he had been trained at Forth Worth's Carter
Community Blood Center to give his sons transfusions. In Texas,
the distances were so great that it sometimes took hours to drive a
hemophiliac to a hospital. Often, what had been only a puffy knee
when the hemophiliac left home had become, by the time he
reached the hospital, a severe joint hemarthrosis that would require
many transfusions and weeks or months of bed, wheelchair, and
therapy before the patient could walk again.

When this family moved to Chicago, home transfusions had
become such an essential part of the family's existence that the
father, being reasonably affluent, had been flying back and forth
to Texas, bringing cryo back to Chicago, where he had been transfusing it himself into his sons. Eventually, feeling that some better
arrangement must be possible, the father had asked Dr. Rabiner to
institute home transfusion in Illinois.

It was easy for Dr. Rabiner to see the advantages. Distances in
Illinois are not as great as they are in Texas, but still he had a
number of patients who lived downstate and who had to travel
more than a hundred miles to reach Chicago. Sometimes these
emergency dashes were made across snowy roads in the middle of
the night. A child in pain, crying in the back seat, a desperate parent
driving too fast—these trips were fearfully dangerous.

Dr. Rabiner knew that there would be problems in starting

such a program, not the least of them being Illinois law, which forbade nonmedical personnel to transfuse patients with blood products. But by calling it an experimental research project and by carefully selecting the parents chosen, he persuaded Michael Reese Hospital to give permission. By the time I saw him, the new program had been underway for over a year.

"We find that the easiest part is training parents to get into a vein," he told me. "Medical students, nurses, even junkies, learn to get into veins. What we had to worry about and watch carefully were the psychological and emotional reactions in this new relationship based on parents sticking needles into their children." Nevertheless, he believed that his experiment was a success. At that point, he had eight families on home transfusions; one mother had successfully transfused her son forty-five times. "We're going ahead and train more families," he said.

That night, flying home, I thought about how much home transfusion could mean to us. Many of Bobby's transfusions were followups that might not have been necessary had he been treated immediately. We would save blood, time, and money. We would be able to travel. (When Bobby broke his arm on the road from Maine, we had found a doctor within forty minutes. But the next time, who could tell how near a doctor would be?)

Most important, we would be able to deal quickly with the "routine" bleedings which had been implacably destroying Bobby's joints. With home transfusion, there would be no indecision, no waiting. A "feeling" would mean a transfusion immediately.

When I got home, Dr. Engel saw no problem and even offered his arm as a practice area. We were temporarily stymied by the Medical Advisory Board of the Hemophilia Foundation in New York, whose chairman worried about parents having to deal with possible allergic transfusion reactions caused by the impurities in cryo. He preferred that we wait until AHF concentrates could be used. But who knew when that would be?

By then, we were unwilling to be held back. We had handled hundreds of bags of cryo in Dr. Engel's presence and only once had there been anything like a transfusion reaction. Dr. Rabiner was using cryo in his home transfusion program in Chicago. And

Dr. Pool herself had just reported in the *New England Journal of Medicine* that she had administered over 4,000 units of cryo without any discernible transfusion reaction. We wanted to go ahead.*

At exactly this moment, the mail brought us interesting news. The previous autumn Sue had spoken at a fund-raising luncheon of the Philadelphia Hemophilia chapter. A copy of their monthly newsletter had just arrived with the announcement that a home transfusion training program similar to Dr. Rabiner's was beginning in Philadelphia. Like Dr. Rabiner, they were going ahead with cryo.

We drove to Philadelphia and, on a warm April afternoon, Sue, Bobby, and I appeared at the Children's Hospital Blood Center. We found ourselves in a large, cheerful room with a TV set, a coffee stand, and a tank of exotic tropical fish. Six people were lying back on deep, padded lounge chairs, talking quietly while giving blood. Other donors, who had finished donating, were licking ice cream cones from an ice cream stand across the street. On the wall, a large sign asked, "Wouldn't Dracula *love* it here?"

In a small treatment room just off this lounge, we met Mrs. Nancy Ramsey, who was to be our teacher. As head of the Children's Hospital transfusion team, she gave thousands of transfusions every year to children with every variety of illness. But her special interest was hemophilia. Her two young sons, Jeff and Chris, were hemophiliacs, and her adolescent sister, Jane, was one of the exceedingly rare hemophiliac females.

The first thing Nancy taught us was how to choose a vein. It varies according to the age of the patient and the prominence of his or her veins, but for beginners she recommended one of the veins on the inside of the elbow or on the back of the hand.

Nancy extended her hand on the table. I rubbe . the area thoroughly with an alcohol sponge, and applied a small rubber tourniquet around her wrist. While waiting for her vein to fill up, she

---

* With the passage of time, most hematologists have overcome their hesitation about using cryoprecipitate in home transfusion programs. Recently, the Medical and Scientific Advisory Council of the National Hemophilia Foundation issued a booklet titled "Home Transfusion for Hemophilia." In the booklet, the Council declares that "cryoprecipitate is truly practical for home use."

explained that the tourniquet must not be too tight or it would cut arterial as well as venous flow. If, with the tourniquet applying reasonable pressure, the veins did not swell, then, she said, you could "insult" them, that is, slap them lightly to provoke additional swelling.

By this time, her vein was ready and she told me to go ahead. With my left hand I took her hand, using my left thumb to press down on the vein I meant to enter, in order to anchor it in place. Then following her calm instructions, I took a child's scalp-vein needle ("the smaller the needle, the less damage to the vein," she said), lined it up along the vein, took a deep breath, and pressed it through her skin. I had seen it done hundreds of times, and the physical sensation was negligible, but psychologically I felt great tension. Quietly, Nancy urged me on. I leveled the needle and its now invisible tip above the vein, and then once again pressed forward and down, hoping to pierce and enter her vein. Had I succeeded, blood would have been forced back through the needle and into the attached plastic tube. But no backflow of blood appeared. I had missed. By now I was deeply worried, but Nancy, with the needle still in her hand, explained that her veins were slippery like spaghetti and could roll away from the needle. She asked me to try again. I did. Again, I missed. Cheerfully, Nancy sent us home, saying she was optimistic for the morrow. The next afternoon, we practiced again, and this time I managed to get into a vein on the back of Sue's hand. Sue tried on me but her angle was too steep, and she went through my vein and out the other side. I became useless as a subject. "I just can't do this again," Sue said, "with you sitting there with a pale face, gritting your teeth." Nancy came, calmly offered her own hand, and this time Sue succeeded.

The following day, Nancy invited us to combine our lessons with a picnic at her father's farm in Chadd's Ford. It was a sunny spring day with the forsythia in bloom. Before lunch we spread out our medical tools on the kitchen table and had another lesson. This time my patient was Bobby. He was very cool and relaxed.

"Come on, Dad, don't be so nervous," he urged. I applied the tourniquet, cleaned the site, unsheathed the needle, touched it against Bobby's skin, and pressed forward. It slid through the skin and then, with a sudden feeling of release, into the vein. Blood poured back into the tubing. "Hey, Dad, you did it!" Bobby shouted. I advanced the needle, threading it along the inside of the vein, then pulled off the tourniquet, taped the needle in place, and unstopped the stopper. Drops of cryo began to fall rapidly into the filter chamber. "See," Nancy smiled. "There's nothing to it." We had chicken salad for lunch, went to Longwood Gardens to see the exhibition of flowers, and came home exhilarated.

Thereafter, we made rapid progress. Dr. Engel was pleased, and after that day he did not insert another needle into Bobby's veins. First, I took Bobby to his office or house as before, but I gave the transfusion myself while he stood behind me.

Then one morning at his office, I gave the transfusion while Lee was in another room, seeing other patients. I missed and went running to him. "What's the matter with you?" he asked. "Are you so good that you're never going to miss? Go back and try again." Later came a night that Bobby had a "feeling" in an elbow. I telephoned Lee. "Bob," he said, "I think you are ready to solo." I asked him to stay near the telephone in case my solo failed. He agreed, and a few minutes later I called him back. "It's O.K.," I said. "Congratulations," said Lee.

Gradually, with Bobby encouraging me ("Try again, Dad. It really doesn't hurt that much"), I built my self-confidence. That summer, we went to Maine, and Nancy Ramsey and her sons came to visit us. One day, she watched approvingly as I demonstrated my improving technique on Bobby. Then she transfused both her sons. An hour later, all three boys were down on the beach, swimming.

From that time on, home transfusion became a part of our lives. By the summer of 1970, when Bobby was thirteen, a home transfusion training program had been established at New York Hospital by Dr. Hilgartner and Ms. Elaine Sergis. There, Bobby learned to transfuse himself. Describing the process, Bobby says:

"After four years of giving myself transfusions, I have been astonished at the reactions of people who have witnessed or helped me. Almost everyone is amazed that I can inflict pain on myself by taking a needle and actually pressing it into my own flesh, that I can stand to do it day after day. Almost everyone tells me, 'I could never do that.' A few hardy souls stay with me during the venipuncture, but many more leave the room with the apology that 'I've always hated needles.' Big strong rough-and-ready men visibly quiver before a little packet of needles, and stare in mild terror at the large syringes I use. Women are generally more helpful, but by far the most delightful companions to have are little children. They stand at a respectful distance, asking intelligent questions: Why do I have to do this? Why don't they? Will they ever have to? Will I always have to? They are aware that a needle can inflict pain, but seeing that I am not scared, neither are they. Their endless curiosity always overrides their fear of needles, the smell of alcohol, or the sight of blood in the tubing. To them, all this is just another interesting facet of life.

"People ask, how can I do it? *They* certainly would never be able to do it, no matter how badly they needed it. Of course they would. Human beings have done far more difficult feats than performing a venipuncture when it became evident that they had no choice. And that is just it. For me, the question of whether it is difficult to stick myself is purely academic: I *have* to.

"Transfusions are an integral, if slightly unpleasant, part of my life, like taking baths or getting cavities filled. Think of it in these terms: Imagine that in order to live a relatively normal life, to pursue your daily activities, all you had to do was stick yourself with a pin or drop a tiny bit of hot wax on your skin every morning. The alternative is for you to spend several days in great pain, and several more in bed, unable to do anything. The slight pain of the hot wax was all that stood between days of anguish and days of joy. Can't you see how easy it is for me to stick myself, can't you see how I welcome it and am thankful for it?"

Today, Bobby handles all of his own transfusions. He travels alone with his medical supplies in his suitcase and his AHF concentrate in a small insulated ice bag. In his pocket, he carries a letter signed by Dr. Engel explaining that he is authorized to carry these materials and use them on himself. He is independent and makes all medical decisions for himself. Some doctors worried that hemophiliacs on home transfusion might overtransfuse themselves, but the opposite appears to be true. Bobby transfuses himself less often, using less concentrate than before. The reason is that he can be precise: he better than anyone knows what is happening inside his body and can choose the moment to act.

Chapter 20

The decision to leave for France seemed, on the surface, impractical. Most of our relatives thought it was lunacy. Why? they asked. Why now, when at last we could think of living more normally? Why, when we could, for the first time, buy some furniture for that empty house which had been for so long "furnished in your mind"?

Nevertheless, barely a year after *Nicholas and Alexandra* was published, we packed up and left for Europe. It was meant to be for a year. It stretched to four. It was not a frivolous decision— quite the contrary. For, more and more, I was concerned that our children were growing up in a narrow atmosphere, too comfortable, too bland. I could see them growing settled in their way of thinking. They had no contact with languages; they knew that other countries existed only because they had geography books. Although they had cousins in Switzerland, France, and Holland, they were strangers to them. They had no sense of this larger family, and even if they had met their cousins, they would not have been able to speak to them. I had spoken French since childhood, and I knew what an extra dimension it had given my life.

I always had wanted for them the widest possible contacts with the most varied people. I wanted them to understand the qualities of all ages, to profit and respect the wisdom of the old, to learn from the man who works with his hands. I have the deepest suspicion and distrust of the truths of "intellectuals." I do not like the snobbism of the intellect, the elitism, the narrow sense of superiority that sometimes accompanies the purely academic mind. There is poetry in the language of a gardener who understands the secrets of the earth. For me, a farmer is a wizard, quite as much as a

physicist. And each nation I have known has seen some of the
special facets of the jewel that is life. More than anything else, I
had dreamed of expansive horizons for my children. I did not want
them to grow up thinking that they, or their nation alone, had
found all the answers.

Bobby and Susy were just at the age when educators say they
are most open to new ideas and the adventure of learning. Yet
people said to us, Why don't you wait? Why not later? Later, I
thought, when they were already teen-aged, they would be too
absorbed in themselves, too locked in their habits. Now was the
time, when they were between fairy tales and reality, to look at
castles, to learn history, to learn languages. And, I secretly hoped,
to mark them for life.

There was another worry that gnawed at me. Bobby was
growing older. He was about to enter adolescence. We had tried
to convince him that his handicaps had nothing to do with his
development as a person, that physical qualities were not essential
to success or happiness. But he was beginning to enter the stage
where sports become a large part of the life of American boys.
More and more, his few friends were talking about the Little
League, the tennis match, the football team. *I* knew how unim-
portant this would be in later life. Who remembers the high-school
football hero? But still, in those years in the suburban United States,
being able to participate in sports was a mark of "manliness." Those
who did not—or could not—participate somehow weren't part of
the group. I did not want that for Bobby. Yet I knew that our
reassuring words that "it doesn't matter" would grow weaker, and
the judgment of the outside world stronger. He had not yet been
really wounded. But how could he, just when it is most natural to
do so, develop independence? His movements were so restricted.
In Irvington, he couldn't walk to the local newspaper store. He
couldn't bicycle, as the other children did. His contacts, his life
outside, depended entirely on his being passively driven everywhere. Soon, I knew, very soon, the moment was coming when all
this would hurt and perhaps damage him irrevocably.

I knew that in France the attitude was different. In the French
school system the emphasis is exclusively on excellence in studies.
Nothing else really counts. In France, I calculated, Bobby would be

honored and accepted for the abilities he had. In France, the boy who concentrates on sports is considered—to say the least—odd. And I gambled that by the time Bobby came home he would *know* inside himself that the American criteria were not the only ones that existed. . . .

I had worried about all this for a long time. For us, travel had not been possible. But now, the opportunity had really come. The new fraction had been developed. It needed only normal refrigeration. We had learned to give transfusions. We could risk living away from our own native medical network. We were freer than ever before, and perhaps than we ever would be. It cost too much, of course. And just when we had some money, perhaps we should have salted it away. But I have always believed that the best investment is in life itself. If the doors were open at last, should we be the ones to close them? Should we try to wrap ourselves in our new security? For me, the answer was no. Hemophilia had too deeply imprinted its implacable truth: There is no tomorrow, only today. Nothing could protect us from the disasters of the future.

We have never regretted our decision. It did cost too much, but it was a golden investment. More than I could have hoped, it accomplished its purpose. By the time we came home all three children were bilingual and had friends throughout Europe. Bobby had grown up. His academic excellence had given him assurance. His qualities had been appreciated. He had traveled alone. He had developed his independence. The cords that so tightly intertwined him with us had been loosened, and this had been done naturally, normally, in the course of growing up. And if the boundaries of his life were still sternly circumscribed, we had been able to push them out farther and farther.

We gave away our cats and put away our clippings. We closed the door of our friendly old house in Irvington and sailed away on the S.S. *France* on August 29, 1968. Thirty friends came to see us off. There was a lot of champagne and Liz Parks burst into tears.

Bobby was just twelve, Susy ten. Elizabeth was only three and a half. Wearing tiny sunglasses and her bright red, white, and blue striped dress with matching beret bought especially for the occasion, she waved frantically to her grandmother and grandfather lost in the crowd on the dock. The sun was brilliant, the skyline of New York knife-sharp against the horizon. And in a swirl of multicolored confetti streamers, with march music blaring from the loudspeakers, the ship backed majestically out into the Hudson River and sailed out of New York harbor.

We had alerted the officials of the *France* about Bobby's condition and the need for refrigerating the cryo we were bringing with us. Despite the gaiety, this trip was a massive gamble, in which we were trusting our new abilities at home transfusion. We had with us a very few bottles of the new Hyland fraction, but we were planning to use cryo, which we were used to, for anything that might occur on the ship and until we could consult with doctors in France. We were also equipped with the usual gaggle of wheelchairs and crutches, medical suitcases and insulated bags that accompanied us wherever we went. One last time, to get us to the dock, a piece of dry ice had even been pried out of the frozen-food depot. The officials of the *France* had promised that upon arrival at Le Havre they would find us dry ice sufficient to make the three-hour trip by train to Paris and the safe haven of another freezer. These preparations had taken endless phone calls and endless explanations, but by the time we sailed the plans seemed foolproof.

The purser came down as soon as the ship had left the harbor to consult with us about the cryo. The cabin steward was called. Everything was explained to him. It must be *frozen*, not refrigerated, we insisted. *Oui, oui, Madame*, we understand (and a look as if to say that they were not, after all, idiots). The steward, along with the insulated bag full of cryo, then disappeared into the bowels of the ship.

All went well for the first two days. But inevitably, one night in the middle of the Atlantic, Bobby's leg began to hurt. Frightened but knowing it had to be done, we decided to give a transfusion. I sent for the steward, but it was impossible to track down anyone who knew what had happened to our cryo. It was our steward's night off, it seemed. After intensive searching he was finally found having a haircut in the ship's barber shop. *Oui, oui*, he remembered. Immediately, he said. We waited. Time passed and we began to grow uneasy. A slightly flustered steward reappeared saying that he could not find it. I said that I would accompany him this time.

Then began a zany search reminiscent of the Marx Brothers—except that it wasn't funny. We ducked in behind one of the service doors that lined the corridors, took the huge clanking freight elevator down, down, emerging on the level of the kitchens. Waiters were still running in and out, finishing dinner. Dodging them, trying to keep our footing on the slippery floor, we searched out one of the directing chefs in his cubbyhole glass-windowed office. No, he didn't know anything about it, but we could look. Where might it be? He hastily abandoned his duties to come with us. I kept insisting over and over that our supplies had to be in one of the freezing rooms at −18° centigrade. Perhaps with the ice cream?

With the anxious steward in tow, trailing behind the chef in his high starched hat and white apron, we hurried back to the elevators. We went still another deck lower. I kept explaining that this was important, that Bobby was bleeding, that we had to find the missing supplies. Down, down. With a heavy clanking of doors, we emerged into the dark refrigerator section. There were several freezing rooms, each forty or fifty feet square. We had to try each one. Each one of them was hermetically sealed like a bank vault and had to be opened by turning a huge wheel. With the chef and the steward we rushed up and down the aisles of each one. First through the ice cream and the butter, then the fish, lying glass-eyed in long rows, then the huge carcasses of meat. Our breath came in clouds, but we never noticed the cold. We rummaged faster and faster through shelf after shelf. Heartsick, I wondered how we would ever find it. How small our little insulated bag would be, compared to this huge mass of food!

The guardians of these vast, floating-below-sea-level stores were dressed in fur-lined jackets, blue work clothes, and heavy boots. At first they were curious at the spectacle of a wild-eyed woman running through their refrigerators with a chef and a steward, but when they heard the word "hemophilia," they, too, joined the search. We finally went down the last aisle of the last −18° refrigeration room. No trace of the missing supplies. The chef was perturbed, the steward frantic. It seemed that he had brought it, as directed, to the chef who had been in charge that day. No one knew where that chef was at the moment. No one had noted where it was to be placed.

And then, one of the refrigerator guardians in his blue work clothes and heavy shoes, as if struck by a terrible thought, exclaimed, "*Les legumes, les legumes!*" ("the vegetables, the vegetables") and began to scurry down a metal circular staircase that went still lower.

Heartsick, I turned to the chef and asked, "What is the temperature for the vegetables?" "Plus four degrees centigrade," he answered. And I knew. A few moments later the man emerged carrying the famous bags. All the cryo was melted—twenty-one precious units, our whole supply for beginning life in France—all ruined. And Bobby was a few decks up, bleeding.

The chef and the steward stood silent. Then the chef shrugged his shoulders and said he was *désolé*, but if he had been informed, he would have seen that it came to the correct refrigerator. The steward was so sad that I felt I had to reassure him. So I told him that everything would be all right. But I wasn't at all sure.

As we made our way back up in the cavernous elevator I turned over in my mind the various implications. Discouraged, I returned to our cabin, carrying the bag full of soggy plastic bags. Bob, who had been impatiently worrying and waiting to begin the transfusion, was stunned when I announced the news.

"All of it?" he asked. I nodded.

All that was left to do was to give the useless cryo a decent burial, which we did later that night, mournfully throwing the bags, one by one, from the top deck into the sea.

Meanwhile, there was nothing to do but try our luck with the new fraction. And so it happened that sometime late at night in the middle of the Atlantic, with nightclub music throbbing and happy couples dancing a little farther down on the same deck, we nervously administered those first units of new Hyland fraction. The ship rolled; Bob tried to steady his hand. The transfusion went well, and by the next morning Bobby's condition improved. He rolled around the decks in his little portable wheelchair. We tried to forget our worries as to what would happen on the other side, now that our entire carry-over supply had been destroyed.

We didn't mention a word about the disastrous kitchen chase

to the ship's officers, not wanting to cause the steward any prob‑
lems for what had really been just another case of misunderstand‑
ing of the intricate problems of our existence. But as we were
approaching Le Havre, the chief purser came especially to our
cabin and announced with great pride: "I wish to tell you, madame,
that the captain of the ship, Monsieur le Commandant himself, has
spoken to Le Havre. There will be dry ice waiting for you upon
arrival. Everything is arranged. You need have no worries."

We had to tell him that there was no need, to thank Monsieur
le Commandant for his concern and his efforts, but that the precious
cryo was at the bottom of the sea.

At Le Havre we managed to cram ourselves into our compart‑
ment on the boat train with our mountains of baggage, heaving
wheelchair and suitcases through the train windows. Late at night,
we arrived at the Gare St.-Lazare. This was the Mecca for which
I had waited and worked so long. Paris, at last. Draped like donkeys
with bags, trying to handle Bobby's wheelchair—and Bobby, who
could not walk, holding tight to Susy and Elizabeth so they would
not get lost—we fought our way through the crowd to a taxi.
And finally too tired and weary to care about the lights of Paris
that at last were twinkling around us, we arrived in the silent,
deserted rue de Messine to face a very uncertain future.

Chapter 21

I had found that first apartment, at 2 rue de Messine, 8e arrondissement, by chance, a few months before. Making a hurried trip to
Paris to reconnoiter the school possibilities, I had found myself in
the middle of bursting bombs, fires, strikes, and barricades. It was
the spring of 1968—that revolutionary time which the French, with
delightful Gallic understatement, refer to simply as "the events."
There were no taxis, no métros, no buses—worse, no apartment
ads: the newspapers were on strike. I was about to give up. Then,
on my last day in Paris, I heard about the apartment while visiting
that hub of specialized knowledge in France, the hairdresser.

To be sure, the apartment wasn't much—a long bowling-alley
hall opening into a series of virtually empty rooms. Our landlord
was a retired French admiral, stingy and hardfisted, who cut
corners by installing skimpy furnishings and charging an outrageous
price. (We had to fight hard to get a stove.) The dismal night we
arrived, we found a few spiky gladioli in a vase in the middle of
the living room floor, but little else. Bob and the children looked
at me mournfully.

In any case, we were not in a position to complain. We had to
organize our lives according to the strict dictates of hemophilia,
and our apartment had two vital advantages: it had an elevator,
and it was only a short, easy walk through the gilded gates and the
pleasant gardens of the Parc Monceau to the École Bilingue (Bilingual School).

My trip in the spring had really been for only one purpose:
to see if I could find a school that would take Bobby. The humiliating experience with the Lycée Français in New York was still
graven on my brain, and despite my hopes, I wasn't at all sure that

things would be different in Paris. Minutely, I checked out the route through the park (very, very good: flat gravel paths, no obstacles). At the edge of the park, I found the antiquated house that served as the school building. Before I went to see the head-mistress, I counted all the stairs (very bad: five steep flights, no elevator). I braced myself for the usual cool and wary reception. To my surprise, the headmistress cut me off in the beginning of my tortured explanations with a brisk, "Calm yourself, madame. Your son, it seems, is a clever boy. He will grow well and strong. Don't worry. Everything will go well here." And that was that.

As it turned out, the adaptation was the hardest for Elizabeth, who at three years and a half suffered greatly at first from being thrown into a strict environment and a foreign language. She began to have nightmares and stopped eating, until I took her to a French doctor who said to me, "Take her out of school for the present. She is being traumatized." We did, for several months, and later all went well. Susy, as usual, applied herself systematically to the new challenge. All of them, to my great delight, began learning their verbs.

The students at the school were mostly foreign. For the very first time in his life, Bobby was no longer "different" because *all* the children at the school were different—the children of foreign service officers and businessmen of many countries. The teachers, mostly French, seemed completely unconcerned about Bobby's hemophilia. I never had to talk to a single one of them. But the most wonderful thing was that, as the days mellowed and the leaves turned golden in the park, Bobby began to walk again, entirely without a brace. He walked with a limp, but he *walked!*

How important living without a brace was to him we never suspected until years later when he wrote this:

"When I entered Bilingue it was an abrupt change for me in many ways other than merely a change of school, or even a change of country. It was the first year that I had ever been to school in which I was not immediately branded as handicapped by the presence of a brace. No longer was this the first premise on which all my relationships and friendships were founded. Of course, the peculiarities of hemophilia were soon evident, but I was allowed to explain it the way I wished, rather than let everyone around me acquire the usual prefabricated misconceptions. In America, my parents had almost always explained hemophilia to my teachers, who nevertheless tended to cling to their original ideas (bleed-to-death-from-a-cut) and, invariably, all this lore—fact and fiction no longer distinguishable—filtered down to my classmates, who did not know how to handle the situation. Soon it became apparent that there was a hands-off policy around me.

"But at Bilingue, this was not the case. I was pretty much allowed to break the news to those around me in my own manner. The result was that instead of becoming the focal point, hemophilia instead became a peripheral factor. For the first time, I fitted in!

"One interesting result of this sudden acceptance was a tremendous desire on my part to conform. After having been painfully different all my life, I was confronted with the opportunity to be 'just like everybody else.' And so I became a superconformist: when the majority wore turtle-neck shirts, I pestered my mother to buy turtle-neck shirts. When the elite went to buy candy at the other side of the park, I was right there, tagging along. The jokes that circulated around the school were dutifully memorized and even the little clandestine groups of scared smokers (of cigarettes) found me among them (although infrequently; the risk was too great).

"All this inevitably resulted in mental conflict (I didn't always believe everything I was saying) and physical stress (I pushed myself beyond my limit in order to keep up). But it was a very valuable experience—this peculiar educational environment outside the classroom."

As soon as we arrived we had made contact with the team of French hematologists to which we had been referred. We visited and talked with Dr. Marie Jeanne Larrieu, a sophisticated woman who worked with the great French hematologist Professor Jean Bernard at the Hôpital St.-Louis; with Dr. Jean Pierre Soulier, a famous research specialist in hemophilia and the director of the Centre National de Transfusion Sanguine; and with Dr. François Josso, who was then the director of the CNTS research laboratories and a professor of hematology.

All of them greeted us warmly, and generously arranged to have the excellent French fraction prepared at the CNTS made available for Bobby's transfusions. Those first months, Bobby was so much better that apart from our first phone calls and visits, we never needed to call. Bob handled all of his transfusions at home.

With a school friend, Schuyler Rumsey, he haunted the stamp market and haggled over prices. Susy spent happy days exploring Paris with her new friends, and even Elizabeth was beginning to chatter in perfectly accented French. It was everything I had hoped for—a wonderful new life.

Bob began working on his book on Peter the Great, isolating himself in one of the maid's rooms under the eaves of our building among the smells of garlic cooking and Spanish voices. I fixed up a corner of the apartment for myself and began to work on my book on the Leningrad poets.

At Thanksgiving, we had a gay celebration with friends. Because our small oven was too small for our huge turkey, I took it in a taxi to the kitchens of the elegant Hôtel George V, where it was cooked in one of their enormous ovens. The friend who had arranged this favor brought it back to us, all steaming and toasty brown, in another taxi. At Christmas we took the children high into the Swiss Alps, where my Dutch cousins and their children were living in an old Swiss chalet that looked out on the Jungfrau. Bobby could not ski, but his sturdy cousins pulled him everywhere on a sled. Once while he was sledding he got slammed in the face in a collision with other children. He bled frighteningly, but a triple transfusion stopped it, and those days were wonderful nevertheless. We all sang carols around the big tile fireplace with the children roosting on its cozy shelves. At New Year's, we gathered by the church and listened to the sound of the bells ringing in relays throughout the mountain valley in the sharp, clear winter night air.

To be sure, there were a few more scares. In January, Bob and I went to Russia and we were awakened one day in Leningrad by a phone call from a journalist friend in Moscow. Tensely she told us that Bobby had been rushed to the hospital in Paris, suffering from a mysterious urinary problem. Afraid that he might be bleeding in the kidneys, we frantically tried to get through to

Paris for information. "Six hours wait," the Soviet operator mumbled grumpily. The USSR is not a place to be in time of emergency. Encased in the cement of red tape and bureaucracy, it is impossible for Soviets to do anything on short notice. It was evening before we were able to get through on the telephone. Bob decided to leave immediately. We rushed down the stairs and barged into the Aeroflot office, which was closing. Everyone had left except for a kindly, sad-eyed blond lady. Bob demanded an immediate change of his ticket to an Aeroflot plane that was leaving for Stockholm early in the morning. Impossible, said the lady; she was not the proper person authorized to change tickets. Her superior had left for the day. Only in the morning. Could her superior be reached? *Nyet.* No telephone. We explained, increasingly agitated. Our son has been taken to the hospital, his case is serious. There is a plane leaving Leningrad tomorrow with empty seats. What can we do?

The sad-eyed lady looked at us. Then, saying simply, "I am a mother too," she did what is unthinkable in the Soviet Union. She acted on her own and sold Bob a new ticket.

The next morning, frosty and clear, Bob took a taxi through the quiet streets of Leningrad and flew out over the Baltic to Stockholm, deep in snow. Then to Paris, gaining hours as he flew westward. He arrived at three in the afternoon, and rushed directly by taxi to the American Hospital. Bobby was in bed after several transfusions, pale but all right.

Still, even these upsets seemed minor compared to what we had passed through before—so much so that we felt we had reached that long-hoped-for plateau at last.

I had forgotten the first rule of hemophilia: nothing is sure.

It was the beginning of spring. That morning we were awakened by gypsy organ-grinders playing and singing in the street under our windows. From our balcony the children gaily threw coins down into their tambourines. The weather had been warm and lovely for a week. In the Parc Monceau the forsythia and tulips were blooming; the chestnut blossoms were growing fat. On the pond the swans proudly showed off their downy new families.

Immaculately dressed French children played sedately in the sand-piles, while benevolent old ladies sunned themselves in their iron chairs and smiled over their knitting. Jaunty, blue-uniformed policemen strolled peaceably, hands behind their backs, eying the mini-skirted girls who hurried through the park on their way to work. It was the beginning of April, in Paris. As I hurried about my errands, shopping for white asparagus, chatting with the butcher, I couldn't help smiling at the buildings with their lacy forged-iron balconies, such was my joy at having finally achieved my ambition, to be at last living in the city I had loved for so many years. Surely, surely our luck had turned.

Then came the telephone call. It was Bobby. "Mom, I had a little accident in school. My leg feels funny. It's not much, but I think I better come home."

The familiar alarms went off.

"Which one?" I asked.

"It's my left leg."

"I'll be right over."

Bob was doing his income tax, straining over the figures and arranging receipts on the living room floor. I said nothing, but ran down the stairs and drove to the school. Bobby was waiting out-side. Quickly I scanned his eyes, his complexion. He seemed all right. Oh, I thought, nothing dramatic, and heaved a sigh of relief.

"How did it happen?" I asked. Bobby suddenly looked wistful. "I fell, Mom, while I was playing at recess." Then his words came rushing out: "Mom, I'm sorry, I really am. I *was* running. But the weather was so beautiful and the sun was shining and I just *had* to run and, well, I caught my toe and fell forward." He looked so ashamed. How well I understood the euphoria of that day! Of course he had felt like running! "Don't worry," I said, "it's not your fault, and it's probably nothing anyway. You just need some rest. We'll elevate it and put some ice on it."

When Bobby walked in the door, on the way to his room, he said to Bob, still hunched over his papers, "Dad, I think I need a transfusion." Preoccupied, Bob answered, "Is it serious? I'm busy now, but I'll do it in half an hour."

Bobby lay down on his bed, we put the leg at rest, and I packed it with ice. It was then four o'clock. Yet in the space of less than

half an hour, the knee was puffing badly. This time I interrupted
Bob and he gave the transfusion. But instead of getting better, the
knee grew even more swollen and painful. Why? He had just had
a transfusion of the new, strong fraction. Perhaps it was not enough?
At six o'clock, only an hour after the first transfusion, Bob gave another, twice as strong as he usually gave. Now, surely, that would
do it. It did not. By eight o'clock Bobby was lying on his bed, toss-
ing from side to side and moaning in pain. The swelling increased,
the bleeding continued unchecked. We were shaken. What was
wrong with the new fraction, our freedom, our miracle, our solace?
Clearly something serious, and we didn't know how to cope with it.

I reached Dr. Josso at home. I was very nervous. It was the
first time we had had to call on him, and now it was at night. To
make it even more difficult, I knew that he was under no obligation to come; he was no longer a practicing doctor, but an eminent
professor in blood research. Yet there was no one else. "Doctor,"
I said, trying to keep my voice steady, "I know it's late. I'm sorry
to disturb you at home, but something is really wrong."

I braced myself for an impatient voice, mentally preparing
myself to plead if necessary for him to come. Instead, a calm and
reassuring answer came: "But, madame, don't apologize. It is
exactly the best time to call. I am much more *disponible* when my
working day is finished. When one is at home, one is entirely free."

"Will you come?" I asked. "I know it's late . . ." He interrupted me. "Of course. Bobby is a good fellow. I will come over
to be with my little friend."

Bobby was screaming in pain. I was desperately worried. Already I knew that we were in one of those unexplored areas where
the disease could buffet us mercilessly with no end in sight. Visions
of new months in casts and wheelchair filled my mind. What
about school? How could we cope? And here we were in France,
far away from all our doctors. We were mad to have tried it. It
was already clear that such a severe bleeding, even at best, meant
three to four weeks of total immobility, hopes dashed, depression,
and the spring blighted. If only that were all! But what if it were
longer? What if our fragile victory were to be shattered entirely?
We should have known, we should have known, I repeated bitterly

over and over to myself as I paced the floor waiting, trying to gain control of my thoughts.

In less than forty-five minutes Dr. Josso arrived at our door. Dressed in an elegant brown suit, composed and charming, he radiated a calm assurance as he crossed our threshold. Tensely I explained the events of the afternoon. Immediately he went in to Bobby. When he saw him there, lying on his bed writhing and moaning, already almost oblivious to us, Dr. Josso's face clouded with concern.

"What painkillers do you have?" he asked. Very gently he approached Bobby's bedside, talking to him quietly, but the knee was so swollen and tight that Bobby would not permit anyone to touch it even with a fingertip. "No, no," he screamed. "Mother, it hurts! It hurts too much!"

"Quickly," said Dr. Josso, "go to the pharmacy and buy some plaster bandages. We must immobilize it; the leg is pulling up."

I saw the leg was already jackknifed and rigid. (Seven more years, I thought. Those endless exercises, Blythedale, those years of therapy, those sand bags carefully measured . . . gone, gone.) "I will try to make a cast," the doctor went on. "I am out of practice, but I will do my best." Swiftly writing out a prescription for painkillers, he pressed it into my hand.

It was nearing nine o'clock. Bob raced to the car to go for plaster bandages. I ran breathless down the stairs and rushed to our pharmacy, which was about to close, and bought whatever they had. My mouth was dry, my hands clammy, but my mind was once again in that clear, deadly clear, state of emergency, eternally ready in my soul and now activated once again. As I ran numbly through the streets, the houses that I had looked at so happily only that morning seemed suddenly cold and foreign.

When I returned, Dr. Josso was already in the kitchen preparing whatever basins he could find. He had removed the jacket of his handsome suit, his tie was off, his sleeves rolled up. He plunged the plaster bandages into the water, quickly improvised a cast, and then, his arms still covered with plaster up to the elbows, carried it into Bobby's room.

But as he approached, Bobby, nearly crazed with pain, tried

to push him away. He gasped hysterically, "No casts! No more casts! I can't stand it!" Susy, in tears, cried out terrified from her room, "What's happening to Bobby!" We tried to hold him, to calm him, but it was impossible. Unhinged with pain, Bobby was at last showing all the horror he had felt, encased in plaster, during all his young years. He had borne it so valiantly, with such strength. He had not complained. Perhaps he hadn't known how. But the suffering and constraint of those years now were making his present pain sharper, his agony more intense. We had to give up. Dr. Josso said, "We must not press it further. If he does not want it, he must not have it." Bobby lay there, exhausted, moaning.

Dr. Josso and I went into the living room and sat silently. I gave him a Scotch, and then another. He had little to say. "His pain is unusual. There is no explanation for it. He may have broken something. He should go to the Hôpital St.-Louis tomorrow for X-rays. We will have to try and stop the bleeding and then see. Give him transfusions three times a day. I will see that you have the fraction." Then he added, "Here are some more prescriptions for drugs. You will have to start preparing him for the night early in the afternoon."

"But so many? What are they for?" I asked, anxiously trying to read this kind but sorrowful face. He was trying, unsuccessfully, to wear that professional mask that gentle doctors wear when they are seriously perplexed but trying not to show it. "Well, this one will work on the knee," he explained, "and this one . . . is for the brain."

His slight hesitation, the drop in his voice, made me ask. "What is it?"

"Morphine," he said. "Synthetic morphine."

"How many times?"

"He can only have this twice . . . or it may be habit-forming. The chemistry of the body of young adolescents is such that any drug taken may be easily habit-forming. You have been wise to keep him as free of drugs as possible." Dr. Josso went on, "I will call Dr. Larrieu in the morning and discuss this with her. We will weigh the dangers and advantages of intervention. We will wait three days."

As he left, I thanked him for coming to us. He said simply,

"There is no need. If one has chosen the trade of helping people and they are in trouble, one must be *disponible. Bon courage.*" It was nearly 2 A.M.

I stayed at Bobby's bed throughout that night. The pain came in waves. I tried to hold his hand, to stroke his head. I could not come near his leg, not even place my hand in the air more than a foot away, or he would scream. The pressure of a sheet was unbearable. And so the night passed until the dawn came gray into the windows and Bobby, nearly unconscious, still cried out.

Early in the morning, Dr. Josso called and advised us that he had made arrangements with Dr. Larrieu for X-rays. The doctors thought that, because of the nature of his fall, he might have cracked a kneecap. It was extremely difficult to move him. The slightest movement caused pain. Somehow Bob and I managed to get him into the car and we began a nightmarish journey through the Paris traffic to the Hôpital St.-Louis, on the other side of the city. Every time Bob had to slow down, or stop for a red light, Bobby would scream out in pain. We were frantic. The traffic was heavy, the ride endless. By the time we reached the hospital Bobby was white and drawn. They took an X-ray but found no cracked kneecap. No one could understand from the X-ray why he should be having such excruciating pain. We had to turn around and go back, with Bobby in agony every time we slowed down. The trip through traffic took almost two hours.

More hours passed with no change. He did not eat, he could not sleep. I began the pills at two in the afternoon. Bob continued the transfusions. Dr. Josso called in the afternoon, sad and discouraged when I told him there was no improvement. I gave the first dose of synthetic morphine. There was no change. Again that night I began my vigil by his bed. I tried everything. I read to him, I talked to him. Desperately, I played all the Peter, Paul, and Mary records we had, in the hope that Peter might again work his magic and sing the pain away. I played the song he had sung, "Freight Train," over and over while I repeated to Bobby, "Don't you remember when Peter sang? Listen to him now. Listen." But the magic did not work and the pain continued. Was it only yesterday, I thought, that the sun was shining? And so, another night passed.

In the morning, the knee was swollen as large as a grapefruit; so swollen that now we could not accurately judge whether it had grown or stayed the same. Pain and drugs gave Bobby double vision. His eyes were clouded and crazed. He still had not eaten or slept and still, despite the drugs, the pain knifed through him.

Again in the morning, Dr. Josso called. He was extremely disturbed over Bobby's continued suffering. It seemed that he could bear it even less than we. I could hear his worry in his voice. "Although it will be difficult, we cannot let him suffer more. I have arranged for a surgeon. If he is not better by tomorrow morning, we shall have to try to intervene." What Dr. Josso was proposing was a controversial surgical procedure in which a needle is inserted directly into the knee joint to draw out the blood and relieve the pressure.

We understood all the difficulties. When aspirating an actively bleeding joint, a surgeon must go in blind. There is a mass of semiclotted material within the knee because of the transfusions. An aspiration must be done quickly, after the bleeding has stopped, but before such clotting has occurred, or there is risk of harming the joint and causing more trauma. It was a last-ditch hope. We had given the two permissible doses of morphine.

Life in our household had stopped. Our *au-pair* girl, Terry Hawley, alone kept things going for the girls. She was subdued and frightened; for the first time since we had found this warm, friendly Midwestern girl in Switzerland, she had seen what the disease could do. She took the girls to walk in the park so they would not have to see and hear Bobby's continued suffering. On the evening of the third day, I again began preparing Bobby for the night. We still could not approach the knee or put a sheet over him. I had tried to sleep, for I had barely rested for three days. Bob made me go out of the house for dinner, but I rushed back, and although he tried to make me sleep, it was impossible. I could hear Bobby calling. So once again, I began my vigil by the bed. I just sat, clasping his hand in the dark, in despairing silence.

Suddenly, in the middle of the night I felt a strange surge of decision. Briskly, I told Bobby that we were going to get up and go into the living room. There, I would prop him up on the couch and find a way to take the pressure off the back of his knee. It

seemed crazy, but during other bleedings before, I had tried this
and it had worked. And something very strong was pushing me.
He cried out, "No, I can't," but I got his wheelchair and lifted him
onto it. It was with great difficulty, for his pain at the slightest
movement was excruciating. We managed, and I rolled him into the
darkened living room. Except for the street lights that shone eerily
into the room, everything was dark and empty and still. It was as
if we were the only two human beings awake in the city.

Quickly, trying to seem in perfect control, I gave him orders:
"Sit there. Let me fix the pillow here. There, it will be better.
You'll see, the pillow will make it better. It's soft." He moaned,
"Leave me alone, leave me alone. I can't." When pain has been constant, it has its own momentum and laws. The vital thing is to
break its ascendancy over the mind. I wanted to give him five
minutes, even five minutes, to break the hold, to distract him.

"Tell me about the moon flight, Bobby," I ordered, harsh as a
sergeant. Bobby had been passionately interested in every detail of
the space program. "I can't, Mom," he groaned. "You know I
can't; it hurts too much."

"Tell me about the moon shot," I repeated. "The moon shot.
I don't know anything about it. I don't understand the moon
vehicle. What does it look like? How does it work?"

"I can't, I can't."

"You have to, Bobby. You know I'm stupid, I don't understand
it. Tell me about the moon shot." My voice grew more and more
insistent.

Finally, in anger, he said, "All right, all right, I'll try. The
moon vehicle has four legs . . ." It was the beginning of a miracle.
His description lasted only a few minutes. I both heard it and didn't
hear it. Then he began to cry and moan again.

But it was enough. Although the pain began again immediately,
the momentum, the total control over his mind, had ceased for
those few precious moments. I knew we had won a tiny victory.

"Bobby," I said, "now you are going back to bed. You are
going to sleep. You'll see."

"No, Mom, no. Don't move me again." Perhaps it was the
silence of the night, the unreal lights in the street, but I knew I
must persist, and calmly, I did. I moved him gently into his wheel-

chair. He cried (was I imagining it was less?), and I took him to
his room, plumped his pillow, and stretched him on the bed. He
was crying hoarsely.

I was spent. In those dark hours before the dawn of that third
night I prayed fiercely for strength. And something very strange
happened, something I have never clearly understood. As if someone were speaking to me I was ordered, "Place your hand on his
knee." I was afraid. I argued, "It is impossible. No one can come
near it, no sheet can touch it." But the mysterious command was
repeated: "Place your hand on his knee." Hesitantly at first, I
obeyed. I began to move my hand closer and closer to the tortured
joint until it was in the air only inches away. Bobby said nothing.
Gently, gently I came down on it and finally I touched it. He did
not cry out. I let my hand rest as lightly as I dared, for only a
moment. I felt a great peace. I *knew* in that mysterious moment
that the crisis had passed.

Bobby slept. For the first time in those three days, he really
slept. I placed a sheet over him and slumped into the chair by his
bed. I wept with joy. He slept only an hour and then woke in pain
again. But the pain was no longer an omnipotent fiend but only
our old familiar enemy which would, with patience, recede like a
terrible tide.

In the morning I called Dr. Josso to tell him. His voice was
joyous and relieved. The surgeon was ready, but now no intervention was necessary.

The recovery was slow. Bobby's immediate recuperative
powers were extraordinary. He ate the next day and was gay and
laughing only a few days after that. For me, it was longer. For
weeks I was depressed, anxious, exhausted. The chestnuts bloomed
but I had no heart to enjoy them. Heartsick, I walked despondently
under their falling blossoms as the spring came and went. Bobby
did not walk until July, three months later, and he has not been
able to run again to this day.

Two years later, Dr. Josso had this to say about the harrowing
knee episode that had shaken us all so profoundly. "I was very
struck by Bobby's episode, and remember it vividly. I have always

been interested by this problem of pain. You do the same thing anatomically to the same person one day and everything is all right; the next day it does not go well at all. It depends importantly on the psychological state of the patient.

"It seemed to me that his extreme pain was unusual. I remember thinking, *Il en a marre* (He has had enough of it). He was unhinged. In such a situation, had he been older, he could have killed himself. Such psychological states are what push hemophiliacs to drugs. The organism is very susceptible to the effect of drugs at such times. The preadolescent organism, we know, is especially susceptible because of its unbalanced chemical state.

"I remember thinking about the cast, well, if he doesn't want one, he shouldn't have it. He was suffering horribly. The fractions could not help. I thought he might have broken something. The extreme pain could not be explained. I thought, the less we touch him, the better.

"When a person is in such a psychological state—if he is tired, or especially upset—he may need an outside influence to break the hysteria of pain."

He sat back in his chair, thoughtfully puffing on his pipe, and he added, "You know, a person can go along for a long time taking everything, but little by little it accumulates, and then comes a moment when he just can't take it any longer. It was such a moment for Bobby. He really had had enough. I saw you, tense and worried. I felt that if I could only have transferred his pain to your leg, it would have been the finest service I could have rendered you both."

Chapter 22

There was a long period of convalescence which lasted almost four months. Most of that time, Bobby had to keep his leg at rest. A removable cast was made. It was a fight, but he wore it. For several weeks, he could not be moved from his bed. After what seemed like a very long time, he was finally able to roll around the apartment again in his wheelchair. There were many relapses, many transfusions, many dashed hopes. Susy's birthday party had to be canceled. She blinked back tears, but quietly accepted her disappointment without complaining.

Again I started my rounds of searching the stores for books, for puzzles. Again, I tried to drop broad hints to acquaintances. ("It's so boring to have one's old gray-haired mother around all the time . . . do you suppose that your Johnny could stop by?") Johnny, I would hear, was too busy with swimming lessons, dancing lessons, outings. The concierge's children came up now and then and looked with great frightened eyes at Bobby's cast.

I wrote to Bobby's teachers. At first they tried to send his lessons. Two of the children offered to bring him his work every day. Valiantly, they got through the first two weeks; after that, their visits became rarer, and finally stopped altogether. Once, to Bobby's great joy, his entire class came to visit. He kept hoping, but they never came back. More and more I felt guilty for having urged this mad adventure upon my family. The French system was no better than the American when it came to coping with lessons at home. And there was no possibility of an intercom. There were no more happy trips to the stamp market, no more "fitting in" at school. We were back where we had been five years before. Bobby's leg was atrophied. Back were all the old familiar problems:

boredom, loneliness, depression. Paris or Irvington . . . it was all the same. We might as well have been on another planet for all that we had to do with the life that went on outside our windows that long and sad spring.

As the days and the weeks passed, Bobby grew more irritable. I grew more desperate to find someone to spell me, to relieve the tedium of seeing the same faces every day. Sometimes my friend Gail Gilbert, the wife of an American investment banker, would come by. Gail brought books, she played games with Bobby. Mostly she just talked to him, and this helped immeasurably. But Gail had three small children and a busy life of her own and could come only very rarely. I blessed her for trying.

There were two other people who did do something: totally different people from opposite poles of experience and from opposite ends of the earth. One was a royal princess from Greece and Russia, and the other was an American abstract painter from Horse Cave, Kentucky.

Thinking back, Bobby says of them: "They were my friends. At that time, they were my *only* friends. The kids in my class were swell, but to make that kind of emotional commitment, coming to see a sick person, being willing to accept that responsibility, takes a very mature person. There have been very few people through my life of my age—of any age—who were willing to make that sacrifice. There were some kids, like Davey and Schuyler, but it was more common in people who had experienced difficult times. With Princess Olga and Joe, it wasn't sympathy. It was empathy. They understood. I don't know why. What common points did a boy of twelve have with them? How can you explain what ties two people together . . . despite years, despite differences in background? Just . . . it was deeper than the surface."

In the first days that followed the crisis, I had canceled all our invitations. One person I called was Princess Olga of Yugoslavia. We had met her and her husband, Prince Paul, a few months before. She was a daughter of Prince Nicholas of Greece and Grand Duchess Hélène of Russia, a sister of Marina, Duchess of Kent, and an aunt of Prince Philip of England.

The day we had met, Princess Olga was dressed in a simple, elegant black dress; her only ornament was a small diamond brooch in the shape of a crown pinned near her shoulder. It was easy to see why she and her sister were considered among the great beauties of their time. Her auburn hair, only slightly graying, was carefully drawn into a soft bun on her neck, in the classically simple style of her Cecil Beaton photographs. She had a long face, with an aquiline, aristocratic nose. Her eyes were blue-green, proud and clear, yet with something shy and wistful in their glance. She had the elegant, elongated look of a lily or a swan; the beauty of another, more refined time. Throughout the lunch, she sat erect with a perfectly straight back, her head held high; her graceful hands with their long slender fingers moved with careful composure. I watched those disciplined, elegant gestures which cannot be learned but are bred into the bones over centuries.

Princess Olga had immediately expressed an interest in Bobby and hemophilia; this is why she had wanted to meet us. As a child, she had played with her cousin, the Tsarevich Alexis of Russia. The morning that I called her, it was to cancel a lunch to which she and Prince Paul had also invited Bobby. He was bitterly disappointed to miss it. As we knew each other so little, I was surprised when in her clipped, reserved accent, Princess Olga asked, "But Mrs. Massie, may I come to visit him?" I said that we would, of course, be honored by her visit.

That afternoon, Princess Olga arrived in her polished gray Mercedes, driven by a silent gray-liveried chauffeur who waited patiently outside. She brought beautifully wrapped, exquisite candies. I ushered her into Bobby's spartanly furnished bedroom and closed the door while Terry and I scurried about trying to find some suitable teacups to serve her. An hour later, I peeked in and saw her sitting regally on the edge of one of our wobbly chairs, teacup elegantly balanced in her hand, wrapped in deep conversation with Bobby. I cringed at the sight of his dirty feet, but she hadn't seemed to notice. Bobby was happy and animated. She was telling him stories of Alexis, her childhood friend.

They were lovely stories . . . about how, on wintry days, she and her sisters went by sleigh from the Pavlovsk Palace to the Alexander Palace in Tsarskoe Selo, where Emperor Nicholas and

Empress Alexandra lived. The children loved to play in the ball-rooms of the palace where the floors were shined mirror bright and were splendid for sliding. In one of the ballrooms a long slide had been erected and the children, sitting on pillows, slid down, scream-ing with delight, and continued to slide halfway across the polished floors, whirling around on their pillows. She told Bobby about Alexis' special little car which he used to get around the palace when he could not walk, and how funny it was to see him riding around with his guardian sailor Derevenko "all stuffed up behind him." "All of us were terribly jealous," she said, "because only he had the right to ride in it!"

Princess Olga came several times during those weeks of conva-lescence and always, it was the same: she would go right in to see Bobby, close the door, and then we would hear laughter.

After that crisis, we became friends. During the four years we lived in France we often went to their small house in the 16e arrondissement. Sometimes we went for tea, Bobby and I, after school. Such marvelous teas they were!—with cakes lighter than air, glazed with chocolate, teas served in silver and porcelain on a polished, inlaid table. We often went to lunch. Bobby remembers every menu.

After lunch, we would all go up to the sunlit drawing room with its flowers and vitrines of exquisite Fabergé objects. On the large writing table that had once belonged to Colbert was the bronze clock that had been at Napoleon's bedside when he died. Bobby, precariously balancing his tiny coffee cup, sat on chairs that had once been Madame Pompadour's, and asked and was told all about the portraits of the various Russian emperors and empresses on the wall. Princess Olga had a wry way of correcting Bobby's manners, very unobtrusively, so privately that usually only she and he could hear. A word from her had instantaneous results and was more effective than a whole lecture from me.

Throughout the years that we lived in Paris, Princess Olga called regularly to inquire about Bobby's health. Many years before, she had lost a young son in a tragic accident. Because of her own son's death, she was deeply religious. She believed in spiritualism. Always, she encouraged and reassured me that Bobby would be better, she was sure of it.

Princess Olga and Bobby have maintained their friendship. Somehow they have continued to find something to share: the young, outgoing American boy and the reserved aristocrat with the formal manners of the nineteenth century. "What always impressed me about her," Bobby says, "is that someone like her—born above everybody, so obviously and so long superior in bearing and up-bringing—could be so understanding despite that . . . well, either handicap or wonderful thing she was raised with."

Handicap or wonderful thing. What Princess Olga impressed upon our children unforgettably were the true qualities of the aristocrat: elegance without snobbism, bearing without arrogance, reserve without inaccessibility—and those gentle manners that have almost disappeared from this earth.

The other friend was a man whose life and manners were as informal as Princess Olga's were formal. Joe Downing is a well-known abstract painter who has lived in Paris for twenty years. One morning, desperately trying to find company for Bobby, on an impulse, I called him. "Joe," I said, trying to make my voice sound normal and not too pleading, "you know, Bobby hasn't walked for a long time. I thought maybe you might come and draw with him for a little while . . . ?" "Fine," said Joe, "only I can't come today; maybe tomorrow." I hung up, sadder than ever. Five minutes later, the phone rang. "Hey, Sue," I heard Joe's Southern-accented voice, "how about if I come over right now?" He had understood.

In what seemed like an extraordinarily short time, Joe was at the door wearing his rumpled tweed jacket and his slouched felt hat. He opened the large pouch bag that was slung over his shoulder and out popped his little dog Suki, a stray he had once picked up and who never left him. He went in to Bobby and, from the same bag, pulled out an ordinary brick. "I found it twelve years ago and I liked its looks," he said to Bobby. "It's the same age as you. Let's see what we can do with it." And that first day, he and Bobby spent several hours meticulously painting the brick until it looked like a valuable Egyptian relic, covered with colorful hieroglyphics.

That was typical of Joe. He always seemed able to find beauty in unexpected places. Wherever he went, however simple his surroundings, the atmosphere was opulent. His living room in a historic but crumbling building in the Marais was lavishly covered with a single magnificent forty-foot Oriental rug. ("I found it at the cleaner's," said Joe. "Somebody had left it.") He always served his guests champagne from magnums in an assortment of glasses— each one different, each beautiful in shape or color, all found individually in a series of junk stores or at the Flea Market. In a corner of his studio, littered with paints and palettes and piled high with his canvases of glowing colors, was a five-foot oak tree that Joe had managed to grow from an acorn. Joe had friends everywhere in Paris, artists and flower-sellers, jazz musicians, concierges and delicatessen keepers.

All this rich sense of life he brought to Bobby. Once the brick was finished, Joe ordered canvases and paints and taught Bobby to paint in oils. Bobby would spend hours deeply absorbed in his work. "Joe showed me that you could create a beautiful life from nothing," he says. "He showed me that you could assemble from what were seemingly random bits about you and put them together and have a wonderful unity. I loved the randomness of his apartment, his painting, his parties . . . they were all typical of him. Joe could live in a ruin and paint beautiful pictures, live in a run-down section of Paris and make it elegant, pick up a dog from nowhere, paint things on an ordinary brick, and out of it all, somehow, he would create beauty. It was the most important thing I learned from him. He was a kind of pioneer—with a lack of commitment to anyone or anything except this process of creating beauty. It was a sort of glorious living, not by any rules or acceptable standards and making it wonderful. It was much much more than just quaint. It was a life to be envied."

And so it was that as the sunny light streamed in our windows and April, May, and June passed by, despite the loneliness, or maybe because of it, Bobby began to develop in new directions. In addition to painting, to my great delight he started to play the guitar. This had long been a secret hope of mine, for I had played the guitar long ago. I had always wanted Bobby to start, because I reasoned that when the legs were immobilized it would be therapeutic to keep both the hands and the brain active. The guitar is demanding, absorbing, precise. And it can be a friend that you can carry with you and talk to when you are lonely. Yet until the time of this crisis he had brushed aside my arguments. But during those months, he gratefully accepted my guitar and began to play. He continued until he had mastered not only the six-string guitar but the twelve-string guitar and the banjo . . . and his music has brought him many friends.

He began to write poetry. This was thanks to a bright young teacher at his school, who, just before Bobby's crisis, had been encouraging his class not to be afraid to open themselves out and to write verses. He had been reading poetry in class and teaching his students the craft of constructing a poem. Bobby began filling neat notebooks, working each day.

>
> My feet are cut.
>> And they bleed
>> But I guess
>> That is what
>> You must expect
>> If you walk
>> In the Field of Reality
>> Where all the
>> Blades of grass
>> Are made of steel
> And you aren't allowed any shoes.

>
>> When I jumped off
>> I thought I had wings
>> Only now do I know,
>> And it is too late.

>
> Relatives are like
> Grains of sand
> On a warm white beach
> But they are as rare
> and different
> As a jewel
> In a bucket of pebbles.

After several notebooks, I encouraged him to send a selection to the Soviet Union to one of my poet friends, Constantine Kuzminsky, in Leningrad for criticism. This poet, who spoke English well, translated them into Russian, and he wrote Bobby the following letter.

I was pleased by your poems—I was shocked by them. Too deep for a boy, well done for a youngster. Even if it is not condition of life to you, you must continue your work. Not for the Future, but for yourself. If I could, I would write music and paint, only to make the soul deeper. To understand. And therefore I bless your work in poetry—but don't play with art. Certainly I have no right to show you your own way. But I believe that you will be serious in this—in art I mean. And therefore I worry that your poems seemed to me so deep—maybe too deep. And it takes the man at whole and you will have to pay a lot for it, you understand me?

Another one of Bobby's poems was written about himself and Joe. Joe wrote to him about it, and in his letter managed to tell Bobby a lot, not only about the art of poetry, but about the art of friendship:

Dear Bobby:
    Your canvas was off to a great start. . . . But I am not writing about that but about your poem. Although of course one should never meddle in another's art, I would like to recommend an important change. The recommendation is motivated partly by vanity; one of the most flattering things that can happen to a man is to figure in a good poem and I naturally want to be at my best.
    You refer to me as a kind painter. This may possibly not be false . . . but it is most certainly not the attribute for which I would most like to be remembered or even noticed. You may be sure that if I had found you a bore, or had my first visit not been a real pleasure, you couldn't have seen the hallway for my smoke. Artists are particularly selfish creatures, and often the better they are, the greater the selfishness.
    . . . In the same way, you may be a sick boy and of course I am terribly sorry you have that to put up with, but most emphatically, it is not that aspect of you that interests me. I long ago gave up seeing anyone except those, not only that I like seeing, but that I like seeing more than others, for life does spin by and

there *are* good ones about. So if I spend some time with you, it is because I want to myself, for myself.

So I think you should find some better qualifying term for me than "kind painter" and better than "sick boy" for you. They are such a small part of each of us.

See you soon,
Joe

It was July before Bobby could take a few tentative steps. We strapped the wheelchair onto the top of the car and left for Greece. We meandered across Europe. Everywhere, Bob gave transfusions. He gave them on the windswept lavender fields of the Vaucluse in France, where we had stopped to visit Joe in his little crooked house tucked away in a hillside town, he gave them crossing the Alps, in a *pensione* overlooking the Grand Canal in Venice, on a ferryboat crossing the Adriatic. In some of these places, I shudder to think of the fuss we would have created had we started looking for a doctor in the middle of the night. "Are you sure he is a hemophiliac? I am sorry . . . our laws do not permit. You must take him to a hospital. In the next city . . ." In hotels, to avoid misunderstandings we always took pains to hide the bottles and needles. (Once, in Naples, the maid came in during a transfusion and began shrieking, "Manager! Manager!" as she fled out the door. Quickly, we disposed of everything except the patient, who was peaceably munching a pear by the time she got back.)

We spent a month with friends on a Greek island; in the house there were sixteen children. The hot sun and the warm water began to take effect. Bobby's leg began to improve. He swam every day, diving off the jagged rocks into the clear turquoise water. With trident and net, he became an expert at collecting sea urchins for our lunches—delicious, delicate morsels that we squirted with lemon juice, scooped out and gobbled up between sips of icy, licorice-flavored ouzo. At the end of a summer full of melons, honey, and sun, he was strong again.

It was September. The first year in Paris was over, but more than a quarter of it had been shattered by illness. Bob's research for his biography of Peter the Great had been much delayed, as had my book on Leningrad poets. So we decided to stay. Anyway, something wonderful had happened. We had found a sanctuary. After the summer, we left the depressing apartment on the rue de Messine and moved to 11 rue de la Cerisaie, in my favorite section of Paris, the Marais. The very name of the street evoked poetry: the Street of the Cherry Orchard, so named because the cherry orchards of Charles V had once been there in the fourteenth century. It was near the Place de la Bastille, five minutes away from the Place des Vosges, a short walk from the beautiful quais of the Île St.-Louis and Notre Dame.

The Marais is a quarter of narrow streets and winding alleys, of secret squares where traveling players give outdoor performances, of wonderful markets; it is full of life, and every house speaks of history. In the time of Louis XIV it was the most elegant section of Paris, a place where noblemen built magnificent private palaces. In the centuries that followed, as high society began to move to other quarters, it lost fashion. The beautiful buildings were left in disrepair and the Marais became a working-class quarter.

In more recent times, artists and sculptors moved in, attracted by the low rents, and set up studios in the old buildings and warehouses. Joe Downing was one of the first. Where artists go, others soon follow. When André Malraux became Minister of Culture, the government began a massive restoration of the beautiful buildings of the Marais. Alas, now the Marais is becoming fashionable again. When we lived there, it still had its earthy atmosphere. On the rue St.-Antoine, in front of the markets, accordionists played, and joking boisterous workingmen in their blue overalls lined up along the marble counters of the bistros for their glass of red wine.

Across the street from the massive green doors that opened into our courtyard, there was a plaque on the wall that read: "In this place, the site of the former Hôtel des Lesdiguieres, the Tsar Peter the Great lived when he visited Paris in 1717." Our house had been there when he was, and had remained. I never opened those massive doors and looked into our courtyard without feeling joy. It was so beautiful. There before me was the cobblestoned courtyard with laurel trees in white pots. In the rear of the courtyard was a graceful four-story eighteenth-century building ornamented with white medallions of cupids. Yet the real wonder was not this lovely quiet court, but the fact that when you stepped into our apartment, suddenly, from every window, you could see trees, flowers, and grass. For beyond the house there was a secret garden. Steps led into it from our living room, and at the back there was a high wall, covered with ivy, that separated us from our neighbors . . . the garrison headquarters of the glamorous elite horse guard of France, the Garde Républicaine. Our second-floor bedroom looked out on their Napoleonic buildings.

We were only a few steps away from the Bastille and the Boulevard Henri IV, one of the busiest of Paris' noisy boulevards. But once inside our walls, no sound of traffic penetrated. It was peaceful; you could hear birds singing. During the three years that we lived in that enchanted place, I never once awoke to a jarring alarm clock. Instead, in the morning, gently into my ears would come the gentle sound of the clip-clop of horses' hoofs. Sometimes the sound of a masculine voice encouraging his steed or singing would waft over the wall.

We shared the Cerisaie with few other tenants. One of our neighbors was an old Alsatian engraver, who always tipped his hat to us in courtly fashion as we passed in the courtyard and who, every Christmas, designed the greeting card for all of us. Another was our landlord, a distinguished white-haired gentleman who lived on the second floor, surrounded with rare old books and objets d'art. The concierge, Madame Rhéto, ran us all. She was a salty lady from Brittany with a highly independent nature. The widow of a country policeman who had come to Paris only ten years before, she staunchly maintained her sturdy country habits, scrubbing the cobbles of the courtyard on her hands and knees. She also was our housekeeper. She ran our household and nagged us and scolded us —and we loved her. She prepared us delicious meals—always without the trace of a cookbook, saying only that she cooked things "by the color or my spirit." As concierge, she knew the most private affairs of everyone in the building; she even knew the special sound of their individual footsteps. I remember one night, as she was working in our kitchen, we heard the great green doors onto the street clang open. Madame Rhéto stiffened, listened attentively, said "those footsteps are not from our house," and scurried out to check on the intruder. As housekeeper, Madame Rhéto was sternly exacting with the local merchants, checking to see, when I shopped alone, if they had really given me the choicest meat, the ripest vegetables. If not, she bustled down to complain. She would walk four extra blocks, past five fishmongers with tables full of fish, to the one farthest down the boulevard, the only one where, in her informed Breton opinion, the fish was *mangeable*. On Sundays, it was my pleasure to shop at the huge open-air market set up on the Boulevard Richard-Lenoir off the Bastille. Stalls of luscious green salads and herbs, tables piled high with apples and oranges, radishes and artichokes, stretched for twelve city blocks. It was such a treat to look at and everything was so succulent that I would always end up buying too much. (This would earn me another scolding from Madame Rhéto for my extravagance.) Then, when there was not another inch of space in my cart overflowing with produce and flowers, I would roll it home to the sounds of the church bells.

At Cerisaie, Bobby had a special room to himself, off another ground-floor entrance. This bachelor independence pleased him enormously, especially because he could leave his room as messy as he liked without risking the wrath of Madame Rhéto. We set up a simple intercom system between the apartment and his room.

We enrolled all three children in a completely French school in the adjoining 5e arrondissement, the Collège Sévigné. Each morning, the three of them took the bus at the Place de la Bastille hard by the canals of the Seine. In winter, they left before daylight and returned long after darkness had fallen. They loved riding in the old Paris buses with their open back-ends, and were dismayed and threatened loudly to demonstrate when those wonderful old buses vanished forever in favor of the modern, closed-in sort which entirely lack the special daring charm of the old ones.

At the Collège Sévigné there were only two or three other foreign students. Nevertheless, the school welcomed our children, including Bobby. Hemophilia was no barrier; again I met the same matter-of-fact, calm attitude. Again I had nothing to explain to the teachers.

The school assured me that if I entrusted the children to them for two years, they would be bilingual. And they were right. But the school program was very stiff. No special allowances were made because the children did not know French well. They were expected to keep up with the French students. That first autumn Susy was reduced to tears every night when she tackled her homework. She was given heavy doses of Daudet, Molière, Racine, and La Fontaine. There were grammar *dictées* every day. But she persevered and even took Spanish, German, and Latin in French, and by the time she left, rose to the top of her class. Only a year later, I would see her curled up with a copy of Balzac or Colette, reading for pleasure. In the lower classes of the Collège, Elizabeth had a superb education. Taught in small classes staffed by an imaginative teacher and two assistants, she learned to read and write in French before she was six, and was reciting and even composing poetry, which she collected and kept in neat little notebooks. Manners were stressed; the children were taught to shake hands with their teacher upon leaving, a wonderful habit which, alas, quickly deserted her when she came home. Elizabeth made many friends among her polite little classmates. One day, a strange thing happened. She had invited a group to her birthday party. One handsome little blond boy arrived with the family maid. As the maid left him, she handed me several elastic bandages and said, "Alexandre is a hemophiliac; if he falls down, would you please wrap his knee?" It was the first I had known that there was another hemophiliac in the school. I told the maid that Alexandre had come to visit the right family.

Physically, the school presented great difficulties for Bobby. It was an old-fashioned building with many steep flights of well-worn stairs and musty old classrooms with old-fashioned wooden desks. The only play yard was a minuscule square of pure cement. Bobby was permitted to use the teachers' elevator to spare him the stairs, and he made his way, on crutches and sometimes even in a wheelchair. When he could not walk, taxis took him to and from school. As the school had only recently begun to accept boys in the upper grades, Bobby found himself with only one other boy in a class of twenty-six girls. During the three years he attended, the masculine population increased, but he was still heavily out-numbered, and thus the center of a great deal of admiring female attention. At twelve, he complained a lot about this; three years later, at fifteen, the complaints suddenly tapered to nothing.

Despite his frequent absences, Bobby rose to be first in his class, and eventually won the highest marks in the school in French grammar. He was able to earn money by helping to teach the English classes at the school. Because of his academic achievements, he became a hero to teachers and students in the school. In France, grades are *all* that matter in school. I had been right about that!

The headmistress of the Collège Sévigné (always known and addressed only as "Madame la Directrice") was a tiny, redoubtable lady straight from the novels of the nineteenth century. She ruled the school with absolute power. Even her little cocker spaniel, Maurice, was important; he served as the official mascot of the school. Maurice's modest little black head, fringed with long floppy ears, was imprinted as the emblem on the school sweatshirt. Madame la Directrice wore mid-length tweed skirts and sensible shoes. Her white hair was tied up in a severe little bun at the nape of her neck. Her little half-lensed, gold-rimmed glasses always rested far down on her nose. Half hidden behind her huge desk, she would peer sternly over these little glasses. Small as she was, she was an awesome personage, and a request to come to her office could reduce students to tears. Although Bobby towered over her, she persisted (as she craned her neck, looking up at him) in calling him *"mon petit* Massie." For some strange reason, this odd couple, Madame la Directrice and Bobby, got on extremely well. This despite the fact that Bobby, full of fiery adolescent emotions and

American idealism, was forever requesting appointments with her in order to make recommendations for school improvements. Once, worried, I asked her if he was not bothering her with his endless stream of suggestions. She answered me primly, *"Non, pas du tout. He understands how to present his case politely."* Two or three times a week, Bobby would enter the inner sanctum of Madame la Directrice and the two of them had discussions: about the prevalence of cheating and the reasons for it, about the formal, rigid nature of the French school curriculum.

Bobby thought there ought to be more school spirit and, after canvassing his fellow students, came to the conclusion that the reason was that, in French schools, there are no extracurricular activities. He persuaded Madame la Directrice to permit him to publish the school's first newspaper. This was a much more daring enterprise than it might sound. The school's reputation was built on its conservative *comme il faut* atmosphere, and French parents looked askance at anything so revolutionary as students actually expressing their opinions in print! But there was such enthusiastic response among the students to having something of their own that three hundred turned up for the first meeting. Bobby, in the course of a marathon series of discussions, had managed to convince Madame la Directrice that there would be no antiestablishment agitation.

When Bobby left the school to return to America, Madame la Directrice had to remove her little glasses to wipe away her tears. And later, when Bobby returned to Paris for a visit alone, she insisted that he stay as a guest in her apartment. The three of them, Madame la Directrice, Bobby, and Maurice the cocker spaniel, had gay little lunches and dinners at the local restaurants in the Latin Quarter, where she plied Bobby with half bottles of Beaujolais Nouveau.

During the three years we spent at la Cerisaie, through our apartment passed a wonderfully varied stream of visitors: artists, dancers, translators, professors, and poets—English, French, Greek, American, and Russian. Bobby says that, during his periods of bleeding and immobility, "it was what kept me alive. More than the beautiful buildings and the French education, it was the thing that was most meaningful to me about our life in Paris: that constant stream of fascinating people coming to our house; the surprise of opening the door and never knowing who would say, 'Hello, I'm . . .' When I was a little boy and I was alone sitting in my wheelchair, I used to make up adventures. But here it all was, and you didn't have to stretch your imagination. It was real."

One of our most interesting visitors and the one who stayed longest was a Soviet poet from Leningrad, Victor Sosnora. In the spring of 1970, Victor was unexpectedly permitted to come to Paris. He arrived at our apartment and stayed two months. During that time, he became a member of our family. The bond that tied us was hemophilia; he himself had had a childhood filled with illness and suffering. It had developed in him, as it has in us, a special shorthand of communication.

Victor was a strange, moody man whose intense nature glowed in his dark eyes. His father, a former acrobat in the Leningrad circus, had been a war hero, a general, and eventually, the deputy Warsaw Pact commander under Red Army Marshal Rokossovsky.

Until the age of six, Victor had lived almost entirely in hospitals suffering from what was diagnosed as tuberculosis of the bones. There had been talk of amputating his hands and feet. During the siege of Leningrad he had suffered from malnutrition, dystrophy, and scurvy. He escaped to the south to live with partisans, only to see them all shot before his eyes. These and other terrible experiences had left him permanently scarred in body and in soul.

For the children, he was a storybook character. Even Madame Rhéto, dubious at first about our strange visitor, finally mellowed toward this gentle man with the melancholy face. We all grew accustomed to his unusual habits. He lived mostly at night. Every day, the routine was the same. He would appear about noon, unshaven, at the kitchen door for his breakfast, a startling mixture which never varied: a raw egg, a tomato, a piece of Roquefort cheese, and a bottle of beer. Then, breakfast over, he would go out into the garden, where he would walk around and around in precisely regular circles for half an hour. Then he would sit a while and listen to the sounds in the air. In the afternoon, I would find him in our garret typing and retyping on the old Russian typewriter we had found for him. After dinner, suitably mellowed, he recited poetry and sang plaintive songs in an oddly touching off-pitched voice.

He was wonderful with the children. Sosnora's poetry is full of fairy-tale images and surreal creatures. He told animal fables and stories of strange creatures. He advised the children, "Man is too arrogant. He thinks himself too important. Who is to say that a man is a higher form of nature than a tree? All things in nature are wiser than man." The children could not speak to him in his own language, so they devised other means of communication. They taught him to blow soap bubbles. Elizabeth drew pictures for him; he would respond by drawing whimsical caricatures of animals and birds. When Bobby could not walk, Victor pushed his wheelchair and helped us to carry him. They played chess, and Bobby taught him to play backgammon. "It was a kind of funny, mute teaching," says Bobby, "but he understood problems better than most people, and he had those extraordinary eyes. It felt as if he were looking right through you.

"Victor made *my* problems seem simple. My problems have been easy in one sense, because they have been physical and I can attribute defeats in life to physical problems that are beyond my control. So, when I conquer physical problems, I conquer many problems and the defenses I have developed—like determination and patience—to deal with physical problems, I can apply to other problems as well. I've got to walk, I've got to keep my bleeding down. That's the most important battle for me. It's really very simple, because I am dealing with something concrete. Not like Victor. He was dealing with much more difficult problems of identity. Victor was so torn. He was in the West, which was a better place physically for him to write and to be—and yet he viewed it with a little bit of contempt, because he saw that for him there was no fruitful artistic study there.

"He wanted so much to be at peace with himself, but somehow I detected that peace would mean an end to his artistic creation and he knew that, too, and that's why he was so torn. There was struggling in him his love for his Russian heritage, his sentimentality —and yet his ruthlessness about institutions and ideals. He was very cynical about some things, very ruthless. I just wish I'd spoken Russian at the time."

Bobby and Victor developed a strange partnership because of two small rabbits, one brown and one black, that we kept as pets in a large cage in the garden. One day we were all sitting in the garden, taking the spring sun, when a sudden silence fell on our little group. We all became very aware of the two little rabbits mournfully hopping about in their cage, perhaps because Victor was looking so intently and sadly at them. We all were thinking the same thing, but it was he who said quietly, "Let them be free."

"All right," I agreed, "but how will we get them back in at night? The rats will kill them if they are left out alone." (A tortoise of ours already had perished in this grim way.)

"Don't worry," he said. "I can get them back in the cage."

So we opened the doors of the cage and the rabbits hopped out happily into the grass and sunlight. Victor instructed the children, "Be very quiet. If you are quiet when they are out and you don't frighten them, in a few days they will be eating from your hand. And if they are not frightened when they are caught, soon they will learn to go back into the cage all by themselves."

That evening before dinner, Victor enlisted Bobby to help him round up the rabbits. Stationing himself behind one bush and Bobby behind another, he gave Bobby a quiet but constant stream of instructions in Russian. Bobby answered him in English. Somehow their coordination was perfect. They approached the rabbits so quietly that, at the moment Victor chose, they were able to pick them up and put them back into their cage. Each night after that it was the same. After only six days we were delighted to see that the rabbits *were* eating from our hands and at night would obediently hop back into their cage.

"We spoke different languages, we were different ages, but for the two of us somehow the rabbits were symbolic," says Bobby. "There they were, living in an enclosed paradise, but being tormented at night by rats. I really hated those rats—sometimes I'd see them and once I cornered one and grabbed a hoe and klonked it on the head and killed it. I viewed them as mortal enemies and, I think, so did Victor. And yet, it didn't seem quite right for the rabbits to live in a cage. That's why I sided with Victor when he wanted to let them go. I was afraid for them, but I had faith and it became very important in my own life to keep those rabbits alive and well and going, despite the rats and the problems and the fact they might run away. The longer we could keep those rabbits free, the longer they could stay alive in the back yard and come hopping up the stairs into the dining room, the longer good was triumphing. Having the rabbits triumph over the rats was a major victory for us both."

Victor went back to Leningrad. He had no children of his own and he always told me he wanted to give something to Bobby. When Bobby was fifteen, Victor managed to send him his own old-fashioned pocket watch with its long chain, the one I had often seen hanging on the wall over his typewriter in his Leningrad apartment. Victor had received the watch from his father on his own fifteenth birthday, as had his father before him.

And that is how it happened that on his graduation day from Hackley School in Tarrytown, New York, Bobby wore the watch that had once belonged to the deputy commander of Marshal Rokossovsky.

Whenever we came back to the United States for a visit, people would ask me apprehensively, "How are the doctors over there? Are you getting good medical care? Shouldn't you bring Bobby back to the United States?"

Actually, in many ways it was *easier* to cope with Bobby's illness in France—psychologically, much easier. The French are an earthy, practical people. They sentimentalize less over children than we do in the United States. When it comes to the problems of chronic illness, they are quite matter-of-fact and unemotional. This attitude may seem cold to some, but it actually relieved me. Everywhere, in the schools, among doctors, I met the same re-action: Well, all right. It's difficult, you have a hard life . . . but then, *c'est la vie*. There is suffering in this world. People have prob-lems. Chronic disease is one of them. No reason to stop living. Fight. *Life* is hard. Just tell us what we need to know and we'll help you if we can.

And there was something else: a healthy acceptance that in life one cannot always expect success. (Don't blame yourself if you fail, they seemed to be saying—that, too, is part of life.) It was amazing how much pressure this lifted from my shoulders.

Was this perhaps a manifestation of an older and wiser society, one that has suffered, gone through wars, known humiliation and defeat? In that context hemophilia was not a striking departure from the happy, healthy norm, only another problem facing the race of men, all God's children.

Whatever the reason, there was an important nuance in the atmosphere, and we felt it. I felt less of a curiosity, closer to humanity. Bobby was not ostracized—in fact, I even think that in

France Bobby never felt particularly handicapped. At that crucial time, when he was just growing into adolescence, the world opened to receive him. I was always certain that once he became a person on his own, once he really knew *who* he was, hemophilia could become but one strand woven into the fabric of his life—not the be all and end all. It is a low self-image that is the real handicap. The French helped Bobby to accept himself and his problems realistically. There was no pity—only, behind their masks of common sense and *logique*, shared sympathy and a willingness to help him fight.

We saw a great many doctors during our four years in France. It was not only Bobby who was sick. Bob suffered a severe case of hepatitis. Elizabeth was to have a very delicate eye operation. We grew to trust and respect the special qualities of French medicine and of French doctors.

As a group, they were outstandingly intelligent and charming people. The medicine they practiced was humane; the relationship between doctor and patient was less that of ruler and ruled than the more reassuring one that exists between partners.

I may be mistaken, but it seemed to me that in France, more than in any other country I know, doctors combined varied disciplines easily, naturally. Very often they knew art and literature as well as they did medicine. Routinely, they knew at least one and sometimes two or three other languages. They consider this essential, so that they can keep up with medical literature in other languages and converse freely with their foreign colleagues.

I was surprised to see how many French doctors are women. These professional ladies see nothing contradictory about the long hours their profession demands and the fact that they happen to be women, wives, and mothers as well. We knew several of them: eye specialists, hematologists, pediatricians. I saw them, in hospitals and laboratories, coolly discussing their complicated cases with scientific intelligence. But once out of their white coats, they would emerge as attractive, warm, and witty Frenchwomen, dressed with flair, worrying about their children, their husbands, their lovers.

There was something very appealing and impressive about

these women doctors—something very sexy, as if their femininity were enhanced by their wit and intelligence. Out of the twenty children in Elizabeth's class at the Collège Sévigné, five had mothers who were doctors, and several others were physicists or chemists. Many among them were married to doctors, probably because, as one of them said, "We are so busy we have no time to meet anyone outside our profession." The one I knew best was Dr. Michele Yannotti, the mother of Susy's best friend at the Collège. It was she who said of French medicine: "I think in France we practice a very human medicine. Americans put a great deal of store on the physical plant. Of course, often they are shocked when they see what seems to them to be our antiquated plant. Because of this, they tend to ignore the outstanding work of research and the great intelligence of our doctors. Our people, I believe, are very well trained."

She was right. Bobby was in three different hospitals in Paris, and French hospitals often do look antiquated. At the Hôpital St.-Louis, the problem was compounded by the fact that the hospital is classified as a historical monument. It was built as a hospital in the time of Louis XIII and it is a magnificent example of seventeenth-century architecture, with an exquisite interior courtyard full of formal flower gardens. Naturally, the rooms are old, but because it is a historical monument, no architectural change is permitted in the original buildings, and new buildings cannot be built higher than two floors. Sometimes the rooms and wards are crowded and look distinctly unmodern. But the care is good, the nursing cheerful and, best of all, the visiting hours are loose and sensible, adapted to humans, not robots.*

Europeans who come here are horrified by the conditions in *our* hospitals and always incredulous at the price they have to pay for medical care. If there is a single message about America that gets through to Europeans who come to the United States, it is:

* We Americans certainly cannot brag about the physical state of our hospitals. Only a few months ago I spent one night in one of New York's most famous hospitals. I was tightly packed into a semiprivate room meant for two in which there were four patients. The paint was peeling off the walls, the night table was dirty and the bathroom filthy. The bill for my room alone (one night) was $120!

"Don't get sick in the United States or you will lose your shirt." So shocking is this state of affairs that the American Embassy in Paris finds it necessary to warn darkly on the application-for-visa form: "There is no medical insurance in the United States and medical care is very expensive."

In France, all medical bills are covered, at least in part, by national health insurance. American doctors have told us, "I don't want to work for the government." Neither do the French doctors, and they don't. They practice exactly as doctors do in America. What the French have is a government-backed system of health insurance in which the Social Security system reimburses the *patient*, not the doctor.

The system is simple. After a medical visit, the doctor gives the patient a small insurance form which he has filled out (usually in an illegible scrawl). This form describes the treatment performed and gives the doctor's fees. The patient pays the doctor. Then the patient takes the form home, fills out his part, and mails it in to his local Social Security center, which refunds whatever the allowance is for that medical procedure. (An efficient feature of the French system is this decentralized administration. These funds are administered by *local* boards.) The responsibility for collecting reimbursement from the government is entirely up to the patient. The doctor does not have to worry about it. Often, as in America, the government allowance does not completely cover the cost of treatment. Expensive doctors will be patronized by affluent patients. But the important thing is that there is a solid floor under all medical costs; the citizen knows that, whatever his income level, medical treatment is available to him.

The single most important feature of the French system is that medical treatment is based not on the income of the patient, but on the *nature of the illness*. This means that all catastrophic illnesses—cancer, heart disease, major surgery, etc.—are completely covered. In America, no one would cover us; private insurance men grabbed their hats and backed out the door when we mentioned hemophilia. In France, a hemophiliac like Bobby is automatically covered one hundred per cent for his care.

France, like every other Western country except the United

States, has long accepted the principle that comprehensive health care is the right of every citizen. No Frenchman ever need fear that catastrophic illness will wipe him out financially. How long, do you suppose, will it take us, in the United States, to catch up?

In hemophilia, of course, medical bills are only one side of the problem; the other is obtaining a sufficient supply of blood. When we got to France, we found that, interestingly enough, among all the other talents for which the French are celebrated, there was still another, much less celebrated talent: the French are really good at collecting blood. Proportionally the French give 25 per cent more blood than the British and 30 per cent more than Americans. This surprising fact is not, of course, only the result of good will. It is also the result of superb organization.

The Centre National de Transfusion in Paris is the center for blood research, blood collection, and fractionation. (All blood in France is automatically fractionated, thereby assuring its most efficient use.) The head of the CNTS is Dr. Jean Pierre Soulier, a world renowned hematologist, and it is under his direction that it has been fashioned into the smoothly functioning, outstandingly efficient blood center that it is.

I asked Dr. Soulier how this had been accomplished and to what he attributed their success. He told me of the center's careful studies of blood-donor motivation, which had precisely identified the fears and hesitations of people giving blood, and about their program of public education. But the most important reason for their success, he felt, was: "We have only one system for collecting blood, the benevolent system. We decided very early, in 1946, to adopt this system exclusively. I believe that the problems in the United States are because you have two systems, the benevolent and the paid-donor, and that these compete with each other. People subconsciously tend to give less if they know that somewhere there are paid donors. In the beginning we, too, had a system of paid donors, but we suppressed it in 1946 in favor of a totally benevolent system. We feel that we can collect much more by basing ourselves solely on the generosity and altruism of the population. There is kind of an esprit de corps. When we go into factories, we find that once a few start to give, they tend to encourage each other."

He stopped a moment, and then went on, choosing his words carefully. "I think the paid-donor system is the best way for an underdeveloped country to begin to build a blood bank. The benevolent system is, in my view, the best for a developed country." He gave only the slightest emphasis to the word "developed," but I understood. It was sobering to find the United States put in the category of an "underdeveloped" country.

Thanks to Dr. Soulier and the CNTS, blood is not a problem for the five thousand hemophiliacs of France—all their needs are covered free. The real problem is that the best center for hemophiliac care is still in Paris. This means that for a boy living in an isolated village where he may be the only hemophiliac, life is still horrendously difficult. The French have tried to overcome this by creating two schools especially for hemophiliacs—the only ones in the world. The main one—the Queue les Yvelines—is thirty-two miles outside of Paris; the other is in the mountains of the Haute Savoie. This isolation is by no means considered the ideal situation, for the trend everywhere in the world is to incorporate hemophiliacs into normal communities and schools, but it has served an important purpose these past years in France, a country where there are still no home transfusions. (The French are trying to bypass this step entirely and are beginning to teach boys to transfuse themselves as early as possible.)

Today, the French medical teams are working hard to incorporate hemophiliacs back into their villages by decentralizing treatment and educating doctors who are afraid or ignorant. Dr. Jean Pierre Allain, the young doctor who is now the resident doctor at the school near Paris, predicts that within ten years the school will be closed. "We hope," he says happily, "there will be no further need for it."

Among all these doctors, the one we knew best was Dr. François Josso. For eight years he directed the Queue les Yvelines school, from 1961 until 1973 he was chief of the Hematology

Laboratory at the CNTS, and today he is a professor of hematology at the Hôpital Necker. It was he, more than any other, whose understanding advice we sought in dealing with all of Bobby's complicated problems. His great tact, his delicate sensitivity to our feelings, were extraordinary.

Among other things, Dr. Josso was the man who had the authority to release to us the vital fractions that Bobby needed for his transfusions. For the first two years in France, we were not covered by French Social Security and therefore we had to pay for the French fraction we used. To supplement our purchases of French AHF, we kept a stream of travelers busy bringing us little bottles of Hyland fraction from New York. We had to pay—dearly —for this, too.

In New York, Blue Cross had begun to pay the processing cost of blood and plasma for hemophiliacs, even when transfusions were given not in a hospital but at home. As the American Hospital in Paris was a participating Blue Cross hospital, it was logical to hope that we might be able to continue the arrangement in France. But logic had nothing to do with it. Bob went to present our problem to the administrator of the American Hospital, which was in Neuilly, on the opposite side of Paris, nearly an hour's drive from where we lived. The administrator had never heard of home transfusions. He was willing to go along but only if he had a letter from Blue Cross, putting it in writing that they approved of the arrangement. "I don't want to jeopardize our reputation," he said.

Bob appealed to Blue Cross, which had already made this arrangement informally with a number of New York hospitals. But Blue Cross refused to put it in writing for the American Hospital in Paris. Bob wrote to the medical vice-president of Blue Cross, Dr. Mark Freedman, reminding him that home transfusion was being enthusiastically endorsed by the medical profession, that it had changed our lives, prevented needless pain and bleeding, and had entirely eliminated doctors' bills and costly (to Blue Cross) hospital bills.

Dr. Freedman's reply is a monument to bureaucratic stupidity. "I agree . . ." he wrote, "that the ambulatory administration of the Anti-Hemophilic Factor is a great advance and makes great sense from the standpoint of overall cost to the community. I must, however, report that under the terms of our contract it is not possible for us to pay processing fees except when blood and blood derivatives are administered in a hospital." That ended the argument. Bob ceased writing letters, but we refused to give up home transfusions. During the years we were in France, we continued to pay our Blue Cross premiums, but Blue Cross refused to cover any of our blood needs.

During this epistolary battle, Bobby, of course, went right on bleeding and we kept right on needing blood fractions. We had no choice but to draw heavily from the CNTS in Paris. As time passed, the bills piled up. The CNTS did not press for payments but we grew more and more uneasy, more and more hesitant to ask for fresh supplies. When the amount rose to 16,000 francs (over $3,000), Bob wrote an apologetic letter to Dr. Josso, explaining our difficulties. This is the graceful reply he received:

> We thank you for the efforts you are making to speed the arrangement of your administrative situation, but please do not worry about the letter which you have recently received from the business office of the CNTS. It is only an administrative document which is designed simply to point up a situation and perhaps in some way help you in your efforts to obtain aid from some kind of organization in the United States.
>
> Naturally, this aspect of the problem remains totally independent of the effort that you are making with us to maintain Bobby in good condition. The fractions of the CNTS will always be at your disposition with an unlimited credit. The only thing that counts is Bobby's well-being. What I absolutely would not want is that this unusual administrative situation should make you hesitate for one instant to come and get your fractions at the Center for the slightest need. Financial problems always finish by resolving themselves in one way or another.

So whenever we needed blood fraction for Bobby, we continued to drive over to the modern green and glass buildings of the Center, behind the Invalides, and Bobby's fractions would be turned over to us, neatly packed in large cartons. That is all that was demanded of us. No asking the neighbors for donations, no embarrassing publicity about helping the "sufferer." We *never* had to beg for blood. The French allowed us our dignity. For that alone I would be grateful to them forever. And eventually, of course, we *were* able to clear up our "unusual administrative situation" . . . but that was thanks to the French. After two years they accepted us into their Social Security system.

It was Dr. Josso who had come to help us through Bobby's terrible knee episode. We never received a bill. We sent him a bottle of Scotch, which we knew he liked, and he replied, "Thank you, dear friends, for your delicate attention which will have, among other virtues, that of preserving my arteries."

It was Josso who, throughout our stay in France, coordinated the advice of all the doctors, referred us to therapists, regularly checked Bobby's joints, recommended orthopedic shoes, watched over Bobby's regular blood tests. For all of this, he never charged a cent.

Dr. Josso was involved in every aspect of the problem of hemophilia, not only in the scientific but in a human way. One of his important goals was educating doctors and medical students. He told me: "By and large, hemophilia is still not very well known in the medical profession. I am a professor, and I am trying to teach my medical students about new methods. Most doctors, you understand, never see any hemophiliacs in all their careers, yet it is a disease in which things are evolving very quickly. The new generation of doctors will know more about it . . . they will be prepared."

On behalf of individual hemophiliacs, he wrote to schools and employers explaining the problem. He counseled hemophiliacs and their families. When I asked him how he felt about the delicate problem of sterilization of hemophiliacs or carriers, he answered: "I believe that this is entirely a question for the individual to decide. Not being a hemophiliac, I cannot decide for him. In any case, for me, there are two sides to my view. As a citizen, I might think that it would be better to have fewer hemophiliacs so that there would be less of a drain on taxes and social funds. But I am also a doctor and I care for people. It is the purpose of a doctor to give to those who are sick the possibility of living a normal life. And what is more normal for a man than to marry and have his own children?

"For me, to inform is the key, the most important thing.

Knowledge is the only way to be really free. If one is not informed, one can never be truly a free man."

Freedom and independence—these were what Josso wanted above all for his patients. He tried to instill these goals into them and their parents. He would say: "A hemophiliac is an absolutely normal individual. He is not sick; he is perfectly healthy. He has the same problems as any other boy but these are multiplied and intensified because of his condition. He must not be treated as a sick person." One day he told me proudly: "Just now we have a group of boys who are between the ages of fifteen and eighteen. They are all alone, on a camping trip in Provence, wandering for a month. They have three tents, and they are traveling with fraction. They did a short course together, then worked at various jobs to get money for their trip, and with the money they earned, they took off. They can help each other if the need arises, but all can transfuse themselves." This achievement gave him enormous pleasure.

He encouraged us in our efforts to keep Bobby in school, to allow him greater freedom of movement, to permit him to start to travel alone. His reassurance was a precious psychological support for us. It was typical of Dr. Josso that when Bobby turned thirteen, he no longer addressed his letters to us, but wrote to Bobby directly.

"Dear Bobby," one letter began, "you will be happy to know that our recent tests have shown that you have no circulating antibody at this time." For him, the most important thing was that as soon as possible a boy must learn to care for himself and to take responsibility for his own life and condition. "For in the end," he said, "an individual belongs only to himself. To be independent, he must be able to take his destiny in his own hands. Le chef, c'est lui. (He is his own boss.)"

Chapter 25

In the third year of our life in Paris, Sue and I became involved in an extravagant folly that consumed time, made enemies, and taught us some bitter lessons about human nature and the charitable urge. Some good came out of it, too—we made new friends and collected some money for hemophilia. But, on balance, we made a major mistake:

We got involved with not one but three premières of the film *Nicholas and Alexandra*.

After I had signed my contract with him, Sam Spiegel had disappeared from our lives. We heard rumors that this or that actor or actress was being hired, we read in the papers that three directors had been fired. People at cocktail parties knew more about what was in the script than we did. Eventually, shooting started in Spain, dates for release of the picture were being set— and suddenly, the question arose: Which charity would be the beneficiary of these film premières?

To us, the answer seemed logical: The book was about hemophilia, the film was about hemophilia; obviously, if there were to be charity premières, they ought to benefit hemophilia. We soon discovered how far out of the real world we were living. Neither logic nor charity has anything to do with it: The awarding of film premières takes place on a cruel, dog-eat-dog battlefield on which every combatant, the charities as well as the film companies, is ruthlessly out for himself.

Sue and I stumbled onto this battlefield armored only in our total ignorance. We had never been to a film première and we had not the slightest idea how to run a charity ball. We had never seen one. We felt simply that what had been done was wrong: In three major cities, London, New York, and Los Angeles, the première of *Nicholas and Alexandra* was to be given to a medical charity other than the Hemophilia Foundation. Confronted with the oddity of a film about a boy with hemophilia being used to benefit other diseases, Sam Spiegel told me, "Charity premières are for publicity. I don't care what charity the money goes to." Faced with the same appeal, the other medical charities reacted like fierce dogs just given a juicy bone. This is ours, they growled menacingly. Go away and find your own.

Looking back, I wish we had given up. But instead, I got mad. Here was a unique opportunity to attract to hemophilia some of the publicity and funds it so desperately needed. By God, I swore, they're not going to get away with it!

I first got wind of what was happening in January 1971, when the Hemophilia Foundation in New York wrote to me, passing along the rumor that Columbia Pictures had chosen Project Hope for the New York première of the film. "Columbia does not want to give it to hemophilia," they elaborated, "because they do not regard it as useful from a promotional point of view to link the movie with hemophilia. They do not feel that people want to go to see a picture about a disease."

Only a few days afterward, an urgent telephone call from the British Hemophilia Society in London brought a different message: The world première of the film in London *would* be for the benefit of a disease—but not hemophilia. Cerebral palsy. The British Spastics Society (an insensitive way to describe cerebral palsy, it seems to me) had been chosen, Columbia explained, "because the Spastics can deliver the Queen." The trouble with hemophilia, in other words, was the same in New York, London, and everywhere. Small in size and influence, it could not attract the glittering names and the publicity that Columbia considered essential.

Still, the film was about hemophilia, and both the London and New York hemophilia organizations asked if there was anything I could do to help. I tried. I wrote to Sam Spiegel, asking simply that wherever he planned to have a première in a city in which there was a hemophilia group anxious to participate on a working basis he make some effort to include them. He didn't answer my letter.

I wrote again, suggesting that it might help with the London première for me to write to the Queen myself, putting the matter before her directly. This time the reaction was immediate. The phone rang. It was Sam Spiegel, enraged. Spitting old Anglo-Saxon words, he screamed that he would "excommunicate" me. "You're paranoid about hemophilia," he shouted. It wasn't my film, he said, it was his film. He could do with it what he liked. That included the premières. "If you want to give your money to hemophilia, that's your business. I'll do what I like with mine."

A few weeks later, however, Spiegel called again. We both had so much interest in the film, he said, it was silly not to compromise. Would I come to London for a talk? I went and we compromised. I would forget about writing letters to royal persons and he would persuade the Spastics Society to give the hemophiliacs equal publicity in London and 25 per cent of the gate. In addition, he agreed to my request that wherever else there was a première, the local hemophilia group would be asked whether it was willing and able to participate.

I thought we might have asked for more, but the British Hemophilia Society seemed anxious to settle. "If there is any hint of controversy, the Queen will withdraw. This will make us very unpopular in influential circles and we will almost certainly be blacklisted as far as future royal patronage is concerned. Taking everything into consideration, this is about the best we can hope for." And so, from that point on, the British Hemophilia Society became a definite part—a 25 per cent part—of the Royal World Première.

But what about New York? Could a similar compromise be worked out? I assumed, following Spiegel's promise, that he would do his best and went back to my own work.

On May 22, a telegram from the New York Hemophilia Foundation dolefully announced that Project Hope, an ultrasocial charity, had indeed been given the New York première. When the Hemophilia Foundation asked to share, a Project Hope executive replied that his organization was "not interested or willing to do this" and offered "best wishes to you in your endeavors to procure a première of another film for the National Hemophilia Foundation." (Thank you, kind sir. Perhaps a film about a wandering hospital ship?) Was there anything at all, the foundation asked, that I could do to salvage the situation?

I tried again. I wrote the five elegant New York women who were the chairladies of the Project Hope première. Not one of these ladies bothered to answer. Instead, I heard directly from the head of Project Hope in New York. "I cannot understand why you have been bothering our very busy HOPE volunteers. . . . I recommend you desist from writing our committee heads as your correspondence with them is annoying and will only be referred to me again . . . there is no likelihood of any change in our plans . . . I consider the matter closed."

Later, to a reporter asking about the controversy, this gentleman huffily declared, "Project Hope never shares. We never have to."

Facing this stone wall, I began to feel other pressures. Columbia called in my agent and warned him that he must get his client's "emotional problem" under control or they might take legal action. My agent and my lawyer invited me to lunch and argued earnestly that any further effort to have a hemophilia première in New York would be a waste of time.

Understanding that they meant well, and knowing that they were probably right, I apologized and told them that I still felt I had to keep trying. "The film," I said stubbornly, "is about hemophilia." They nodded their heads, looked at me sadly, and wished me well.

Keep trying! Bravo! But what exactly was I going to *do?* Fortunately, at this point the New York Hemophilia Foundation, which at first had worried about the risks of getting into a fight with Columbia and Project Hope ("We have to raise money in this town"), began summoning up its courage. People were getting angry. (There was even a proposal to picket the Project Hope première with hemophiliac boys in wheelchairs. Happily, this kind of talk soon faded.)

There was, we discovered, a positive alternative. As a result of all the fuss, Columbia had granted the foundation the right to buy all the tickets in the theater for the night following the première. (It was strictly a business arrangement: Columbia extracted the full price, $4.00, for each seat in the house. From its limited funds, the foundation paid $6,000 for fifteen hundred seats.) Why not start from here and try to make the second night a big success, perhaps even bigger than Project Hope's? I discussed it with the foundation and I talked it over with Sue. It wasn't an easy decision for us. We were living in Paris, trying to write books. There were the everyday demands of family life and the extra strains of Bobby's problems. Logically, it just didn't make sense. But logic had no more to do with our decision than it did with Sam Spiegel's. We decided to do it.

And that is how, quite preposterously, Sue and I became co-chairmen of a major New York charity benefit called "The Author's Première for Hemophilia," scheduled for the night of December 14, 1971.

To everyone's amazement, once we had agreed to run the New York première, we wanted to run it. This made the Hemophilia Foundation extremely nervous. After all, we had no experience whatsoever in this kind of enterprise. They had assumed that, once we became co-chairmen, we would retire gracefully into figurehead-dom and turn the actual mechanics of the evening over to a professional public relations organization. This is the normal way charity balls are handled, and there are several firms in New York who specialize in this business. Their reward is either a substantial fee or a percentage of the gross—usually 15 per cent. To us, it seemed like too much.

The foundation, again following time-hallowed custom, also wanted the evening to be in honor of Somebody, probably a Giant of Industry. The Giant sits on a dais, he is given a plaque, he and his company are flattered, and they contribute. Better yet, all his business contacts are dragooned into coming and contributing, too. (One can imagine the Giant's displeasure if he stares out over the assembled guests and notices that X or Y, with whom he was about to place a large order, is missing.) It was quickly spelled out to me that if we wanted "a strong Wall Street group" to come, it would depend on getting a prominent guest of honor—not on the cause, not on the children who are sick and need care. I envisioned a room full of men sitting, eating, sneaking peeks at their watches, thinking about the next day's business and, at the earliest opportunity, hurrying for home.

It seemed demeaning to everybody concerned. Sue and I wanted people to come because it meant something to them; we wanted to send them home thinking about hemophilia. So we decided to run the evening ourselves.

Who might help us? I wrote to Ladybird Johnson. She said she would be happy to be listed as an honorary chairman. I wrote to Mary Lasker, the great medical philanthropist, whom we had met through Mrs. Johnson. Mary agreed to become another honorary chairman. I wrote to Prince Vassily of Russia, Tsar Nicholas II's nephew and the senior member of the Russian Imperial family living in the United States. Prince Vassily agreed to be an honorary chairman and to come.

I cabled Janet Suzman, Michael Jayston, and Tom Baker, who played Alexandra, Nicholas, and Rasputin in the film, and whom we had already met. They were being flown to New York by Columbia for the Project Hope première. All three immediately agreed to come to ours. (Columbia later growled that, if it wished, it could forbid the stars to attend our première. "Their itinerary is completely under our control," the studio threatened. "If we want them to, they'll be on a plane out of New York the morning after they've done their bit at Project Hope." Michael Jayston's response to this was rich and earthy.) Two generous people immediately helped in the most tangible way, by buying a number of tickets. Mary Lasker bought twenty and our friend Dick Dowling took thirty. At least we would not be sitting alone in the theater.

We were encouraged. But the key to success in the cold, ruthless business of charity is a list of Important People. We had no such list. Rather pathetically, we began making a list of our friends. We went through old address books, searched through old diaries, found names scrawled on yellowing slips of paper. We made a list of 123 people we thought might remember us: high school friends, college friends, Rhodes scholar friends, Sue's old admirers; colleagues from *Collier's, Life, Newsweek, U.S.A.*1,* and the *Post;* my agent, lawyer, and publishers; our doctors, bankers, and insurance men; our neighbors, our congressman, our Russian friends, translators, folksingers. . . . Their response was overwhelming. Public relations firms who organize benefits normally send out 1,000 invitations to bring in 200 people. Our letter to 123 friends brought us 250 people.

But we needed more—more publicity, more glittering names. A *New York Times* reporter, experienced in this business, was appalled at our lack of society support. She gave us her own list, and then she introduced us to Oscar and Françoise de la Renta.

Suzanne Massie: I was delighted by this introduction. Just like millions of other readers of the fashion pages, I knew that Oscar de la Renta was a superfamous New York fashion designer. His name and that of his elegant wife, Françoise, are household words for all the faithful readers of *Vogue, Harper's Bazaar,* and *Women's Wear Daily.*

The de la Rentas know *everyone, everywhere.* Through the drawing rooms of their lavish New York town house, filled with soft pillows and orchids, passed the tinsel aristocracy of the Beautiful People. But Oscar also happens to be a generous man with a good heart. His passion in his private life is an orphanage for abandoned boys in his native Santo Domingo; he helped to create it and has supported it for many years. When he learned from Virginia Lee Warren, a *New York Times* reporter, of the effort we were making on the première, he said, "Tell Mrs. Massie to call me." I did, ready to hang up at the first icicle in his voice. Immediately he said, "How can I help?" and I found myself telling him our problems as if he were an old friend.

Despite the fact that many of their famous friends and many of Oscar's noted customers were deeply involved in the Project Hope première, Oscar and Françoise threw themselves into swinging the Right People for Charity Balls our way. They charmed friends into agreeing to be patrons, gave us names and addresses for invitations. They invited us to dinner constantly to meet their friends. They took three tables (thirty tickets) at the première itself. In a remarkably short time, they turned the struggle into a

Fashionable Event, one that People Were Talking About. And so
it happened, according to the laws of that special society, that suddenly the second night became the right place to be seen.

Robert Massie: Briskly, Françoise began putting together an
honorary committee for our invitation. She collected names from
among her friends as if she were collecting exotic flowers from
some rare greenhouse. Every morning she would telephone and
say, "Diana Vreeland has agreed. Gloria Vanderbilt Cooper has
agreed. Ceezee Guest and Irene Selznick have agreed. I'm hoping
Ethel Kennedy will agree."

At the same time that Françoise was gathering society names
to form an honorary committee, Sue and I were putting together
a committee of three dedicated women who would do the un-
glamorous work. All were volunteers, none had any experience in
managing charity balls, and all got involved because they cared
about hemophilia. The leader of this group was Elaine Hart, a
lab technician at New York Hospital who had worked for Dr.
Hilgartner and had known Bobby since he was ten. Elaine took
a leave of absence from her job and worked without pay on the
première for three months. Helene Weld, a doctor's wife, took
over dealing with the hotel, and our friend Janet Dowling handled
publicity.

At this point, even with the de la Rentas behind us, it was hard
to be optimistic. We were absurdly late. It was already mid-September. Project Hope's invitations had been mailed out in June; our
invitations still hadn't been printed . . . they hadn't even been
designed. Ladislav Svatos, who designed the book jacket, offered
to help, but he needed the text. Where was the party after the film
going to be? How much was it going to cost?

Where was easy—most of the hotels were already filled up:
only the St. Regis was left, and Sue took it. *How much* was more
of a problem. The normal price of a ticket to a major charity dinner
or ball in New York is $100 per person. Against all advice, we
set two prices, $100 and $50, the only difference being that the
$100 ticket holders would become patrons and be listed in the
program. Our theory was that everyone would give according to

his ability. It didn't work out that way; many wealthy people were happy to come for only $50, and some people of modest means struggled to pay $100 because they knew it would mean a lot to hemophilia.

Meanwhile, we were living out of suitcases like a family of gypsies. Our house in Irvington was rented, and we had no place to live in New York. Our apartment, our work, and the children's school were all in France. School was beginning, so we separated briefly: Sue and the children returned to Paris; I stayed behind in New York continuing my frantic dance, writing letters, seeing people, telephoning.

Finally, two weeks later—my suitcase stuffed with lists and files, notes falling out of my pocket—having made thirty-one phone calls that day and gone to the Bronx to pick up AHF concentrate for Bobby, I staggered to Kennedy Airport and collapsed into a charter flight 747. Somewhere in mid-air, consulting my fellow passengers, I discovered that the plane was bound for Brussels, not for Paris. In Brussels airport I found that I was ten francs ($2) short the cash necessary to buy a plane ticket to Paris. One minute before the plane left, I borrowed a ten-franc note from a suspicious Frenchman, threw it at the ticket agent, and dashed for the plane.

Trying to run a film première in New York while living in Paris was zany. In the previous three years, we had had perhaps three transatlantic phone calls. When we heard that America was calling, we trembled; it meant some family catastrophe. Now almost every day when the phone jangled, the children, becoming blasé, shouted through the apartment, "Dad, it's New York again."

And, of course, life continued normally. Bobby, whose ankles were showing signs of hemophilic arthritis, could no longer walk to the bus stop and take the bus to school. He had to be driven back and forth. In October, he had twenty-four transfusions.

Along the way, however, two strokes of good luck gave us a boost. Mrs. Johnson decided that she would fly up from Texas for the evening; this raised us many notches in the public eye. And the Sunday *New York Times* did a full-page article on the battle ("It is a story of cynicism, probable deception, anger, blasted hopes, recrimination, frustration, depression, a wild gamble . . ."). Immediately, Elaine Hart's mail gushed with ticket requests and Sue began to wonder whether the New York City fire laws would permit us to squeeze 525 people into the St. Regis, instead of the 480 whom originally she had rather wistfully hoped for.

By November, money was flowing in and we seemed on the way to success. Then, within our own ranks, we began to have trouble. Back in New York, one of the Hemophilia Foundation executives was turning everything upside down. As most of the problems had to do with the hotel, the seating arrangements, and the evening program, we decided that Sue should go home to try to salvage our plan and straighten things out.

Suzanne Massie: Packing furiously, leaving last-minute instructions for a bewildered Madame Rhéto, I rushed to Orly and flew to New York. I went directly from the airport to Elaine Hart's apartment, where I met the executive of the foundation. The atmosphere was chilly. I found that in the weeks since Bob's departure the ground had indeed shifted. Less than three weeks remained before the evening and all our carefully laid plans were awry. The idea now was to try to squeeze into the evening the maximum number of speeches, get the maximum amount of mileage from famous guests, pile on the maximum weight of exhortations about "sufferers."

I was handed a "suggested" program ("Sue Massie introduces minor celebs . . . Bob Massie introduces major celebs . . ."). It looked like more than an hour of droning and meaningless pats on the back. Then I was attacked on another front: our seating arrangements were all wrong and had to be changed. The St. Regis Roof has two rooms, one large and one small, separated by a long hall. I was told that everybody had to be crowded uncomfortably into the big room. The decoration chairman was nearly in tears. All her plans with the restaurant manager of the hotel had been changed over her head. The manager was beginning to lose his imperturbable calm. Whose orders was he to follow? What was he to tell his captains? Fire laws did not permit such crowding. . . . We, who had been trying to sell tickets to raise money, would have to send them back. All this, the better to hear speeches and because, as I was threatened, "no one will want to sit in the back room." People would feel like "second-class citizens" and would be so furious that they might possibly never contribute to hemophilia again. It was hard to believe that people actually were that petty, but with horror, I began to see that it might be true. Elaine Hart reported that she had been besieged with calls. X had to sit there, Y hated Z, and so forth. Somehow, everyone had to be placed in the correct pecking order around Mrs. Johnson or some other Important Person. Some people made it clear that they were accustomed to having the best table wherever they went, and they had better be given the best table *now* . . . or in the future they would go to some other charity event.

Seeing all this for the first time, I despaired. These "affairs" (a word I loathe) seem to bring out the pettiest side of human nature. Entangled in the minutiae of useless detail and minor jockeying for power, people seem to lose sight entirely of the goal itself —alleviating pain. How hypocritical, how dulling of the real instincts of charity it is to appeal to people's cupidity (tax deductions) and snobbism (some charity balls and charities are better to be seen at than others). Do such piecemeal fund-raising efforts do anything to uplift the spirits of those who go? Do they do anything for the diseases they are ostensibly to help? I wondered. If so much effort is to be expended by so many people, is there no way to direct it toward a broader, more humane and profound solution to our nation's health needs? Because, from these superficial exercises comes no real sense of involvement, no caring, no sense of brotherhood in pain. On the contrary, they tend to discharge any sense of direct responsibility, by assuaging with a small gift of money the sense of guilt that lurks in those who are both wealthy and healthy. Needless to say, the sick themselves are always kept conveniently out of sight. Their need is so real, so poignant, that it might intrude on the festivities. It is easier to pretend that they don't really exist, and if they do, that they are being cared for adequately somewhere, by others. But alas, too often, when contact is excluded, so is real compassion.

I was sickened by all this. I wanted to flee. Privately I decided that I would never, ever, have anything to do with such events again. But this time, we were embarked. Determined to try to make this one evening be different, I dug in my heels and insisted that everything be put back the way it had been originally planned. No speeches. No phony pats on the back. The tables were to stay put. As for the seating, all right, we would make every effort not to insult any of the complainers. Every one of them would sit in the main room with our most honored guests, Mrs. Johnson and Mrs. Lasker and all the socialite celebrities. We, the Massies, would sit in the back room with our personal friends, because we knew they wouldn't mind. (I was to despair over human nature when, only ten days later, as this news got around, some of the very people who had been clamoring loudest that they would be second-class citizens if they were seated in the back room, decided that now they, too, absolutely had to be in the back room instead! They stayed out front.)

I had less than six days in New York to make all the final arrangements. The theater seating posed its own pecking-order problems. Who would sit on the center aisle? Who on the side? Nobody wanted to sit in front or in the very back. But somebody *had* to. For me, the most important thing was that many hemophiliacs were coming, some in wheelchairs or with crutches. If anybody should be comfortable, *they* should, even though most could afford only the least expensive seats. I went to the darkened, empty theater and sat in every section in order to judge for myself, then counted the stairs and checked on their steepness. With the hotel manager, once again I puzzled over lists and floor plans dotted with round tables and finally managed to distribute 504 people in places made for 450.

I found our friend Peter Yarrow, who offered to sing along with Paul Stookey and even came up with a balalaika orchestra to play during the evening. Then, just before leaving New York, I was having dinner with the de la Rentas when Oscar turned to me and asked, "But what are you going to wear?" and I realized suddenly that I had had no time to think about that. Overriding my objections, he insisted that I come to his showrooms the next morning.

When I arrived, shy and ill at ease, I found that Oscar had already chosen a dress. It was a yellow Paisley-printed silk, woven with gold that shimmered when I moved, because he said on that evening I should wear something in which I could be seen. I was a bit overwhelmed by it. But when a god of fashion picks out what is *you*, what can you do but be grateful? He scrutinized me intently and then decided it needed something more flowing around the neck. "Anyway," he said practically, "it may snow. You need a scarf." He rummaged around in his office, and finally came up with another piece of the expensive material. He ripped into it decisively with his hands. Then he said contentedly, "Now we have a scarf," and ordered it hemmed. More scrutiny. "Earrings," he mused. They were brought, and when he had examined the effect he put them in my hand. He told me that everything would be ready on my return. Thus buffeted by the world and soothed by Oscar, gathering up my lists, I flew back to Europe. Bob and Bobby were already in London. The London première was two days away.

Robert Massie: Since the previous spring, when I had gone to London to compromise, we had heard little from England. Everything seemed normal, everyone relatively happy. Then, one day in October, we received a printed invitation to the London première. Under a handsome Romanov crest, it announced a Royal Command Performance "In aid of the Spastics Society." There was no mention of the Hemophilia Society.

My compromise with Spiegel had specified an equal sharing of publicity. I telephoned the British Hemophilia Society. Yes, they were very upset. But what could they do?

As it happened, we were having lunch that day with Princess Olga and Prince Paul. We told them about it. "Write to Dickie," they advised. I did.

Earl Mountbatten wrote back promptly. He had called Buckingham Palace, reconfirmed the arrangements originally agreed on, and declared that, when he escorted the Queen to the première, he would mention my letter to her. He concluded, "I am very sorry about this as I entirely see your point of view and indeed I share it. Let us hope that the final compromise arrangements will at least give the British Hemophilia Society a worthwhile place in the evening even though it is not all that you originally hoped for."

Soon afterward, hundreds of posters went up on London

billboards and daily newspaper ads began to appear. "In aid of the Spastics Society and the Hemophilia Society," they proclaimed.

As the date approached, a new embarrassment arose to vex and frustrate Columbia. The central figure in the London première was to be Queen Elizabeth II, a cousin of the Romanovs (or as *Variety* put it, "Queen to See Pic of Her Ill-Fated Kin"). Unfortunately, seven days before the première, the Queen developed a temperature, a rash, and then spots. Doctors hurried to Buckingham Palace, examined their royal patient, and met the press. "Her Majesty," they announced gravely, "has chicken pox." While the British people worried mildly about their monarch, Columbia Pictures turned purple. It was on the promised "delivery" of the Queen that the Spastics Society had won the première. Then there was all this trouble with hemophilia. And now, for God's sake, chicken pox. . . .

The Queen recovered nicely but not in time and so Columbia settled for Princess Anne. A Royal Highness, but still not the same as A Majesty.

Suzanne Massie: After two trips across the Atlantic in less than a week, after the bitterness and wrangling in New York, my nerves were so jangled that my memories of the London première are as disjointed as colored pieces of confetti tossed to the winds.

I remember that Susy and I woke early in a cold, foggy Paris, kissed a tearful Elizabeth good-bye, and hurried at 8:30 A.M. to the hairdresser. Monsieur Louis was waiting for us. Not trusting the English hairdressers, he had come in especially on his day off to make certain that we would look our best. It was to be Susy's first big evening. She was thirteen and very excited. Louis spent most of the time with her, consulting very seriously about the clothes she was to wear: a high-necked white ruffled lace blouse (mine) and a black velvet skirt (cut down from one of my old evening dresses for her tiny waist). Then, with elaborate, inimitable French art, his skilled hands carefully braiding her long blond hair with red ribbons. When he was finished, she looked like a budding Gigi. Sitting in the plane, she tried to hold her head straight, so as not to ruffle her hair, a gesture so unpracticed, so new, that it touched me deeply. I saw for the first time the promise of the lovely young woman she would be in a few years. The dress I wore that night had a special meaning for me. I wanted my friends in Russia to share this night with us. One winter night a group of us were together in a shabby Leningrad communal apartment—an apartment with a toilet and kitchen shared by ten people. In a room lit by an overhead naked bulb, my friends had proudly produced a petticoat made of iridescent rose silk trimmed with black lace from the days of St. Petersburg at the turn of the century. Where and how they had found it in the harsh reality of the Leningrad of today, I cannot guess. They insisted that then and there I put it on. I did, and whirled around in it while they clapped. They were happy and proud to give me something beautiful, something, they said, "you can wear in the West."

I had kept it, preciously saving it for a great occasion. In time for the London première, a retired eighty-year-old Alsatian seamstress had made it into a gown with a black French lace top. That night, surrounded by royalty, by the aristocracy of England, I was wearing the converted petticoat from the days of Nicholas and Alexandra's youth. Somehow, it seemed like closing a circle.

Miraculously, that night Bobby's joints were all fine. He was wearing his first tuxedo, and even in my distracted state I was struck by how very handsome he looked, how suddenly grown up. We were preparing to rush out into the street to try to find a taxi when a smooth, chauffeur-driven Rolls drove up to the door. Friends had hired it for us so that we would arrive in style.

When we arrived, there was the strange rock-music-like sensation of the klieg lights playing over the marquee of the theater, the first shock of seeing the curious lined up on the streets, the cameras flashing inside, the cordons roping off the crowd, the red carpet. I saw Janet Suzman in a daring electric-blue gown with a dizzyingly plunging neckline and Sam Spiegel in Gucci moccasins and a blue velvet dinner jacket. Then down the line came Earl Mountbatten with Princess Anne, sparkling in a white gown sewn with brilliants. I was struck by her tiny waist, her straight back, and her flawless, magnificent complexion.

As we climbed to our seats high in the balcony, far below on the stage the Queen's Trumpeters, all scarlet and gold, were already on the stage playing heraldic flourishes.

Then the large figures were moving on the screen, figures of real people I knew—Janet, Michael, and Tom—but somehow now terrifyingly transformed. Their faces were enormous. It moved me, it upset me. I remembered those dark nights in Irvington, lying in bed thinking, exhausted with worry but unable to sleep. To have these ghosts, these ideas, come to life on such a scale awed and frightened me. For some moments I had no sense of what was real and what was not. This emotion was so strong that I could not absorb the film. Not until Nagorny, the faithful sailor, was taken out to be shot, and I saw the tears of Alexis, did I begin to weep, and then I sobbed to the end of the film. At the end, when the lights went up, people we know turned around to see what our reaction was. Shy and embarrassed, I turned away my tear-stained face.

Robert Massie: After the film, Sam Spiegel gave a private supper party for two hundred people at Claridge's. At the ballroom door, we were handed a shiny red book, embossed with the Romanov double eagle, which listed the guests. They included:

1 Princess (not Princess Anne, but a lady named Princess Lowenstein-Wertheim)
2 Princes
1 Duke
2 Duchesses
2 Marquises
1 Marchioness
1 Marquesa
3 Earls
4 Countesses
1 Baron
3 Baronesses
9 Lords (some confusion here, as in Britain this is a courtesy title for a nobleman whose rank may be Earl, Viscount, or Baron. The red guidebook did not specify.)

20 Ladies (even more confusing, as the courtesy title "Lady" can
   be applied to the wife of an Earl, Viscount, Baron, or Knight;
   or to the daughter of an Earl, no matter whom she marries)
4 Baronets
4 Ambassadors
6 Movie Stars (from the film only Janet, Michael, Tom, and Jack
   Hawkins were there. The four girls who played the daughters
   were asked to come after dinner, to dance. Roderick Noble, who
   played the Tsarevich Alexis, wasn't asked at all.)
3 Movie Producers
3 Authors (Sue, me, and the beautiful biographer, Lady Antonia
   Fraser, already counted as the daughter of an Earl and the wife
   of a Knight)
1 Billionaire (a Mr. Getty)
1 Doctor (who had nothing to do with Cerebral Palsy but was the
   Columbia Pictures doctor)
No Spastics
No Hemophiliacs

Of course, it was Mr. Spiegel's private party.

The morning after the London première, Sue and I put our
suitcases side by side; out of hers and into mine went a stream of
notes, memos, and seating diagrams. Then we were off to the airport; she and the children flew back to Paris, I was off to New
York. Our own New York première was still two weeks away, and
I was going to see that all of her plans and diagrams were imple-
mented, and to help with any last-minute problems.

There were plenty of them. Elaine Hart was ready to start
sending out tickets to the theater according to Sue's seating plan.
I was helping her. But every time it seemed that we had a row of
seats assigned, the telephone rang and somebody wanted to make
a change. It was always urgent, a special case, "potentially a very
big donor." At one point, we were informed that an enormously
wealthy woman, a famous patron of the arts, had suddenly decided
that she wanted to come and had offered a big donation on condition that she sit next to me. I reacted instinctively: No, we weren't
selling seats that way. On reflection, why object to this kind of

nonsense? We were trying to raise as much money as possible for medical care. In effect, the whole enterprise was a form of insanity forced on us by our backward system of medical care in America. With a stroke of her pen, this lady could have given us many times the amount we raised with our whole year of work. I should have been willing to have her sit next to me—on my lap, if that was what she wanted. In any case, I refused. The lady came and sat with some people she knew. She paid for her ticket but skipped making a donation.

Then, when it seemed that everybody in New York wanted to come to our première, the lesser Romanovs began to desert. From the film première in England and from a press preview screening in New York, word had come that the film contained objectionable scenes about the family. Two days before the première, I had a call from a woman who, the summer before, had married one of Nicholas II's great-grandnephews. "This is Princess Romanov," she announced to Elaine Hart, who had answered. I took the telephone. "Unless you stop the picture, we are going to sue," she warned. I gave her Spiegel's telephone number. She called him. "I didn't make this film for your family," Spiegel growled at her. In the end, they didn't sue but they stayed away.

Travesty piled on top of twaddle: suddenly, I learned that Sam Spiegel and most of the Columbia Pictures brass *wanted* to come to our première. Mrs. Johnson, Mrs. Lasker, and a lot of other important people were coming, it was their Big Picture, and it would be embarrassing for them if they weren't there. They demanded ten tickets.

Our answer was No. There simply wasn't room. Already, in obedience to the fire laws, we were returning checks.

The next request was even more surprising: Could Sam Spiegel come by himself? "If he comes, I won't come," threatened Elaine Hart. "I think he shouldn't come," I told Columbia. "I can't promise that, late in the evening and filled with champagne, one of our guests won't come up to Mr. Spiegel and be rude." ("I will personally lay him out," a normally gentle Philadelphia teacher had promised.)

Sam Spiegel didn't come.

When it finally arrived, the evening of December 14 was rainy and cold. As it turned out, a major fire in New York the night before had stolen all the TV cameras away from the Project Hope première, so they all came for ours. Crowds of people were standing in the rain behind the police barricades. Mrs. Johnson arrived in a white lace dress covered with a maroon cape, accompanied by Mary Lasker and Lynda Bird Robb. I escorted Mrs. Johnson through the lobby and down the aisle. I took her ticket and tried to catch an usherette to help us find her seat.

"Listen, can't you see, I've got a party already," she said.

"But this is Mrs. Lyndon Johnson," I appealed.

"O.K., O.K., I'll be with you in a minute."

In mid-aisle, we waited.

Suzanne Massie: I was numb with fatigue that evening, but I remember the warm feeling of sitting in the theater surrounded by family and friends. Behind Van Cliburn was Elizabeth, dressed in her best and nestled in the comforting lap of her dear friend Mrs. Connors. Excitedly, she asked questions all the way through the film. Finally, before the end, she fell asleep.

By the time it was over, it was snowing, just as Oscar had predicted. Bob had had to leave with Mrs. Johnson, so a husky friend, Willis Wood, like a blocking back, cleared a path for Elizabeth, Mrs. Connors, and me through the crowd back to the limousine. At the hotel, lifting the sleeping Elizabeth high in the air, he forced another path to the elevators. She never woke up.

Familiar faces whirled past me, familiar hands shook mine. I never had time to eat, but I noticed, with a kind of stunned surprise, that everything was moving as planned. The flowers were in place, the candles flickered welcomingly. The St. Regis waiters were executing all those listed plans as if they were a well-choreographed ballet. Past me whisked the vodka bottles and the cutlets with sauce smitane. And then, amazingly, it was already one o'clock and the best moment of the evening arrived: Bobby began to sing with Peter and Paul.

Only a few days before the première Peter and Paul had hit

on the idea of Bobby playing with them. The three of them had managed to get together for only one rehearsal. Bobby was playing the banjo to their two guitars, and they sang the song that Peter had composed only a few months before, "Weave Me the Sunshine." It could have been written for the occasion:

> They say that the tree of love
> Shine on me again
> Grows on the banks of the river of suffering
> Shine on me again . . .
>
> Weave, weave, weave me the sunshine
> Out of the falling rain
> Weave me the hope of a new tomorrow
> And fill my cup again.

To see Bobby standing there with total confidence in front of the large crowd, to see those elbows and arms that had been rigid and crippled strumming furiously, to see him standing straight and vigorously pounding his foot, joining in full voice with his two admired heroes and friends, was one of the great moments of a lifetime. Vivid in my mind was the memory of Peter sitting in the wheelchair by Bobby's bed during one of his nights of pain. Was it possible that it had only been five years before?

The people in the room were rapt. Then they joined in the singing. They sensed that it was a magical, deeply personal moment. I kept moving in closer and closer, standing so I could hear better, and a man, with tears running down his face, grabbed my hand tightly and said, "We're going to do something for hemophilia in my state, I promise you, we are." (And they did.)

And then it was over. Bobby, who had invited Maria Shriver, his Paris classmate, for the evening, was so worried about his promise to Mrs. Shriver to get her home at the promised hour that there was no time to sing again in the big room. Franklin Schaffner, the director of the film, offered him his limousine, and Bobby sped off. Anyway, Peter refused to do it again. "Something really happened," he said. "We shared something great and we couldn't duplicate it."

In fact, no one else but our family could know what a triumph that song had been. It was what the evening was all about: not business, not "charity," but medicine, persistence, faith and friendship; a lonely, proud, and happy moment. I forgot all about the Chinese gods and exulted, just that once.

People stayed very late, but about 2:00 A.M. they began to leave. We drifted down to somebody's hotel suite for more late talk. Finally, around 5:00 A.M. we went to bed. On our pillow was a note:

> Dear Mom and Dad:
>   It was *wonderful!*
>   Love,
>   Susy [signed with drawing of a horse]

Robert Massie: The gross income from the Author's Première in New York was $68,000. But expenses took half of this and, in the end, the Hemophilia Foundation received $34,000. Most of this was given as a research grant to Alan Johnson to continue his work in finding a more powerful AHF concentrate.

Happily, the fight in London and New York produced a snow-ball effect in other cities. A gala for hemophilia was held in Toronto under the chairmanship of Susy's godmother, Kay Breithaupt. There was a hemophilia première in Philadelphia, with Sue's parents acting as honorary chairmen. My mother helped to organize a hemophilia première in Nashville. There were others in Atlanta, Dallas, Detroit, Chicago, Miami, and Denver.

There was only one major première in which hemophilia played no part. That was in Los Angeles. This, too, was arranged by Sam Spiegel. The local hemophilia chapter had written to him years in advance; he rejected them and then gave the première to St. John's Hospital, a fashionable hospital used by movie stars. The chapter appealed to me to fly out and help them hold a press con-ference denouncing Spiegel's action. I couldn't; I was just too tired.

Nevertheless, around the world, the various hemophilia founda-tions and societies collected perhaps $250,000.* If we had not made our fight, I don't think any of them would have got anything.

---

* This figure does not include an anonymous gift of twenty-five thousand pounds (about $60,000) that came the following spring to the British Hemo-philia Society. As in Victorian novels, the society was sternly warned not to attempt to learn the identity of its benefactor. Being a romantic, I like to think it was the Queen.

In any case, after the fight was over, we didn't want to think about it. Within a month, it seemed that it had taken place years before. Even now, sifting through the piles of fat folders, rereading the letters, memos, and notes, I am amazed at how much work we did in a single year—how much emotion was burned, how much time was lost. Worse, the disgraceful state of affairs that made this kind of effort necessary continues to exist in America. Which patients are properly treated still depends on which charity has a more glittering ball committee. Health and medical care continue to be charitable donations, graciously bestowed by one group of citizens on others less fortunate.

For Sue and me, this effort was worth making. We made it—and the amount of money we raised in New York is not enough to keep two severe hemophiliacs like Bobby on prophylactic transfusions for one year.

Suzanne Massie: The première story had a completely unexpected happy epilogue in Paris. For us, the French première was a joy. We simply received an invitation and were accorded the greatest luxury of all, just to go and look.

The person who singlehandedly engineered this triumphant ending was Marie Hélène de Rothschild, wife of Baron Guy de Rothschild, the head of the legendary House of Rothschild. In the sophisticated world of the Tout Paris, a few ladies are given the titles of "locos" or locomotives—those who make everything run. Marie Hélène is chief among them. Living like a queen—ruling over castles and houses, stables and estates—exquisitely dressed by the greatest couturiers of France, she shines in the social firmaments of Paris, Marbella, London, and New York. The perfect social butterfly—or so it seems. Actually, Marie Hélène suffers from a mysterious illness of the bones which causes her great pain. Behind the scenes she has helped medical research in many fields. Over the years she has helped to create the Fondation de Recherche Médicale.

We had met casually once or twice. One November evening in Paris when we were deeply embroiled in the problems of both the English and the American premières, we were invited to a dinner for the visiting de la Rentas. On one of the plump, pillow-filled couches sat two counts, d'Estainville and Montpezat. They asked what was going to happen with the première in Paris. I explained, briefly, what had happened in London and New York. I thought their interest was only polite. But the French have a characteristic I have always admired. Although they often give an impression of cynicism, in reality they have a very clear sense of justice and injustice—with no equivocating. "No," said the elegant d'Estainville, "but it is grotesque—the whole book is about hemophilia. It is from your life." Marie Hélène de Rothschild, who overheard us, quietly moved closer and asked, "May I join the conversation?" She sat there, hands demurely folded, and listened. Then she said decisively, "*Oh, non!* It shall not happen this way in France." And turning to the two counts, she said with a smile, "*Eh bien*, we shall organize this together, won't we? We will do something." (Even if nothing were to come of it, I was grateful for the momentary compassion that had moved her to express the intention.)

On our way home, Bob told me he had learned that Sam Spiegel was coming to Paris the following week to make arrangements for the Paris première and that it was to be for the French branch of the Kennedy Foundation for Mental Retardation; the key figure in arranging this with Spiegel had been Sargent Shriver, the former American ambassador to France.

We were both depressed by this news. Here in France, where so much had been done to help us with hemophilia, the one gesture we could make in return was once again to be prevented. Bob tried to protest. He spoke by phone for almost an hour with Mr. Shriver in New York. He went to see the ladies involved. Everyone was sorry, but no one was willing to give it back to hemophilia. We could not take on another unequal struggle; we couldn't fight the Kennedys as well as Sam Spiegel. This time we gave up.

Yet, to our surprise, when we returned to Paris in January, we found that the plans for the première were already firmly launched —in the hands of Marie Hélène and for hemophilia.

For all her social activities, Marie Hélène de Rothschild had never run a charity gala in her life. In France, unlike America, the charity gala is relatively rare and it is not the usual way of raising funds for health needs. For one thing, the French have their efficient government health insurance program. For another, and perhaps more practical reason for the realistic French, donations to charity are not tax deductible.

Yet at the eleventh hour Spiegel had had to reverse himself and give in to this determined blond woman. In the face of his growls, Marie Hélène had coolly told him that if the première did not benefit hemophilia, she would torpedo any other kind of gala. He knew that she could and would.

The honorary committee she had collected in less than a month was truffled with elegant names. She herself was the president, two French ministers (Health and Education) were patrons of honor. On the list of the committee were the names of Princess Grace of Monaco, Prince Paul of Yugoslavia, the Duchess of Windsor, assorted important counts and countesses, barons and baronesses.

Along the way, Mr. Spiegel tried to wiggle out of the whole idea of a charity première by saying that he would have only an invitational première. "Fine," answered Marie Hélène, "let us do it that way. But we will invite for hemophilia." So the première was by personal invitation only, of Baroness Guy de Rothschild and Mr. Sam Spiegel. Instead of charging admission, Marie Hélène hit on the ingenious plan of selling the theater programs for the benefit of hemophilia, at 500 francs ($100) apiece.

There was a golden carrot to encourage sales. In each program was printed a lottery number; of course, one had to buy the expensive program to get it. Straining to describe its opulence, *Jour de France* called it a *"tombola* (lottery) *rothschildienne."* Among the donated items were a dress each from the five great couturiers (Dior, Cardin, Lanvin, Saint Laurent, and Ungaro), a magnificent ranch-mink coat from Chombert, four cases of magnums of Moët et Chandon Brut Imperial 1964, cases of rare Mouton-Rothschild wine, an original lithograph by Salvador Dali, and six and a half pounds of caviar. The Countess of Brandolini persuaded her brother, Fiat magnate Giovanni Agnelli, to donate a car, and then turned around and persuaded a friend at Renault to do the same. Harry Winston donated a diamond pendant worth $6,000.

Marie Hélène convinced Maxim's to lend her the restaurant for the evening. She called in a designer and had plates, goblets, and tablecloths designed for the occasion. The Rothschilds themselves donated the wine. At each step along the way, she was interviewed by the breathless Paris press. She missed no occasion to point out sweetly in print that Mr. Spiegel had felt that hemophilia was *"pas assez élégant"* for a première.

For weeks, Marie Hélène worked furiously, often from her bed. By devoting herself and driving her friends, by working from six o'clock in the morning throughout the day, every detail of the complicated arrangements was perfected. In the end, Mr. Spiegel himself was persuaded to donate the theater and pay for the dinner at Maxim's for the 350 invited guests.

On the evening of April 13, 1972, in front of the Marigny theater just off the Champs Élysées, klieg lights burned down on the two gift cars displayed outside the theater. Crowds of curious people lined the street watching the limousines roll up. As the rich and the famous placed their patrician toes on the earth, photographers' bulbs flashed like fireflies.

Inside the theater doors stood a smiling Baron Guy de Rothschild, with a group of elegant friends. Clutching armfuls of programs, they politely but firmly extracted five-hundred-franc bills from those entering. Like brightly plumed birds, the most beautiful women of Paris fluttered in the lobby and halls of the theater, their dresses reflecting the arts of all the greatest couturiers of France. The couturiers themselves arrived. Cardin, Saint Laurent, Lanvin.

The House of Christian Dior had designed a special blue-and-white silk scarf for the occasion, printed with the Russian double eagle and inscribed in French and Russian. Molyneux launched its new perfume, Vivre, for the occasion. These favors were distributed as presents. Every seat in the theater was taken. In the middle of the theater, the row of honor was banked with red roses, white lilies, and chrysanthemums. Marie Hélène sat in the middle, flanked by two ministers of France.

After the film, it was on to Maxim's. On the red-carpeted stairs leading to the second floor, the gypsy orchestra of Reginskaya, one of Paris' most elegant nightclubs, was playing furiously as guests arrived. All the dining rooms and even the dance floor of Maxim's were filled to bursting with tables. Baron de Redé supervised the seating arrangements, which had been minutely planned by Marie Hélène. Seating at Maxim's is governed by occult laws; there is always one table that is considered *the* one. Marie Hélène was, of course, sitting at this table; and in the places of honor near her were the Minister of Health, the great French hematologist Jean Pierre Soulier, Henri Chaigneau, the head of the French Hemophilia Society, Bob and I.

Soft pink lights glowed at every table, golden goblets and golden service plates gleamed on tablecloths of red and gold damask. The red and gold menus announced that we were to be served two kinds of vodka, Château Duhart-Mouton-Rothschild 1966, and Maxim's own special Brut 1964 champagne. Dinner included pâté of eel of the Neva, borscht, quail with raisins Tartar style, and finished with a velvety charlotte russe.

Marie Hélène was still there at 4 A.M. with a small group. Finally, she walked out the door and stood under a predawn but still starry Paris sky. Quietly she said good-bye, waved, and stepped into her limousine. The next day she had to take to her bed again with a relapse of her mysterious malady.

The evening raised over $65,000—clear; there were no expenses. The French Hemophilia Society was overwhelmed. Half of the money was put in a permanent fund to establish an international prize to be awarded every two years for research in hemophilia.

Since that time, our paths have not crossed. Yet I believe that, given the challenge, Marie Hélène would react again as she did for us. Generous and cunning, compassionate and tough, I am certain that, if necessity dictated, Marie Hélène could run General Motors. In any case, we will never forget that, for a question of justice, alone, she took on Sam Spiegel and won. Few people would fight so hard, fewer still would have the skill to succeed.

As the French say, *Chapeau*, Marie Hélène, to you, and to your friends.

Chapter 26

During those years 1969–72 at la Cerisaie, Bobby grew into adolescence. More and more he gained independence and confidence;
socially he blossomed. He excelled in his studies. He became the
president of a church group called Agape, made up of a hundred American teen-agers. Together they held weekly meetings,
planned a folk service, and held retreats where they engaged in long,
soul-searching conversations. With his English teaching money,
Bobby bought a banjo and a camera. He started earning money
taking photographs of his schoolmates and learned to develop and
print pictures. He took fencing lessons and, thanks to his summers
in Greece, became an excellent swimmer. He began to travel alone.
(The first time was an agony for me. I resolutely closed my mind
and pretended that he was still in Paris.) At fifteen, he went to
England, where he lived with the treasurer of the British Hemophilia Society, Ken Polton (himself a hemophiliac). In London,
Bobby worked in the St. Thomas' Hospital office, filing medical
records. He transfused himself and under the English National
Health Services, he was provided with free cryo for his transfusions.

He made many friends. One of them was the novelist James
Jones, who lived not far from us on the Île St.-Louis. I admired Jim
enormously, but he awed me, and I shyly observed him from afar.
But Bobby somehow established a warm communication with this
intensely committed man, and Jim was a wonderful friend to him.
Bobby wrote this about their meeting:

> When I was in bed for a long time, I read. People would bring me
> all sorts of books, and I usually read every single one. But gen-
> erally I would get involved in an area, or with an author, and I

would read everything about it or by him. There were the Geoffrey Household, Alistair Maclean thrillers; C. S. Forester and the entire Hornblower series; Gerald Durrell and his animal stories. I was very thorough. So it is no wonder that when I received another batch of books my curiosity was sparked by a new sort of book: a book about war. It was an old paperback copy of *The Thin Red Line*, so badly glued together that when I opened it the first six pages fell to the floor. It was an incredible book, so vivid that I lost track of all time.

A month or so later we went to a party. Many interesting people were there and I felt a little out of place. So I sat on the sofa to listen to my father, who was talking to a very interesting-looking man. They started talking about *The Thin Red Line* and, finding common ground, I mentioned that I had read it, that I had liked it very much, and I began to describe it to the man.

My father smiled and said: "Bobby, you don't need to. This is Mr. Jones, and he wrote it."

Over the next two years Jim Jones and I became good friends. I loved to go to his house, which was actually two buildings, stitched together by a peculiar series of stairs and hallways, on the Île St.-Louis, overlooking the Seine. I loved sitting in the living room, toying with a Roman short sword or an empty hand grenade, eating ripe plums and playing chess. And best of all, I loved sitting around on Sunday evening, after a spaghetti dinner, when the large, circular, green-felt covered table was placed in the center of the room and the traditional poker game began. The stakes were high and it was serious business. Irwin Shaw and a host of other regulars would come to win (or lose) four or five hundred dollars in an evening. I would sit on a high bar stool watching carefully, fixing a drink from time to time for anyone who could relax enough to realize that he was thirsty.

Jim was a wonderful friend for me to have, for he is a unique combination of outward toughness and inward sensitivity. He is *tough* too: the poker-playing, pistol-shooting ex-G.I. who makes his own bullets, smokes $2 cigars, and finds highly graphic nicknames for people he doesn't like. For me, he was a combination of John Wayne and Popeye. He had been there, seen it all; a life I knew that I would never know.

But Jim is also a sensitive man who can see right through almost everyone he meets. He cares deeply about his writing, about his books. His living room is half art gallery and half library, the latter portion being filled with books on the Civil War and American history. He does everything with great determination and does not qualify anything for anyone.

Why do I like Jim? Because he has had many problems, and he knows what it is to be different. And yet he has turned his differences into uniqueness; now every detail in his life reaffirms that success over his earlier problems. He understood something that I had yet to learn: that life is filled with senseless actions . . . and one should enjoy it for its own sake.

But, sadly, during those same years that life was growing better and fuller psychologically, medically things were getting worse. Just after the new school term had begun at the Collège Sévigné, when Bobby was just fourteen, Susy remembers coming home from school on a sunny afternoon in late September: "I saw Bobby, so pale . . . so very pale. I was worried; no one was home. He said it was nothing. As soon as you came home, everything started happening." He had a headache, a simple headache. But almost immediately we knew it was not simple. He lay there on his bed in the darkness, the shades drawn. He was white, his eyes strangely glazed. I took his temperature. Nothing. I asked him what he had eaten. Nothing abnormal. But something was very wrong. I started calling. No Josso—away. Dr. Larrieu, away. Dialing faster and faster, I finally connected with Dr. Soulier. "You know what it is as well as I do," he said. I did. It was a cerebral hemorrhage. With the smooth functioning of years of experience, calmly, quietly, speedily, we gathered him up, resting him on the back seat of the car. We drove through the streets of Paris, along the canals to the Hôpital St.-Louis, trying not to panic, trying to pretend that the world was the same—that suddenly unreal world of passers-by hurrying home for dinner. We missed a turn, frantically circled our way back through one-way streets. The guard lifted the barrier, and I saw the gardens, red with salvia in the sun. The doctors were ready, with their bottles, their needles, their tests. Bobby could not sit up. Pain was coming in sudden blinding waves.

Quickly, a transfusion was started. "We must do a spinal tap," said the doctors. But this could not be done without ascertaining precisely what pressure was on the brain. An ophthalmologist was immediately called, but he had to make his way across Paris traffic in the rush hour. While we waited, I nervously paced back and forth in the halls. I passed the office of the doctors, and I saw one of them standing with her back to me, leaning against the glass with her head bowed. From that discouraged pose, I knew. They did not know what it was. They did not know what would be the outcome, any more than we did. Dr. Josso arrived; he and three other doctors clustered around the foot of Bobby's bed. They talked. They looked brave. They were terribly worried. Josso scratched the bottom of Bobby's feet. No reaction. Tapped his knee. No reaction. "Where are you, Mother?" said Bobby with his eyes wide open staring at me. "I can't see you." And I thought, Is it possible? After we have fought so hard. Are we going to lose him now—this calm sunny afternoon, with so little notice? How is it that although I have been prepared every day, I am *not prepared?*

Finally the ophthalmologist arrived. He peered into Bobby's eyes. No pressure. They went ahead with the spinal tap. Bobby could see again. The pains subsided. The doctors ordered transfusions every four hours and began to run tests. If it was not a cerebral hemorrhage, what could it be? Perhaps a sudden attack of spinal meningitis? It was important to ascertain this—a cerebral hemorrhage could have repercussions in the future; an attack of meningitis was *preferable:* the course and prognosis would be clearer. Unfortunately, the symptoms are almost identical clinically. While the doctors tested and gave transfusions, Bobby remained in the hospital for a week, in a ward with three Frenchmen all with serious bleeding problems. Nevertheless they were gay, they cracked jokes and told stories. After a few days, Bobby was cheerful; but, inexplicably, he still could not sit up. Jim Jones came to visit. He brought books about sharks and told Bobby about his skin-diving adventures. Madame la Directrice rushed over during her lunch hour and brought fruit syrups in a little wicker basket.

At the end of the week Bobby was better—but the cause of his mysterious attack still could not be ascertained. The doctors decided to release him and keep him under observation. It was over, but we never did learn precisely what had caused it.

And, discouragingly, after a period of relative calm, Bobby's joints once again were beginning to bleed, seemingly without apparent cause, in a vicious cycle we could not break. More and more during that winter, he began missing school. More and more he was using crutches. One knee would swell and get better only to have the other begin. One elbow would bleed and then the other. It was mysterious, inexplicable, frustrating. Some of it we could attribute to the extreme trauma of adolescent growth: Bobby was swiftly growing taller and heavier; joints already damaged were less able to bear his weight. This in itself could cause bleeding as the increased weight caused small blood vessels to rupture. Yet no matter how many transfusions we gave, he kept right on bleeding. We began to spend more and more time with doctors, there were more and more perplexed conferences. Nothing seemed to break the cycle.

The doctors began to worry seriously about the presence of an antibody. In 5–10 per cent of hemophilia patients, for reasons still unknown, a circulating anticoagulant acts as an antibody to the infused Factor VIII. This drastically reduces the effectiveness of a transfusion. The development of such an antibody is one of the greatest fears of hemophilia doctors; it leaves the hemophiliac almost helpless. For many years doctors have worried that giving too much plasma or fraction might stimulate this antibody. This is why, when Bobby was a young child, no matter what was happening with his joints, we were told to give a transfusion only *after* a bleeding started and were specifically prohibited from giving preventive transfusions. Today, it is beginning to appear that perhaps the presence of the antibody is genetically predetermined and is not the result of overtreatment. No one really knows.

During these months, Bobby was tested and retested for the presence of an antibody. None was found. Still, his knee did not recover, but remained swollen and bent. The doctors recommended a knee aspiration. He was sent to the school for hemophiliacs at Queue les Yvelines; on March 1, 1971, he described his visit to Dr. Hilgartner in New York:

Dear Dr. Hilgartner,

After many months of trying to arrange to visit the hemophiliac school at Queue les Yvelines, I was finally obliged to go there for medical reasons: a very swollen left knee which had failed to go down even after repeated transfusions, cortisone, and a week's immobilization, was aspirated by the doctor who takes care of the hemophiliacs. It was a small operation; my knee had to be anesthetized, and I received two transfusions (making a total of 1200 AHF units) during the operation. There was a little difficulty in that the liquid was deep, and so it took longer than usual, though he drew about 40 to 50 cc. from my knee. The results were astonishing: today my knee is straight (at least more or less straight), the swelling is almost completely down, and I should be back on my feet sometime toward the end of the week.

Aspiration is rather common practice here, so I gathered, and the doctor says he has done more than two hundred over the last few years and they have never had any bad effects. It seems to work perfectly.

There are over a hundred hemophiliacs in this school, ranging from five to about fifteen years of age. They sleep in dormitories with five or six beds each, they have a pottery workshop, classrooms, a dining room, a movie or TV room, a small lounge with a ping-pong table, a woodworking shop, and even a small room which the teen-agers decorated themselves, and is now a sort of bar where they can get Coke, lemonade, and beer. There is, of course, also a well-equipped infirmary with a dentist and several transfusing rooms. There is even a special room where they make casts for all the boys, and each boy has a rack where he keeps six or seven casts for various parts of his body until he needs them. It is, above all, very well organized. At the moment, they are in the process of building a swimming pool next to the main building, which will be heated so I guess therefore will be used all year around.

Generally speaking, all the boys seem very happy and I understand that there is a very long waiting list of applicants trying to get into this school.

Dad has given me about 20 transfusions in the past two months (about half of that was for this knee) and I stuck myself for about 7 of those. I still have a little trouble getting into the veins in my hand, which seem to run away from the needle, although it is getting rarer for me to miss. Dad almost never misses, except he is still a little uneasy about threading the needle once it is in the vein.

If you have anything you want me to say or do, please just let me know, and I'll do it as best as I can.

My father sends you his very best, and so do I.

Yours sincerely,
Bobby Massie

Yet only a few weeks after this optimistic letter, Bobby was bleeding in his knee again. The doctors conferred. Perhaps we were no longer dealing with "normal" hemophilia bleeding. Evidence was now appearing that permanent, irreversible damage to the joints had been done by Bobby's repeated hemorrhages. In a normal joint, and in Bobby's when he was a little boy, the opposing surfaces of the bones constituting the joint are lined with a layer of cartilage, a glassy-smooth tissue. The joint itself is enclosed by the synovial membrane which secretes a fluid, a substance of egg-white consistency, which acts as an additional lubricant to the joint.

In hemophilia, all of this engineering marvel is destroyed. Repeated bleeding into joints produces enzymes that act like acid, chewing up and eating away the cartilage and eventually attacking the bones themselves. When this happens, the hemophiliac has what is very like arthritis, except that he has it in adolescence, not in middle age or old age as do most arthritis victims.

After repeated bleeding and healing, the synovial membrane becomes distended, filled with bloody fluid, fragile blood vessels, and scar tissue. Any undue exercise, motion, or stress can tear it. And when a joint is puffy and painful you are never quite sure whether it is blood . . . or blood mixed with synovial fluid . . . and in what proportion.

In Bobby's case, the doctors decided that we were dealing with a badly inflamed synovial membrane. With this condition, AHF fraction could stop bleeding temporarily but not long enough to allow healing. And every bleeding episode was further eroding Bobby's damaged joint. We had exhausted all the normal ways of treating him. We had no choice but to try something drastically new.*

Bob wrote to Dr. Hilgartner:

> We have heard about something new . . . osmic acid. They are recommending for Bobby an injection of osmic acid which neutralizes? destroys? the synovial membrane so that it becomes less troublesome. I was told that this is now being done rather regularly at the Queue les Yvelines. So far, they say they have observed no harmful side- or after-effects and that the only qualification is that after a period of a considerable number of months, another injection may be necessary to reneutralize the membrane. This, I was told, is an application to hemophilia of a technique followed in various kinds of severe arthritis.

As in all new procedures, there were risks and we delayed. But by April we could wait no longer. After the terrible knee episode in the spring of 1969, X-rays had revealed a growing lesion in Bobby's left knee. Two years later, the hole was much worse, more than two inches in diameter. The knee was being worn away. Further deterioration had to be stopped or Bobby would lose his knee altogether.

We went to the Hôpital Cochin for a conference with Dr. Menkès, the arthritis specialist who was to perform the injection. It was a highly experimental technique. Soberly the doctors explained to us the percentage of success and failure. The amount of acid injection had to be precisely gauged—too much and it could eat away the remaining cartilage. Dr. Menkès held the X-rays of Bobby's knee up to the lighted board and we could see the extent of the damage. In the room, there was total silence . . . a shocked silence which Bobby broke. Sitting in his wheelchair, looking at the board, he too understood, so he said lightly, "I'm sure glad that's not my knee you're looking at." We all laughed . . . hollowly.

The procedure was painful. A syringe of liquid was injected

---

* The effects of repeated untreated hemorrhages on joints are nightmarish. When, in 1971, world hemophilia specialists convened in Teheran for an International Hemophilia Conference, they were taken to a village where they found two hemophiliac brothers, one thirteen and the other fifteen: one was locked in a sitting position, the other in a standing position.

directly into the knee, causing exactly the same kind of pain as a knee hemorrhage. Once again, Bob and I divided our time between two hospitals. Elizabeth's eyes were being operated on. For two days she was blind. I sat by her bedside and watched her, lying still, a small wraith in her little white nightgown, heavy bandages over her eyes. Outside a violent spring storm once more blew away the chestnut blossoms.

Bobby stayed in the hospital three days, then came home and remained in a wheelchair another two weeks. But then, incredibly, the swelling went down and stayed down. For the rest of the spring and through a good summer, he was able to walk. The number of bleedings in his left knee dropped from ten the previous winter to only three in the next few months. At last, we had done something right!

Then came the first rainy days of the autumn of 1971. Up to that time, Bobby had been walking to the bus at the Place de la Bastille a few blocks from our house, and then walking from the bus to school, another block. Suddenly, one day he could no longer cover even this short distance without pain. This time, it wasn't his knee, it was his ankles. We tried special orthopedic shoes, custom-made, to lessen pressure and help to support weight. We tried exercises to strengthen the muscles. We tried giving him cortisone, which acts on the synovial fluid in the joints. But cortisone taken regularly can have serious side effects and it could be taken for a short term only.

The doctors put aside their fears of an antibody and, ignoring the cost, prescribed prophylactic transfusions. This meant Bobby would have preventive transfusions two or three times a week, whether he was bleeding or not. In enormous quantity, the CNTS provided fraction. But we were too late. The damage was permanent.

And, less than a year after the first injection of osmic acid, the number of Bobby's knee bleedings began to rise again: the shriveled synovial membrane had once again grown larger and was causing trouble. In addition, Bobby was now bleeding regularly into his right elbow. So in the spring of 1972 he had two kinds of injections. This time, for the elbow, we tried something new: radioactive gold.

Then after being injected with radioactive gold for his arm at the American Hospital, he went back to Cochin for a second injection of osmic acid into the knee.

That was to be the last of Bobby's French hospital stays, for that spring we had decided it was time to go home.

Bob was chafing at becoming an expatriate. He wanted to work in his own home, in his own country. Bobby wanted to graduate from high school in the United States. An autumn atmosphere had come to la Cerisaie. Our landlord had died, Madame Rhéto was growing old and was going into retirement. I could see . . . I knew . . . an era was coming to an end.

We had accomplished what we had set out to do. The children were bilingual. They loved France, they knew their cousins. They were marked.

But I did not want to leave. I cried a lot. I knew how I would yearn for the look of old stones—their poetry, the igniting of the imagination and dreams that no amount of concrete and glass will ever evoke. I knew how much I would miss the excitement in the air and in the streets, the feeling of being warmed and glad to be alive . . . the wonderful sensation that tomorrow, if not today . . . tomorrow, something exciting will happen. All this was in Paris. And there was no use telling myself that obstacles were good and that our departure would lead me to something better. I knew that it wouldn't, that a precious part of life that could never be repeated was being left behind forever.

After all the glitter of four years in Paris, when we left France only this unlikely pair came to see us off: Madame Rhéto, our salty Breton concierge housekeeper, and Mikhail Chemiakine, a painter friend recently emigrated from Leningrad. On the boat train Misha, who had not slept the night before, blinked his eyes behind his heavy black-rimmed glasses and yawned. Madame Rhéto was tremulous and talkative. On the boat, we all got tipsy on champagne and there was an overwhelming sense of good feeling and the pain of departure. Misha took me aside and put something into my hand, saying, "It is our Russian custom to give an icon on departure to protect and keep you." Madame Rhéto burst into tears and lost her hairpins kissing me good-bye. I kept one for good luck. And then we parted.

They stood on the pier as we looked down on them from the immense height of the decks of the *France*. Elizabeth waved until her arm got tired and we sent down balloons; before we even knew it the gigantic ship had swung around and was headed out to sea.

As soon as we were well underway, I went to the steward with our bottles of AHF fraction. This time I had to be sure that it was placed in *normal* refrigeration—not in the freezer, or it would be ruined. I went with the steward myself to sign it in with the chef. It was the same chef. He remembered our frantic chase and I had a difficult time convincing him that this fraction absolutely had to *ride with the vegetables* and *not* with the ice cream. He shrugged his shoulders at the mystery of it all, but he agreed. Several times during the trip I went down to check and I saw our bottles resting happily amid the green and juicy watercress of France.

School had already begun when we returned to Irvington in the fall of 1972. We hurried Elizabeth into the third grade at Dow's Lane school. Susy, bilingual in French, with two years of Latin, two years of German, and a year of Spanish, became a high school freshman. Bobby, who should have been a junior, persuaded Hackley School to allow him to enter as a senior and do two years' work in one. This meant taking a heavy academic load and graduating at sixteen. But he wanted to do it so that he could take a year off and have flying lessons. We all began to call this special year Bobby's "Super Year."

He plunged in with his new classmates in September. Immediately, his joints and his arthritis began to react. He went on crutches every day and still missed so many days that we had to have the telephone company come back and reinstall the intercom he had used in the sixth grade. In November, he went to Florida to watch the lift-off of Apollo 17, the last of the manned moonshots. He came home excited—and depressed. While there he had talked to a group of cadets from the Air Force Academy, many of whom hoped—as Bobby once had hoped—to become astronauts. "When I saw those guys, I knew that I could have done it," Bobby said. "And then I looked at my crutches and I knew, once and for all, that I would never be able to do it."

Bobby used the Hackley pool faithfully. The coaches helped. One day, he came home very pleased. "You know, Dad, the coach said today that if I were going to be here next year, I'd be good enough to make the swimming team!"

In the spring he took the lead in a school play, *Blithe Spirit*. At the end of the year, Bobby graduated with the highest academic average in his class.

Bobby's post-high-school Super Year was delayed—in fact, it was almost canceled—by a serious knee hemorrhage. We had gone back to France to spend the summer of 1973; Sue and I were working on this book. We were in a little farming village on the great rich plain that rolls northwest from Paris toward Normandy and the sea. We were living in an old farmhouse with high walls around the garden. Only Bobby and Elizabeth were with us—Susy was living one of her dreams: riding horses in Kentucky bluegrass. Bobby was strong; he liked to take bicycle rides by himself on the country roads that laced the golden wheat fields. Twice a day, we played ping-pong. In the farmhouse, tucked away in a cupboard, was a badminton set. One day, Elizabeth found it and begged me to set it up. Foolishly, I agreed. Bobby began to play; foolishly, I agreed to that, too. Competing vigorously, playing well, he lunged this way and that.

The following morning his knee was badly swollen. It was too much for me. I knew why it had happened—perhaps—and yet there was no way of knowing. I knew who was responsible—Bobby, Sue, me—and that none of us really was. Unable to work, I grabbed my pipe and went for a walk through the village streets out into the fields.

There was a dirt road at the edge of town which wandered off into a wheat field. As the days had passed, I had walked there often. The wheat which was green when we arrived, turned gold and then, just before it was cut, white and dry. Sometimes, a solitary horseman would ride down the road, turning out into a threshed and empty field, urging his horse to a gallop, sitting far back in his saddle in the French fashion.

It was a splendid place with the majesty of the sky and the wheat fields, and the simplicity of the dirt road.

That morning, as I walked along, I was thinking about myself. Why does this have to happen—to me? Will it ever end—for me? If only Bobby had listened—to me. If only Sue had reinforced my hesitations. Somehow, it was all directed at *me*. It wasn't exactly a plot, there was no motive, but somehow I had become the victim.

Not the only victim, of course: Bobby and Sue were suffering too. The pain you feel for Bobby is not to be compared with the pain he feels in his leg. The despair you feel over him is not to be compared with the despair he feels for himself. And this thought increased my own despair. As I walked, I could feel my brow knotted, my teeth clenched.

How can we deal with this, I asked myself. In most way⸱ Bobby is grown. He hates the constant surveillance, the negative glares and murmured cautions I give him when he starts doing something that might cause bleeding. I hate it as much as he does. If only I could watch and say nothing, put it out of my mind as all parents do with children beyond the age of toddlers, as I do myself with Susy and Elizabeth. But it is deeply ingrained, so deep that it may never completely disappear. And episodes like this reinforce and strengthen this instinct. Why didn't I forbid him to play badminton? I could see the torque it put on his knee when he lunged to swat the birdie. Perhaps because he has done other things that might have hurt him and haven't. He plays a miniature softball on our lawn in Irvington. We even played a little basketball one afternoon after swimming at Hackley. And these didn't hurt him. Besides, who knows whether it was the badminton this time? He might have got away with it. Perhaps he can judge better than I can? He has such a good time. "Bobby, you mustn't . . . Bobby, don't you think . . . Bobby, if I were you . . ." It's a role and an image I would give anything to shed. But I can't.

So I hang back, biting my tongue most of the time, but still riding him so often that it must seem to him to be constant. But I am caught. If I do tell him every time, it frays both our nerves. If I say nothing, and something like this happens, then I feel responsible: Why didn't I stop him? Why did I allow this?

Why worry about it? Why not let him take over the decisions? He is old enough and experienced enough now to understand the relation of cause and effect. He knows better than I do what it means to have a swollen joint and to spend days unable to walk or to play his guitar. Why can't he make the decisions? Why not let Bobby run his own life?

Perhaps we should. But two things keep me involved. One is the irreversible nature of what is happening to his joints. We have made

so many mistakes in the past; we have so often let joints go untreated or improperly treated that I feel we must do everything
possible to save what remains. When Bobby wants to play badminton, I think of his joints. They are *his* joints, but I feel responsible for them. I feel almost that I want to protect them from
getting worse . . . whether he likes it or not. This is one of the
problems.

The other is the amount of blood fraction we use. Perhaps I
shouldn't think of this, but I do know how lavish we are, relatively
speaking, in our use of this precious material. Of course, it shouldn't
be so precious and we should not be unique in our intensive use of
it. Somehow—by collecting and processing more blood—it should
not be in such scarce supply. Somehow—by a change in philosophy
—mine, other people's, society's—I should not feel guilty that we
use so much. I should not count the cost. It is, after all, used
legitimately and for a high purpose. Society wastes infinitely more
on things that have no purpose or even an evil purpose. And yet,
when Bobby goes into a bleeding episode and starts to use large
amounts of fraction, I feel somehow guilty. As if someone is going
to appear and demand an explanation, which, if not overwhelmingly
persuasive, will result in the decree, No More Fraction for You.
It is a nightmare I frequently have in daylight hours.

All this whirled through my head as I walked down the dirt
road. A strong wind was blowing; I had to lean forward to keep
going. Finally, I reached a point where four fields came together.
On a little patch of grass, I sat down. It was a juncture in space.
Overhead, an immense blue sky with white clouds moving swiftly
sent shadows racing across the fields. On one side behind me was a
wide field of wheat, white dry, ready to be cut. It seethed in the
wind as millions of kernels at the heads of the stalks rustled against
each other. On the other side was a field of corn. Most of the stalks
already were taller than I am, but the ears still were thin; it would
be another month before they ripened. In front of me lay two
empty fields. One was fallow, with some faded chaff washed into
the mud. The other already was freshly plowed; I had watched the
farmer churning the earth with his tractor a few days before.

I looked down the long furrows toward our small village a mile
away. The church tower, seven hundred years old, rose over the

red tile roofs nestling beneath for protection, built and consecrated by man, protected by God. I looked at the four fields, each at a different stage, in a great cycle of use, planned by the farmer, nurtured and blessed by God. I put my head down on the earth, and I looked up through the grass at the blue sky. I began to feel that I, we, all of us, were part of it. Part of this cycle. We would be born, grow, be fruitful, live, and when the time came, die, so that others could live. It was part of an enormous cycle, all of it protected, nurtured, and blessed by God. We had a part to play, as the village people centuries ago who built those houses and that church, as the farmer who this summer had planted and would reap this wheat and corn. It could not be done without our effort. But there would be help, as the sun and the rain were given to help the wheat and the corn. The knee would get better, Bobby would walk again, we would continue to struggle and to search, he would make himself a life, we would live the rest of ours, all somehow always—whether we realized it or not—protected, nurtured, and blessed by God.

With this renewed surge of hope, I wrote to Los Angeles Orthopaedic Hospital. They agreed to take Bobby immediately for a program of joint rehabilitation. He and I left France early and, one morning in September, I took him in his wheelchair to Kennedy Airport and put him aboard a jet for California. He stayed with my old Oxford friend Dennis Stanfill and his wife, Terry, who drove him every day to the hospital. It was an active exercise program, covered by a daily transfusion of AHF concentrate. Starting with mild isometric exercises in the exercise room and swimming pool, he proceeded gradually to more active exercises, using weights and pulleys. From the beginning, Bobby was enthusiastic about the hospital. He wrote:

"To give you an idea of my progress: Russ (the physical therapist) said that I worked harder and did better than I ever have, and I worked out on the treadmill with weight attached to my splint, something that I never could have done before. I am lifting ever increasing weight and have reached the maximum on several of their machines. I am swimming all day long. I have lost weight although I eat large meals, and I can do thirty pushups without being short of breath. When I return, I will put you all to shame, I will be in such good shape . . . and I still have a whole week more! As for my knee—because all these other things are secondary—I have worked it as hard as I can every day and it is *definitely* much stronger. I hope to be lifting weights with it by the time I leave— an incredible improvement, considering it was impossible for me to lift its own puny weight when I first arrived. I have acquired a reputation for working hard, and I intend to live up to it to the last day."

"I am very tired," he wrote later, "but I put my whole heart into it; indeed they have to keep me from doing too much! I can honestly say that this place is unique; it is highly organized without being cold, strict without being inflexible, compassionate without being pitying, and highly optimistic without being unrealistic.

"I have to go . . . dinner, and I wouldn't want to miss that! I am having a good time because I have something concrete to grapple with for the improvement of my knee, and because I am in control of the situation psychologically. I have enormous respect but am not overawed by the doctors here. Secretaries don't push me around with things like 'wait here' (for an hour or two). I've made many friends and have learned a lot of things that I wouldn't have known if I hadn't spoken to people and roamed around the hospital in my spare time. And I know when to be quiet and listen to nurses complaining to each other, or watch a three-year-old boy have a transfusion that he is scared of, or watch once strong men who have been bedridden for months learn slowly to walk again."

Despite his enthusiasm, there was one thing about Orthopaedic Hospital that bothered Bobby greatly:

"There is an ever present emphasis on one's ability to pay. It is no one's fault. This hospital is run on charity and fees, and it is in the red. They have had some bad experiences with uncollectible fees, and now they have been warned by the financial section that this better not keep happening so they are doubly careful. Everyone agrees that it shouldn't be that way, but again, no solution. The care here is excellent. It makes the weak strong, the depressed optimistic, and it gives a new meaning in life to those who are usually given up as hopeless. And the fact that this depends on the haphazard of charity, and that those who cannot financially qualify cannot benefit from it, is *immoral*. It is an outrage and a disgrace to the country."

The bills *were* astonishing. Eighteen dollars for each half hour of therapy in the pool with the therapist and five other patients; and Bobby had two of these pool sessions per day. Twelve dollars for each half hour of therapy in the exercise room; two of these exercise sessions per day. Plus dozens of other charges, including ten dollars for each of his daily uses of the treatment room where, without assistance, he gave himself transfusions. The total for seventeen days' care was $1,699.

Again, Blue Cross refused to pay more than a fraction of this bill. Yes, they admitted, all of Bobby's treatment had been within the four walls of Orthopaedic Hospital, but technically, they argued, Bobby was an outpatient.

When Bobby arrived, the hospital was short of beds and reluctant to surrender one solely for insurance purposes. So, believing that I was doing the right thing for Bobby (who was happier not sleeping in a hospital bed), for the hospital (by saving a bed for someone who really needed it), and for Blue Cross and my fellow subscribers (by saving them the additional $1,700 a bed would have cost), I decided that Bobby should sleep with the Stanfills and come in every day for treatment. And so Blue Cross rejected our claim. I protested, and for a year correspondence and telephone calls flowed back and forth between me and Blue Cross. I argued that a system of health care insurance that required that the patient be given the most expensive possible care in order for his coverage to be valid was illogical and an unfair additional burden for Blue Cross subscribers. Eventually, Blue Cross agreed and paid Bobby's entire bill.*

The important thing was that Bobby was better—unbelievably better. When we met him at the airport, the boy who hadn't walked for two months that summer, whom I had put on the plane in a

---

* Of course, there are some bills that Blue Cross pays promptly. At the same time they were refusing to pay for Bobby's treatment, Blue Cross paid for a dinner for the medical staff of a hospital in the Bronx. The bill was $1,354. "Blue Cross routinely pays for food expenses of hospital business meetings," an official explained.

That same year, Blue Cross paid $14,800,000 for free medical services given to physicians and their families and other "courtesy" patients at ten New York hospitals. Paying for such "courtesy" services is also routine.

wheelchair three weeks before, now refused to wait while I went for the car in the parking lot. Grabbing his suitcase and walking beside me without a limp, he said, "You don't understand, Dad. Everything's changed."

In part, it had. He continued to have bleedings; only a few weeks later another bad knee kept him in bed for almost a month. But the Los Angeles experience had given him an enormous boost. It strengthened his body. It taught him how to exercise. And best of all, it gave him the knowledge that somewhere there was a place that could turn things around dramatically; a place to which, if he needs to, he can go back.

Once Bobby could walk again, his Super Year began. He got a part-time job working as a tape-deck technician for Paul Stookey. In a corner of the basement, we built a darkroom where Bobby spent hours working in the reddish gloom to develop and print his own pictures. And although I winced inwardly when I saw him doing it, he took an ax and saw, and began to clear the dense brush that had grown up in the patch of woods behind our house. "It may seem strange, Dad," he explained, "but this is just as important to me as music or photography or anything else."

The summit of the Super Year arrived when Bobby began to live out his childhood dream of space and flight. Two or three times a week, he drove to Westchester Airport for flying lessons with Al Hill, his experienced, low-key instructor. Finally, one day, Al said, "Bobby, let me out. This time, you go around by yourself."

"You mean solo?" Bobby asked, first incredulous, then over-joyed.

"Yep," Al said.

Al dropped out onto the runway, Bobby closed the door, gunned the motor, and roared down the runway into the air. "I couldn't help it," Bobby said later, "but my radio button was off and as I lifted off the ground, I just shouted 'Yippee!' It was the greatest feeling of my life."

The month of January 1974 brought a long string of beautiful, blue flying days. Bobby had lessons scheduled every day and hoped, before the end of February, to have logged enough hours to take his VFR pilot's license test. Suddenly he was suspended from any further solo flying until a medical board reviewed the question of his hemophilia. I telephoned the FAA flight surgeon's office in Oklahoma City, explaining that Bobby was swimming 1,000 yards a day, lifting 140 pounds, pushing 80 pounds with his knees; he was far more physically qualified than some of the middle-aged ladies who were flying at his school. The FAA answer: No exceptions until they discovered what hemophilia was.

More letters and telephone calls. Hematologists and ortho- pedists wrote to the FAA that hemophilia was not going to bring on dizzy spells or any other kind of sudden incapacitation. They urged that Bobby's medical certification be restored.

By March, when his FAA permit was reissued, Bobby had gotten a job as an intern in the Washington office of Senator Henry M. Jackson.

For five months, Bobby became highly visible rolling in his wheelchair down the long corridors of the Old Senate Office Build- ing and the Capitol. Lawmakers and Capitol policemen soon got used to the sight of Bobby collapsing his folding wheelchair to take it on the trolley railway that links the buildings on Capitol Hill. He kept a supply of concentrate in a small icebox in the office, and when he needed a transfusion he gave it to himself. For the first time in his life, he was adequately covered by private health insurance— the policies available for government employees are infinitely better than those available to most of us.

Interns are supposed to soak up atmosphere and lore by going to hearings and Bobby did plenty of that. He became a fixture at Senator Kennedy's lengthy hearings on health legislation. As part of his job, he was asked to look for a job in the government for a Russian-speaking student from the State of Washington who had become a quadriplegic after a trampoline accident. One day, he went on the regular White House tour in his wheelchair. When he came back, he wrote to the President telling him how difficult such tours were for handicapped people and suggesting, "The problem would be better understood if a staff member would simply attempt to get around for one full day in a borrowed wheelchair."

Bobby's major Washington project grew out of this book and an experience he had trying to get AHF concentrate from a sub- urban Bethesda hospital. He read what I had written about the Red Cross and Hyland Laboratories in 1968. And then, one day, trying to get some Hyland AHF he was told that the company shipped to small hospitals only when it had a surplus; its bigger customers, with whom it could sign an annual contract, were serviced first.

He began to dig for the facts about the way commercial pharmaceutical houses collect and distribute blood. When he was finished, he wrote a report. He hopes—and I hope, and all hemophiliacs should hope—that it will provoke a congressional investigation into this continuing scandal. The harder Bobby worked, the happier he was and the less trouble he seemed to have with hemophilia. "Things are hopping," he wrote. "I am working longer hours and I am going to bed at 8:30 P.M. so that I am rested. It isn't easy. Very spartan. But I love it."

In the fall of 1974 Bobby entered Princeton. He was also accepted at Yale and, in a letter to his godfather, Jack May, he explained his choice:

> I went up to Yale. I spent two days rolling around the campus in my wheelchair. I mapped out a typical freshman day, investigated the pool, the infirmary, the dining halls, and other places that I would be heading for with some frequency. It was a nightmare. The walkways were almost designed to snare wheelchair wheels. The curbs were high, almost insurmountable. The classrooms and campuses were separated by moats filled with mechanical crocodiles: city buses, trucks, and cars. The gym was far from any college I could have lived in and the infirmary was nearly off the campus map!
>
> When I went to Princeton, I was shown a dorm that was literally in between the gym and the infirmary. I could swim every morning without moving more than a hundred yards! I could eat in the same building. There are few steps, few curbs, and few cars. In almost every single physical way, the Princeton campus might almost have been designed for a hemophiliac.

Once on the campus as a freshman, Bobby fell in love with Princeton. He is taking intensive Russian (the next time he sees Victor Sosnora, they will be able to talk) and a serious course in drawing (to carry on what he began in Paris with Joe Downing). He zips around the campus on an electric battery-powered cart. He keeps his AHF fraction in his room and transfuses himself. Every day he does physical therapy and swims for two hours. Steadily, his endurance is rising: 40, 50, 60, 70, 80, 100 laps a day. "The best thing," he says, "is to see my therapist's face when she looks at my legs. She is really pleased . . . so am I."

With exercise Bobby can build his muscles and protect his joints. But the joints can never be restored. He has permanent, painful arthritis in his knees and ankles and sometimes in his elbows. Some mornings, when he wakes up, he can barely walk. He hobbles across the room, soaks in a hot bath or shower for fifteen minutes, and then, with his joints warmed up, can begin to walk. During the day, he cannot sit for long periods in class without his joints becoming stiff and painful.

Arthritis hurts because the bones in the joint, stripped of their protective coating of cartilage, are grinding and scraping against each other. There is nothing he can take for the pain. Aspirin, which most people with arthritis take, contains analgesics that, in addition to helping pain, also impair clotting. Other, more effective drugs could be addictive. In the long run, he may be given a new, artificial knee; experimental work on artificial joints is going on in Sweden. But for the moment, most American orthopedists believe that even a painful real knee is better than an insensate artificial one. "Come back in about fifteen years and perhaps we'll give you a whole new knee," the doctors said at Los Angeles Orthopaedic Hospital when Bobby was there. Until then, the best that Bobby can do is keep trying—by home transfusion, prophylactic transfusion, and proper exercises—to keep his joints from deteriorating further. Neither unlimited money nor unlimited concentrate will buy back ruined cartilage and bone.

But there are thousands of younger boys in America who are just beginning the long struggle with hemophilia. Despite the fact that it is possible for their joints to be preserved, they are going to be allowed to suffer what Bobby has suffered. Somewhere, there is a blond, blue-eyed five-year-old, like Bobby, whose joints are still nearly perfect, who is running across the grass as Bobby used to run, and who, ten years from now, will be in a wheelchair.

Unless we—all of us—do something to help him.

Over the past eighteen years, Sue and I have done everything we could to help Bobby. He has done everything possible to help himself. Doctors, teachers, friends have done everything they could for him. But this country, the United States, the richest on earth, has done nothing.

The United States is the most backward of all the "civilized" nations in its attitude toward chronic illness. Countries much poorer than we recognized long ago that the medical and emotional problems of chronic disease are enough for a family to deal with, and they found ways to spread the crushing financial burden.

The United States spends money lavishly. It has given away over $100 billion in foreign aid. Since the year of Bobby's birth, the United States has spent $2 trillion on defense. Even now we are preparing to order 244 B-1 bombers, costing $76 million apiece, and a new fleet of submarines that will cost over $1 billion each. We spend $1 billion a year for treatment of drug addiction, which, however grim, is a self-inflicted disease.

Why do we spend money for drug addicts and not for the chronically ill? Because drug addiction is socially disruptive. Would the United States have been quicker to do something for Bobby and other hemophiliacs if they had taken to the streets to menace citizens with knives to get the money they need to buy the antihemophilic fraction their bodies must have?

It has been said that you can tell a lot about a nation's values by looking to see how much its people choose to help less-favored elements in society. And which less-favored elements they choose to help. Our society has become an enormous economic engine, the world's greatest producer of goods. Thus, the needy people we choose to help first are people who are suffering economically. If you lose your job or can't get a job, our society regards this seriously and worries about it greatly; you become an important economic statistic ("Unemployment is up to seven per cent!"); and emergency meetings are called at the White House. But if you are chronically ill, you are not a part of the economic engine, nobody gets excited, no meetings are held, and no money is forthcoming. In the United States, we succor the unemployed and ignore the sick. In terms of health, the nation's philosophy is the Survival of the Fittest.

In fairness, it has to be said that most Americans are astonished and horrified to learn what hemophiliacs face in this country. Is it really true, they ask in disbelief, that *nothing* has been done for hemophiliacs? Haven't hemophiliacs been covered by some part of our crazy patchwork of Crippled Children's programs, vocational rehabilitation programs, or economic opportunity programs?

The answer is, up to now, no.

States exclude hemophiliacs from their Crippled Children's programs because they believe that a child with a blood disease cannot be classified as a "crippled child." Vocational rehabilitation administrators reject hemophiliacs, saying, "They are not suitable for vocational rehabilitation because hemophilia is an unstable disorder." Federal Economic Opportunity administrators say, "We don't have anything in the Poverty Act or the Economic Opportunity Act for this kind of child."

For years, the federal government has talked about doing something to help. In 1968, Dr. Brinkhous told me that Wilbur Cohen, Secretary of Health, Education, and Welfare, was studying a plan for coverage of catastrophic illness, including hemophilia. Six years and four secretaries of HEW later, nothing has happened.

Meanwhile, of course, some Americans do receive free federal health care: all members of the armed forces and their dependents, all wards of the United States, such as Indians and Eskimos, lepers, narcotic addicts, prisoners in federal prisons, and presidents of the United States. And, slowly, the federal government has begun to help the old and the poor. Between them, Medicare and Medicaid now cover 38 per cent of the American people. The rationale is that these are people more likely to be ill and less able to pay the high expenses of modern medicine. But what about those citizens who are already permanently ill and whose medical bills are permanently astronomical?

One explanation may be that the poor and the elderly can vote, while many of the chronically ill are children and cannot. But there is more to it. A majority of the American people have always favored a national health care program of some sort. In 1949 a *Fortune* magazine poll found that 74 per cent of the people favored

President Truman's proposed program of prepaid health care. To-day, more than two out of three Americans favor national health insurance.

What has prevented it? There is a villain: the American Medical Association. Down through the years, doggedly arguing that medical care is not a right of citizens but a privilege extended by doctors, the AMA has damned national health insurance as "socialized medicine." Today, as some form of national health insurance becomes increasingly likely, the AMA continues to fight a dogged rear-guard action. Endowed with a staff of 1,000 and a budget of $36 million (think what this amount of money could do if it were spent on blood: it is much more than half the amount spent on the entire Red Cross blood program), the AMA pours money into the campaigns of congressmen who support what the AMA calls grandly, "the free enterprise system in medicine." It opposes any form of national health insurance tied to Social Security, arguing that this would lead to a further inflation in already soaring medical costs.

This argument is dishonest. The AMA has never opposed soaring medical costs. It has taken no steps to lower the bills charged by doctors, or hospitals, or pharmaceutical companies. The AMA fought Medicare for years, but as soon as it found that the program was loosely administered, and that most doctors' bills could be generously large, the AMA fell silent.

What the AMA objects to is not government paying soaring medical costs, but government trying to control those costs by regulating the American health industry. The national health industry is the third largest in America; it spends $105 billion annually. It involves all of us, all our lives, as actual or potential consumers. And yet, the AMA insists that we, the consumer, and the government on our behalf, have no right at all to say how medical care shall be dispensed or to whom, or what it will cost.

Instead, the AMA argues, American medicine should function as a free enterprise system. This argument, too, is false. A free enterprise system assumes a free market of suppliers and demanders. It is based on the ability of the demander—the public—to say, "No, I won't buy your product. The price is too high." In medicine, there is no free market. The relationship between supplier (the doctor) and demander (the patient) is entirely different: the doctor has technical knowledge and overwhelming psychological domination over the patient. When a doctor prescribes a drug, the patient can't say, "No, I want to shop around for a cheaper drug." Or when a doctor orders tests in a hospital or calls in a specialist, the patient cannot say, "No, all that will cost too much." And, in our case, when Bobby needs a transfusion, we can't haggle with the drug companies over the price of each bottle, threatening to walk away if the price does not come down. So it is an insult to the intelligence of all of us for the AMA to talk about "free enterprise" in medicine.

As a justification for its philosophy and behavior, the AMA boasts that American medicine leads the world. In research, technology, and care for those who can afford it, American medicine can be superb. But its miracles are poorly distributed. The United States ranks thirteenth in infant mortality, and eighteenth in life expectancy for males (behind such countries as Bulgaria, Hungary, and East Germany). American medicine does lead the world in one respect: making money. Money for doctors, for drug manufacturers, for private insurance companies. Physicians are the highest paid of all American professionals. The average income of doctors in private practice, after deductions but before taxes, is $42,700 a year.

It disturbs me to write in this way about American doctors. I was brought up to respect doctors as I respected ministers and teachers. But the image of the American doctor as presented by the AMA has blurred that respect. What confuses me is that the doctors Sue and I have known as individuals are a sensitive, compassionate, and sacrificing group of men and women. Why, then, is the collective image of the American doctor so tarnished with nasty traces of greed? I want to believe that all doctors are motivated like Dr. Margaret Hilgartner, Bobby's hematologist at New York Hospital. Once, when Bobby was nine and in the hospital for tests, she was telling him about her own three children at home and how busy and complicated her life was.

"But why are you here?"

"Because I want to help you," she said.

A hopeful sign is that, gradually, the tyranny of the AMA is crumbling. Today, only 55 per cent of America's 355,000 medical doctors belong to the organization.

But the AMA still wields great power and in its fight it still receives support from politicians. In 1973, President Nixon picked up the refrain: "We want the doctor to work for the patient, not for the government." None of the current national health insurance proposals suggest that American doctors work for the government. Doctors in France, where Bobby's costs were covered under national health insurance, were not working for the French government. And even in places where doctors do work directly for a government, does this mean that patients are less well cared for? Do British doctors not work for the patient? Do U.S. Army and Navy doctors not work for the patient? What made President Nixon's statement almost Kafkaesque was that he spoke on the doorstep of Walter Reed Army Hospital, where he had just had his annual medical checkup. It was free to him, performed by army doctors, "working for the government."

Meanwhile, with no national health insurance in our country and private insurers unwilling to give them adequate coverage, what do American hemophiliacs do? Some sink under the emotional and financial weight. Some hustle blood for drinks on Miami's skid row. Some go abroad for the medical treatment they cannot afford at home. In 1968 at a hospital in Oxford, England, I met an American judge, a hemophiliac, who needed a hip replacement. Because he could not pay the costs of this operation in America, he had arranged to have it done in England. The judge was in the hospital for three months, had complicated surgery and innumerable transfusions of cryo and AHF concentrate. The cost to him: Zero. This was a special case. Britain's National Health Service normally will not cover treatment of chronic illnesses of visiting foreigners. But the spectacle of American citizens forced to flee the richest nation on earth to seek medical care shocks foreign doctors and occasionally they try to help.

Some states have begun to help hemophiliacs. Michigan has the most long-standing and generous program, providing free to all nine hundred hemophiliacs living in Michigan AHF made in state-funded laboratories. A dramatic episode occurred in 1972 in Pennsylvania, where the governor learned that the father of a hemophiliac, supporting a family of five, was being required to quit his job and go on welfare in order to receive state coverage for his son's hemophilia. A few weeks later, the law was changed and money appropriated directly for hemophilia care. In most of these states, the sums granted are a pittance (Virginia appropriated $50,000 to be spent over two years). But they are a step forward.

Recently, the federal government seemed about to take a major step. In March 1973 Senator Harrison Williams of New Jersey introduced a hemophilia bill into the Senate. He emphasized the crucial point: "Hemophiliacs are not born crippled and . . . permanent damage can be prevented if financial conditions permit them to take advantage of newly developed forms of therapy." This bill would have helped hemophiliacs in several important ways. It would have established new treatment centers like those which already exist in most large cities. It would have encouraged blood fractionation by funding new equipment for blood collection centers. And—by far the most important feature of the bill— it would have provided direct financial assistance to hemophiliacs and their families to purchase AHF. The government would not pay the entire bill; it would step in only after the individual had reached a certain level of out-of-pocket expense; that level to be determined by the individual's own financial situation. Senator Williams estimated that his bill might cost $125 million to $150 million per year.

Senator Williams and his staff fought hard for the bill. But such is the pace with which American government moves on these matters that it took eight months before one day of Senate committee hearings could be held. Another year elapsed before the full Senate voted. When the vote finally came, it was unanimously favorable, although heavy cuts were made in the appropriation (down from $125 million–$150 million to $20 million per year).

And then, in November 1974 the bill went to the House of Representatives. Apparently, a majority of the members of the House committee considering the bill did not want to accept any hemophilia bill at all. In joint House-Senate meetings, Senator

Williams fought even harder. Finally, the House agreed to appropriate $8 million for the first year. But the money is not to be spent on transfusions. It is for treatment centers and fractionation facilities only. The key provision of the bill, which would have provided direct financial help to hemophiliacs to enable them to buy AHF and pay for transfusions, was killed.

Explaining their action, the members of the House said that they did "acknowledge the great need for personal health services for the victims of hemophilia and hope to address hearings to this need in the context of health services and national health insurance next year." More hearings, more talk, maybe next year. Meanwhile, each day, each week, each month, more hemorrhages are occurring, more joints are being damaged. Louis Friedland, the present chairman of the National Hemophilia Foundation, appealed to the senators during the hearing: "The concentrate is there. The procedure [home transfusion] is simple. There really is no way you can say to a kid that the government is not ready this year or next year, so in the meantime sleep in those braces. 'It hurts a hell of a lot, we know, but in two or three years we will get to you.' We just cannot do that." But that is exactly what the members of the House of Representatives—and we, the American people who elect them—are saying.

Sometime in the nineteenth century, we Americans decided that the success of our democracy rested on the general intelligence of the citizenry. The public good demanded public education. Today we all consider this an inherent right. For those who wish them, we also have private schools, but none of us, not even the most conservative, advocates abolishing the public schools.

We have never done this with health, although one could logically argue that good health is an even more basic requirement for the "pursuit of happiness" than a good education. Somehow, we have let ourselves be frightened away from a form of insurance that we need almost more than any other. We insure our cars, our houses, our silver, our boats; the government insures our jobs, our bank deposits, and our old age. But because of one small, highly effective lobby, we cannot insure our health. Yet who can tell when he, or his child, will be sick? How does one know that he will not suddenly be faced with a catastrophic illness? And not just one catastrophic illness, but a permanent catastrophic illness?

Bob Stone, the director of Blythedale Hospital, where Bobby went for early orthopedic therapy, shakes his head. "It is incredible, *incredible*, that in a country of this much wealth we leave catastrophic illness to be handled by those who can least handle it. It is as if we turned to the guy whose house has just burned down and said to him, 'Too bad, but it's un-American to have insurance.' It can happen to *anyone*. How can we say that we will extend medical aid to someone over sixty-five, but if someone incurs catastrophic illness that is *his* problem. It is a national problem, not a problem for the individual. No one knows when it might happen to him. I mean, there but for the grace of God, goes *anybody!*"

Chapter 28

Robert Massie: As a biographer, I have my own peculiar personal standard for judging famous men. Along with the careers and accomplishments for which the world hails them, I judge them also as fathers. Along with saving nations, making wars, making peace, how much did they care about their children? How well did they succeed in equipping their children for life and sending them prepared out into the world? By this admittedly idiosyncratic measure, there are reclassifications to be made. Giants of our time like Churchill and Roosevelt shrink to normal size, perhaps even less than normal. De Gaulle grows larger. Even when he was most preoccupied, this austere colossus always managed to spend time with his mongoloid daughter, Anne. Playing records, singing to her, even dancing before her, he made her smile. When Anne was born, his wife Yvonne wrote, "Charles and I would give everything: health, fortune, promotion, career, if only Anne were a little girl like the others." When Anne died, de Gaulle stood by the grave and, taking his wife's hand, said, "Come, now she is like the others."

I love my own two daughters no less and no more than my son. I delight in their beauty, their intelligence, and their grace. I cherish every small, intimate detail of their lives. But there is something a little different in a man's feeling for his son; it reaches into the future and becomes a link with the past. Onto these younger masculine shoulders go hopes unfulfilled, dreams unrealized, a sense of continuity, of contribution; in a word, perhaps, the wisp of immortality at which we all are clutching.

My own father died before I could know him. I was an infant; I have no memory of him at all. He was stern, even puritanical, but he was admired by everyone who knew him. In life, he had many disappointments. He was born in China, where his father was an Episcopal missionary. In the First World War, he was a captain in the army and he wanted desperately to go to France. But he was kept at home, training other men. He started a school for boys, the Massie School, near Lexington, Kentucky. It lasted ten years, then closed when its backers were ruined by the Depression. My father took a job selling life insurance. A year later came cancer and death. He was thirty-nine.

I never knew this man, my father. But the link between us is there. When I reached twenty-one, my mother wrote me a letter congratulating me on my birthday. In it she said, "Above all, I know that your father would have been very proud of you." I have never had any praise that meant so much.

I believe that in life it is not what happens to us that makes us what we are. Over this, we usually have no control. It is how we react to what happens that matters. I believe that my son has reacted well to life.

Bobby, I am proud of you.

Suzanne Massie: Our life has changed now. It is already hard to think of those days—almost as if they had happened to someone else. After Bobby left for Washington, I would glance into his room. It looked odd, so lifelessly neat—strangely empty and yet still full. There was the bed I had so carefully chosen—a bed in which to spend days and days. Nearby, on the floor, the wooden bed tray that Bob had lovingly designed and made for him to draw and play on. On the walls, the jaunty Currier and Ives engraving of George Washington I'd found for him one Christmas, the wooden whale, the photograph of the children in Maine, the sampler embroidered by Bob's grandmother. Above the desk there was a poster of a precariously balanced orange cat that read gaily, "Hang in There Baby." On the mantel rested the sea urchin shells, the rock collection. In the corner, gathering dust, was the transfusion rack that Susy used to love to jump on. A French beret was dangling rakishly on it. All abandoned now.

The burden has shifted. It happened almost imperceptibly. One day I realized that it had been weeks since I had had to remind Bobby to do his exercises, that we hardly ever had to say "no" anymore, that he was picking up his own fraction. More and more, I found, it was he who was comforting me. Then he went away, and when he called, each time, his voice sounded deeper and more confident. One weekend he came home and I looked at him and I saw: he had grown into a man. His shoulders and arms were muscled and strong from exercise and swimming. His hair, once so sunny and blond, had darkened into a warm brown, his features were firmly etched. His eyes, blue-gray, have something sad and deep in them . . . even when he laughs and smiles, which he does often. He is a bit arrogant, I am afraid, a little too pompous, with a will that can wear away granite. But he is generous and idealistic, and that is precious. He cares for others.

His left knee is destroyed. He will have to fight pain for the rest of his life. We did not win the battle. It left us all wounded.

Everything that he is, everything that we are now, is because of hemophilia. Our life cannot be separated from it. We would not even be ourselves without it. So how can it be judged? Was it good? Was it bad? I don't know. It just happened, and everything else happened because of it. The answers we sought have only deepened the questions. His is now the burden and the responsibility. For him there will be new battles, new windmills, new doors. Where will they lead him?

Robert Massie, Jr.: I have had a great deal of trouble drawing memories of hemophilia from the past. I don't know why. It has been suggested that some of the memories are so terrible that my mind has blocked them off, buried them, so that they only disturb me in dreams. But I have no such dreams and when I search back through all the childhood memories, I find nothing but home-movie trivia. I see birthdays, a clay squirrel made in kindergarten, third-grade girl friends, Christmases. . . . Sandwiched in are cameo shots of me sitting in an orthopedic appliance manufacturer's outer office for hours, memories of time passed in bed and on therapy room tables, smells and sounds normally alien to small children, hospital emergency wards and waiting rooms. But they don't stand out. Why?

Perhaps because for me it was a normal life. It never really occurred to me that I ought to be different from the way I was. Oh, there were times when I would pray to God to have me wake up the next morning able to run and walk, but I knew that the doctors' offices, the shots, the braces, and the humiliation were all there to stay.

People have asked me to describe the first time it dawned on me that I was different, the first time I realized that I was not like the others and that I never would be. I thought very hard, trying to find some shadowy wisp of memory, but I found nothing. It seemed to me that such an important moment would not easily be forgotten . . . and yet there was nothing. It finally occurred to me why.

I *always* knew I was different. I knew that I couldn't climb the tree house at nursery school. I knew that I was somehow special. Arrangements were always being made. I had dry ice and no friend of mine did. I had plasma bags and tubing and bad knees and traction, all things I was well aware were not a part of my friends' lives. I had to be careful when others didn't. I was always having adventures. Rushing to the hospital in the middle of the night, I can remember pretending that I was a secret agent, ingeniously escaping my would-be captors by posing as a sick little boy wracked with pain. Blood-bank laboratories were converted into Frankensteinian laboratories, where wondrous potions would emerge from my ingenious chemical combinations, capable of wiping out or saving millions, depending on my mood. And my wheelchair, wondrous contraption that it was, object of admiration to all my friends, could become a James Bond machine (complete with laser, oil slick, and two-way radio) or a private rocket ship to go from Earth (or my room) to the moon (or the kitchen). The wheelchair even became a weird musical instrument as I plucked the spokes of the wheels, convinced that I had created a new artistic medium. All this and more could occur in an afternoon—indeed, in the time span from *The Roy Rogers Show* to *Sky King* and *My Friend Flicka*.

I knew that I was different. What disturbed me, as the years went by and the thought gradually dawned on me, was that somehow to be different was to be wrong, was to be out of place, was to be rejected.

People around me began to say things like "I'm sorry." People were either nervous or suspiciously nice, patting me on the head whenever I came within arm's reach. It became apparent to me that these people in the supermarkets, the waiting rooms, the new schools . . . these people were *sorry* for me. They *pitied* me!

One day years later I walked into an elevator in the U.S. Senate office building and was confronted by a pleasant young elevator operator who, having seen me, in the same morning, in a wheelchair, on crutches, and then on foot, was understandably curious. She asked about it.

"I have hemophilia," I said. "It gives me trouble in my legs. The wheelchair helps if I have to walk a long way."

Expecting a simpler answer, the girl blinked and stared at me. "You have what?"

"Hee-mo-phil-ia." I explained it to her a bit more ("It's-not-bleeding-to-death-from-a-scratch-but . . .").

This apparently satisfied her until we arrived at my floor, when she looked at me again and very slowly and sincerely said:

"Listen, I want you to know that I am very sorry you have this . . . disease. I am very sorry that this misfortune has come over you."

I was amazed. No one had ever expressed sympathy so openly to me. Never before had anyone used the word "misfortune" . . . but that's what they all were thinking! I realized in an instant that what everyone who had ever expressed that sort of sympathy was actually saying was that if they could change things, they would. That they viewed my problem as a misfortune . . . something that ought not to have happened.

But I am pleased with the way I am, for I feel that I have the potential within me to lead an even more beautiful life than I have up to now. I am not afraid of adversity, having suffered setbacks and bounced back. I think that my character has been improved by my difficult childhood. I have gained resilience, will power, determination, and appreciation for what I have, not regret for what I lack. How can I—or anyone—wish that the most important thing that ever happened to me had not happened? It is like saying that I wish I had been born on another planet, so different would I probably be. Put it this way: I wouldn't have it any other way.

Because of hemophilia, I have been able to see both sides. I realized this vividly when I went up to visit Harvard just after I had come back from Orthopaedic Hospital. I wanted to see the Harvard swimming pool, and when I went in they were having practice. It was a big pool with seven or eight lanes. In the pool were many long-legged swimmers, so powerful, so physically perfect, all six feet, five inches, just going back and forth, churning up and down the lanes like speedboats, with the coaches hanging over them.

Watching them, I thought about a little boy I had just met at Los Angeles Orthopaedic Hospital. Jamie was born with *osteogenesis imperfecta*. He was nine years old and he had had twenty-seven operations. One of his legs was amputated at the knee, the other at the ankle.

He was in terrible physical shape and was in whirlpool baths to cure the amputations. I could take it, but I knew that anyone who had not had medical problems would have been upset to see him. When he sat on a chair, it looked as if he didn't have any legs at all. But Jamie was a very spunky boy and liked to swim when he could; he drew pictures and was a wonderful person. So when I was swimming in October, November, and December in the Hackley pool, I would think of Jamie as he swam, and then I would think of those Harvard guys as they swam, and I would think of myself as I swam. I realized that the Harvard men would feel nothing but pity for Jamie, and Jamie would not understand the Harvard men at all. But, amazingly, I felt at home with both kinds of people and yet somehow was not in either place.

And suddenly, I had a revelation of commitment to try and bring these two worlds together, because I have a unique experience in both. I saw myself as bridging the gap. So when I would get tired, I'd think, "You're bridging the gap. You've got to work harder." And that's why I swim more laps each time, first 60, then 80, then 100.

At a hemophilia symposium I attended, one doctor stood up and spoke about a "phenomenon" he had witnessed during his years of dealing with children with chronic diseases and their families.

"You know," he said, shaking his head in bewilderment, "I have even heard parents say how wonderful it is to have a child with hemophilia because it has given them a greater feeling for others who suffer in this world and because they appreciate life more." He paused to allow the absurdity of that statement to sink in. Then he continued, "It is amazing how these parents, desperately searching for a single redeeming feature in the affliction, will rationalize."

Rationalize! Am I rationalizing? Am I deluding myself with thoughts that I am better off this way in order to quell the True Me who is longing to play football? Am I enshrouding myself with legitimizing reasons for my existence? Am I fabricating compensations, as I did when I gave away my sought-after syringes (they became superior squirt guns) to my childhood friends?

To say that would be to say that I have come through the pain and troubles of my first eighteen years with nothing to show for it. To believe that would be to believe that I learned nothing of human nature and kindness through all the years of hospitals, that my parents were unable to impart more than an average sense of faith through all my setbacks. If this were true, if having vanquished braces, bleeding, pain, self-consciousness, boredom, and depression, I have not added in any way to my appreciation of this life that has been given me, then that indeed would be a misfortune to be pitied.

Appendix: The Genetic Transmission of Hemophilia

Genes have the unique double role of transmitting genetic information to the next generation and informing the cell in the current individual exactly how to make specific proteins. Although usually any one gene is copied exactly in succeeding generations, occasionally an error in copying occurs. Such a change is called a mutation. Once a mutation has occurred in a reproductive cell it may be passed down in the family and, because this mutant gene no longer carries the correct specifications for protein building, individuals who inherit it will lack a particular normal protein. Hemophilia is an example. In hemophiliacs, a clotting factor, which is a protein, is missing or abnormal because the correct instructions for its formation have been lost.

Two of the forty-six chromosomes in every human being are the so-called sex chromosomes. Women have two X chromosomes and are said to be XX. Men have a single X chromosome plus a Y chromosome and are said to be XY.

A baby's sex is determined at the moment of conception when it receives one sex chromosome from each parent, one of the mother's two X's and either the father's X or his Y. Thus either one of the mother's X's linking with the father's single X creates a girl:

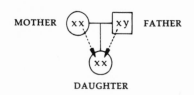

while either one of the mother's X's plus the father's Y creates a boy.

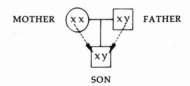

The key to hemophilia is that the defective gene is found on the X chromosome. Thus when a faulty X chromosome is present in a male, that male will be a hemophiliac:

and when a faulty X chromosome is present in a female, she will be a carrier of hemophilia.

The carrier will not normally show symptoms of the disease, i.e., her blood will clot, because her one good X chromosome will provide her with sufficient clotting ability to avoid bleeding.

In conception between a normal male and a carrier female, four different possibilities arise: a hemophiliac son, a normal son, a carrier daughter, and a normal daughter:

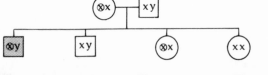

| The hemophiliac son has received his mother's bad X chromosome and his father's Y. | The normal son has received his mother's good X and his father's Y. | The carrier daughter has received her mother's bad X and her father's X. | The normal daughter has received her mother's good X and her father's X. |

Thus, with each conception and pregnancy, if the mother is a carrier (as we learned that Sue was when Bobby's hemophilia was diagnosed), the chance is one in four that the baby will be a hemophiliac boy.

Finally, when hemophiliac males become fathers, the genetic pattern dictates an ironic reversal: none of their offspring will be hemophiliacs (unless by rare chance he should happen to marry a carrier). Their sons will all be normal boys, but their daughters will all be carriers. This is true of Bobby: if he has children, none of his sons will be hemophiliacs, but all of his daughters will be carriers.

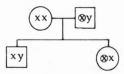

All sons will be normal. The father's Y is normal and both the mother's X's are normal.

All daughters will be carriers. No matter which of the mother's good X's they have, they will all have the father's bad X.